Palliative Medicine

A case-based manual

SECOND EDITION

Edited by

Neil MacDonald

Director, Cancer Nutrition–Rehabilitation Program, and Professor of Oncology, McGill University, Montreal, Quebec, Canada

Doreen Oneschuk

Palliative Medicine Physician, Associate Professor, Division of Palliative Medicine, Department of Oncology, University of Alberta, Edmonton, Alberta, Canada

Neil Hagen

Professor, Division of Palliative Medicine, Department of Oncology, University of Calgary, Calgary, Alberta, Canada

and

Derek Doyle **(International Editor)**

Vice-President of the National Council for Palliative Care, President Emeritus of the International Association for Hospice and Palliative Care, and formerly Medical Director, St Columba's Hospice, Edinburgh, UK

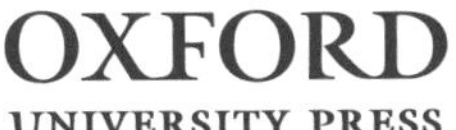

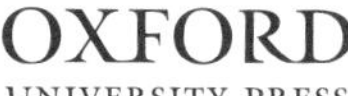

Great Clarendon Street, Oxford OX2 6DP

Oxford University Press is a department of the University of Oxford. It furthers the University's objective of excellence in research, scholarship, and education by publishing worldwide in

Oxford New York

Auckland Cape Town Dar es Salaam Hong Kong Karachi Kuala Lumpur Madrid Melbourne Mexico City Nairobi New Delhi Shanghai Taipei Toronto

With offices in

Argentina Austria Brazil Chile Czech Republic France Greece Guatemala Hungary Italy Japan South Korea Poland Portugal Singapore Switzerland Thailand Turkey Ukraine Vietnam

Oxford is a registered trade mark of Oxford University Press in the UK and in certain other countries

Published in the United States by Oxford University Press Inc., New York

First published 2005

Reprinted 2006

A catalogue record for this title is available from the British Library

Library of Congress Cataloging in Publication Data
(Data available)

ISBN 0–19–852832–9 (Pbk.) 978–0–19–852832–6 (Pbk.)

10 9 8 7 6 5 4 3 2

Typeset by Cepha Imaging Pvt. Ltd., Bangalore, India.
Printed in Great Britain
on acid-free paper by Biddles Ltd., King's Lynn

Foreword

Oh, I have suffered with those I saw suffer

William Shakespeare (1564–1616) *The Tempest*

Caring for people at the end of life is seldom easy for the family or the doctors. Often it tests a doctor's knowledge, skills, humanity, and even his or her faith or philosophy of life. Many will know only too well what Shakespeare meant by suffering in the presence of another's suffering. It is more than sympathetic suffering. They will remember the occasions when they knew that they could have relieved pain more effectively; when they could have explained things better; when they felt embarrassed and inadequate on being asked about existential matters. Their suffering was as nothing compared with that of their patient, but they suffered nevertheless. To make it worse they knew that their lack of knowledge or skill could have been avoided.

If perhaps they feel some guilt that they never took 'care of the dying' seriously in medical school, they can console themselves with the thought that the fault is not all theirs. Care of the dying or, to give it the name first coined in Canada and now used worldwide *Palliative Care,* should be taught in every medical school, demonstrated at every bedside, and made examinable in every medical school and Royal College of Surgeons and Physicians. The fact that it is not given such a high profile and priority demands attention.

We are, after all, not talking about a rarity, something seldom likely to be encountered in medical practice, something that can and should be left to 'experts' or 'specialists'. All of us will die, 50 per cent of us from a chronic illness whose endstage may last for months if not years, characterized by a spectrum of physical, psychosocial, and even spiritual suffering that can scarcely be imagined, but yet has been well researched and recorded in the literature. How bizarre, how obscene, that so much medical training is devoted to conditions which most of us may never encounter whilst palliative care—getting alongside the dying patient and easing the kaleidoscope of his suffering at that time—is all but ignored.

Devising a curriculum, as has been done in several countries, is a first step towards improving the situation, but unless there are tutors, mentors, examiners, and books written especially for learners, palliative care skills will continue to be learnt by trial and error, and only occasionally absorbed by osmosis from charismatic teaching and sensitive bedside demonstrations. Young doctors will continue to describe their experiences of caring for dying patients as the most frightening yet rewarding of their short careers. They will continue to recount how lonely they felt, how helpless, how unsupported by some of their seniors.

This book is not a curative for this sad situation, a scenario that is replicated round the world. However, it will go some way to removing the sense of helplessness we have described. Whereas in the past, doctors have lamented 'I didn't know what to do or where to turn', they will now know where to turn. Tutors will have first-class teaching material for tutorial groups and discussions, based not on theoretical knowledge but on real-life cases. Edited by Canadian physicians with worldwide reputations for clinical skills in palliative care and teaching, and with contributors all equally distinguished in this field, this is a book which manages to avoid being yet another therapeutics recipe book. It captures something of the complexity of palliative care—the constantly changing patterns of suffering, the often unfathomable depths of existential pain and human relationships, and the ever-changing relationship between patient and physician. As the illness progresses the physician's role changes almost imperceptibly from that of the skilled diagnostician and clinical pharmacologist to the friend whose willingness to share his humanity with someone on life's last lonely journey becomes the most important feature of the relationship. Something of that mystery is to be found in this book which it is my honour to commend to colleagues in Canada and the world.

Derek Doyle OBE
Edinburgh, Scotland
Retired Consultant in Palliative Medicine
Emeritus President of the Internal Association for Hospice and
Palliative Care

Preface

We learn from our patients.

In the second edition of *Palliative Medicine—a case-based manual* we intend to reinforce your personal experience with the collective wisdom of colleagues who have integrated their clinical acumen, research findings, and informed literature review in chapters considering the major problems in palliative care.

Reflecting the broad mandate of our field, this edition contains new chapters centring on chronic non-malignant illness. In addition to many new authors we have added chapters on informatics and on research issues in palliative care.

The book offers a panoramic view of palliative care with a Canadian bent. Although it is directed to resident physicians and senior medical students, we believe that the topics presented also provide the busy practicing physician with a concise authoritative approach to specific patient issues. *Palliative Medicine—a case-based manual* is not a textbook in the usual sense. Yes, as in other palliative medicine texts, one can learn details of opioid usage, guidelines for communication, and specific information on other challenging areas in our field. However, our main purpose is to mirror 'real time' patient–family–palliative care team interactions by presenting difficult cases and following the patients through their course of illness.

Patient–family causes of distress are often multifaceted, as are their solutions. For example, one cannot consider dyspnoea without discussing opioid use; communication and ethical considerations are closely linked, as are psychosocial issues with all 'physical symptoms'. Therefore readers will note a degree of what we hope is reasoned duplication on similar clinical scenarios in a number of chapters. We believe that, as a result, we more closely reflect actual patient–physician contacts. We also realize that our chapters are used as 'stand-alone' teaching exercises. Whether it is for the individual reader or the small group teaching exercise, we wish to have all aspects of the problem under consideration in the chapter which is discussing it.

Away from consulting rooms and the bedside, *Palliative Medicine—a case-based manual* can be used by training directors in their group discussions, by team training sessions, and as preparation for students as they sit and discuss clinical challenges among themselves and with their mentors. Perhaps the book will encourage physicians to bring their own cases to group discussion. We hope that *Palliative Medicine—a case-based manual* will be provocative and, in some sections, even contentious—a book that helps to stimulate enthusiastic discourse. Of course, we want it to find favour among our palliative care colleagues, but we wish to reach a broader audience, including trainees and physicians who bear responsibility for the relief of suffering in people with a wide range of chronic illnesses.

We express our thanks to the numerous Canadian palliative care physicians who have contributed to the second edition of *Palliative Medicine—a case-based manual*, and to the Canadian Society of Palliative Care Physicians for their continued support.

We owe a special note of gratitude to Derek Doyle, our international editor, whose wise guidance has informed every aspect of our work.

N.M.
D.O.
N.H.

Contents

List of contributors

Kim Blake
Associate Professor,
Department of Pediatrics,
Dalhousie University,
IWK Health Centre, Halifax,
Nova Scotia, Canada

Eduardo Bruera
Professor of Medicine,
Department of Palliative Care and
Rehabilitation Medicine,
University of Texas
MD Anderson Cancer Center,
Houston, Texas, USA

Michéle Chaban
Social Worker,
Mount Sinai Hospital,
Clinical Thanatologist,
Education Consultant,
Toronto, Ontario, Canada

Srini Chary
Lecturer,
Department of Family Medicine,
University of Saskatchewan,
Palliative Care Physician,
Saskatoon Health Region, Saskatoon,
Saskatchewan, Canada

Susan Chater
Palliative Care Program,
The Ottawa Hospital;
Assistant Professor,
Department of Medicine,
University of Ottawa,
Ottawa, Ontario, Canada

Harvey Max Chochinov
Canada Research Chair in
Palliative Care,Director,
Manitoba Palliative Care Research Unit,
CancerCare Manitoba Professor,
Department of Psychiatry,
University of Manitoba,
Winnipeg, Manitoba, Canada

Garnet Crawford
University of Manitoba,
Faculty of Medicine, and
Department of Family Medicine
(Section of Palliative Care Medicine)
Winnipeg Regional Heath Authority
Palliative Care Sub-program Winnipeg,
Manitoba,
Canada

Millie Cumming
Clinical Associate Professor,
Department of Family Medicine,
UBC, Consultant Physician,
Palliative Care Program,
St. Paul's Hospital,
Vancouver, British Columbia,
Canada

Paul Daeninck
University of Manitoba,
Faculty of Medicine, and
Department of Family Medicine
(Section of Palliative Care Medicine)
Winnipeg Regional Heath Authority
Palliative Care Sub-program Winnipeg,
Manitoba,
Canada

Ingrid de Kock
Assistant Clinical Professor,
Division of Palliative Care Medicine,
Department of Oncology,
University of Alberta;
Palliative Care Physician
Capital Health Regional Palliative
Care Program
Edmonton, Alberta, Canada

Dominique Dion
Clinical education coordinator,
Département de médecine familiale,
Université de Montréal;
Hôpital Maisonneuve-Rosemont and
St Mary's Palliative Care Service,
Montréal, Quebec, Canada

Michael Downing
Clinical Assistant Professor,
UBC Faculty of Medicine, Division of
Palliative Care; Adjunct Assistant Professor,
UVic School of Health Information Sciences
Medical Director,
Victoria Hospice Society Victoria,
British Columbia, Canada

Derek Doyle
Vice-President of the National Council for
Hospice and Specialist Palliative Care
Services; President Emeritus of the
International Hospice Institute and formerly
Medical Director,
St Columba's Hospice,
Edinburgh, UK

Deborah Dudgeon
W. Ford Connell Professor of
Palliative Care Medicine Professor of
Oncology and Medicine,
Queen's University,
Palliative Care Medicine Program,
Kingston, Ontario, Canada

Sharon Duncan
Clinical Instructor,
Department of Family Medicine UBC,
Consultant Physician,
Palliative Care Program,
St. Paul's Hospital,
Vancouver, British Columbia, Canada

Robin Fainsinger
Associate Professor,
Division of Palliative Care Medicine,
Department of Oncology,
University of Alberta; Clinical Director,
Capital Health Regional Palliative Care
Program, Edmonton, Alberta, Canada

Wilma Falconer
Nurse Consultant,
Palliative Care Service,
McGill University Health Centre,
Montreal General Hospital,
Montreal, Quebec, Canada

Gerri Frager
Associate Professor,
Department of Pediatrics,
Dalhousie University; Medical Director
Pediatric Palliative Care,
IWK Health Centre Halifax,
Nova Scotia, Canada

Jacqueline Fraser
Clinical Assistant Professor,
Department of Family Medicine UBC,
Consultant Physician,
Palliative Care Program,
St. Paul's Hospital, Vancouver,
British Columbia, Canada

Bruno Gagnon
Assistant Professor,
Department of Oncology,
McGill University Physician Consultant,
Palliative Care Service,
McGill University Health Centre,
Montreal General Hospital,
Montreal, Quebec, Canada

Romayne Gallagher
Clinical Professor,
Division of Palliative Care,
Faculty of Medicine,
University of British Columbia,
Consulting Staff,
British Columbia Cancer Agency,
Vancouver Home Hospice Program
Physician, Vancouver,
British Columbia, Canada

Neil Hagen
Professor,
Division of Palliative Medicine,
Department of Oncology,
University of Calgary,
Calgary, Alberta, Canada

Jennifer Hall
Associate Professor Family Medicine,
Dalhousie University,
Saint John's,
New Brunswick, Canada

Pippa Hall
Assistant Professor,
Department of Family Medicine,
University of Ottawa,
Program Director,
Palliative Medicine Residency Program,
SCO Health Service, Ottawa,
Ontario, Canada

Mike Harlos
Professor, Faculty of Medicine,
University of Manitoba,
Medical Director,
Palliative Care,
Winnipeg Regional Health Authority
Winnipeg,
Manitoba, Canada

A. Nina Horvath
Assistant Professor,
Department of Family and Community Medicine,
University of Toronto, Palliative Medicine
Consultant at The Temmy Latner
Centre for Palliative Care and
Sunnybrook and Women's College
Health Sciences Centre,
Toronto, Ontario, Canada

Tom Hutchinson
Palliative Care Program,
McGill University Health Centre;
Professor, Department of Medicine,
McGill University, Montreal,
Quebec, Canada

Alejandro R. Jadad
Director, Centre for Global
eHealth Innovation,
Canada Research Chair in
eHealth Innovation Rose Family
Chair in Supportive Care.
Professor, Faculty of Medicine,
University Health Network and
University of Toronto,
Toronto, Ontario, Canada

E. Anne Langlois
Assistant Professor,
Department of Family and
Community Medicine,
University of Toronto,
Palliative Medicine Consultant at
The Temmy Latner Centre for
Palliative Care and Mount Sinai Hospital,
Toronto, Ontario, Canada

Bernard Lapointe
Chief, Palliative Care Division,
Sir Mortimer B. Davis–Jewish
General Hospital,
Montreal; Associate Professor,
Department of Oncology and
Department of Family Medicine,
McGill University, Montreal,
Quebec, Canada

Elizabeth Latimer
Professor, Department of Family Medicine,
McMaster University,
Hamilton Ontario. Palliative
Care Program,
Hamilton Health Sciences Centre,
Hamilton, Ontario, Canada

Peter G. Lawlor
Associate Professor,
Division of Palliative Care Medicine,
Dept of Oncology,
University of Alberta, Director,
Palliative Care Program,
University of Alberta Hospital,
Edmonton, Alberta, Canada

Pauline Lesage
Attending Physician,
Department of Pain Medicine and
Palliative Care,
Beth Israel Medical Centre;
Associate Professor,
Albert Einstein College of Medicine,
New York, USA

S. Lawrence Librach
Director, Temmy Latner Centre for Palliative Care,
W. Gifford Jones Professor
Pain Control and Palliative Care,
University of Toronto,
Mount Sinai Hospital, Toronto,
Ontario, Canada

Daphne Lobb
Clinical Instructor,
Department of Family Medicine UBC;
Medical Director,
Palliative Care Program,
St. Paul's Hospital, Vancouver,
British Columbia, Canada

Leah MacDonald
Palliative Care Physician,
University of Manitoba,
Winnipeg Regional Health Authority
Palliative Care, Winnipeg, Manitoba,
Canada

Neil MacDonald
Director, Cancer Nutrition–Rehabilitation Program, and Professor of Oncology,
McGill University, Montreal,
Quebec, Canada

Susan MacDonald
Associate Professor of Medicine and Family Medicine,
Memorial University of Newfoundland; Divisional Chief of Palliative Care,
Health Care Corporation of St. John's, St. John's,
Newfoundland, Canada

Dwight Moulin
Professor,
Departments of Clinical Neurological Sciences and Oncology,
University of Western Ontario and Medical Director, Supportive Care,
London Regional Cancer Centre,
London, Ontario, Canada

Balfour M. Mount
Eric M. Flanders Professor of Palliative Medicine,
Department of Oncology,
McGill University. Attending Physician,
MUHC Montreal,
Quebec, Canada

Doreen Oneschuk
Palliative Medicine Physician,
Associate Professor,
Division of Palliative Medicine,
Department of Oncology,
University of Alberta, Edmonton,
Alberta, Canada

Jose Pereira
Alberta Cancer Foundation Professorship of Palliative Medicine,
University of Calgary,
Palliative Care Consultant,
Calgary Regional Palliative Care Program, Calgary,
Alberta, Canada

David J. Roy
Director, Centre for Bioethics,
IRCM Research Professor,
Faculty of Medicine,
Université de Montréal
Editor-in-chief,
Journal of Palliative Care

Valerie Nocent Schulz
Palliative Medicine Consultant,
Assistant Professor,
Department of Anesthesia and Perioperative Medicine,
University of Western Ontario,
London Health Sciences Center,
London, Ontario, Canada

John F. Seely
Palliative Care Program,
The Ottawa Hospital;
Professor, Department of Medicine,
University of Ottawa,
Ottawa, Ontario, Canada

Kurt Skakum
Assistant Professor,
Department of Psychiatry,
University of Manitoba,
Palliative Care Program Affiliation:
CancerCare Manitoba,
Winnipeg,
Manitoba, Canada

Yoko Tarumi
Physician Consultant,
Regional Palliative Care Program,
and Clinical Assistant Professor,
Division of Palliative Care Medicine,
Department of Oncology,
University of Alberta,
Edmonton, Alberta, Canada

Anna Wreath Taube
Associate Professor,
Division of Palliative Care Medicine,
Department of Oncology,
University of Alberta,
Palliative Care Consultant,
Regional Palliative Care Program,
Edmonton, Alberta, Canada

Anna Towers
Associate Professor and
Director, Palliative Care Division,
Departments of Oncology,
Medicine and Family Medicine,
McGill University; Director,
Palliative Care Division,
McGill University Health Centre,
Montreal, Quebec, Canada

Raymond Viola
Palliative Care Medicine Program,
Queen's University,
Kingston, Ontario, Canada

Paul Walker
Assistant Professor of Medicine,
Department of Palliative Care and
Rehabilitation Medicine,
University of Texas
MD Anderson Cancer Center,
Houston, Texas, USA

Sharon Watanabe
Associate Professor,
Division of Palliative Care Medicine,
Department of Oncology,
University of Alberta and
Medical Director,
Tertiary Palliative Care Unit,
Grey Nuns Community Hospital and
Director of Symptom Control and
Palliative Care,
Cross Cancer Institute,
Edmonton, Alberta, Canada

Natalie Whiting
Palliative Care Physician,
Peterborough Regional Health Centre,
Peterborough; Assistant Professor,
Queen's University, Kingston,
Ontario, Canada

Chapter 1

Communication in advanced illness

Balfour M. Mount

Attitude

To enable each student to:

- Understand the wide spectrum of patient–family responses to the news of a diagnosis of a potentially fatal illness (anger, questioning, withdrawal, blame, etc.).
- Recognize the personal difficulties clinicians may have in delivering such 'bad' news.
- Recognize the importance of both verbal and non-verbal forms of communication.
- Use open honest communication to facilitate the therapeutic efficacy of the physician–patient relationship.
- Demonstrate respect for family structure and roles when sharing information and arriving at decisions.
- Understand the value of a family conference for conveying information to all family members, for identifying vulnerable family members, and for dealing with family conflicts. In particular, to recognize a 'conspiracy of silence' which can have devastating effects on the equilibrium of the family.

Skill

To enable each student to:

- Demonstrate techniques for communicating distressing information to patients and families.
- Ensure that the setting provides as much privacy and dignity as possible.
- Encourage the patient to share information with a family member, or in the case of an incompetent patient, encourage the family member to share information with at least one other relative.
- Provide understandable information.
- Convey hope by emphasizing what can be done.
- Use touch appropriately to convey caring.
- Listen to and interpret anger with concern and understanding.
- Welcome questions and concerns that patients and families may have in order to assist them with appropriate decision-making, including the possibility of obtaining a second opinion.
- Use techniques to ensure that you are hearing the patient's and family's primary areas of concern.

Knowledge

To enable each student to:

- Describe the range of possible responses patients and families may have to 'bad' news.
- Describe the goals of effective physician–patient communication.
- Describe strategies to maximize good physician–patient communication.

Mr A.G., a 70-year-old retired auto mechanic, has been referred to your clinic. His complaints include persistent moderately severe back pain, general malaise, insomnia, and a 5 kg weight loss. He states that it is at least 6–8 months since he last felt well, adding that initially he had gone to his chiropractor who treated him with a series of weekly back manipulations. With failure to improve, he had then consulted his family physician. Physical examination and radiographs of his lumbar spine were unremarkable. Noting a past history of recurrent work-related back problems, the physician made a diagnosis of low back strain and gave him a prescription for acetaminophen 325 mg with codeine 15 mg, one or two tablets every 4 h as necessary, telling him to avoid lifting. When his pain continued despite this regimen he wanted to see another physician. This is the reason for his visit to you.

On further questioning, Mr G. admits to recent mild nausea and loss of appetite. He denies abdominal pains, change in bowel habits, and blood in the stool. Physical examination is normal. An ultrasound of the abdomen is obtained. It demonstrates an 8 cm mass in the body of the pancreas. On a return visit you inform Mr G. of the findings and recommend hospital admission and biopsy. He replies, 'It isn't serious, is it?' He then adds with evident anger, 'I sure as hell don't want any trouble turning up now after you doctors have been fooling around for almost a year without finding anything!'

Question 1. What do we know about patient wishes and physician skills concerning discussions aimed at delivering bad news?

The literature is sobering. In a multicultural study of palliative medicine specialists and their advanced cancer patients in Europe, Canada, and South America (Argentina and Brazil), all physicians said that they would like to know the details about *their own* life-threatening illness, yet only 93 per cent of the Canadian physicians, 26 per cent of the European physicians, and 18 per cent of the South American physicians thought the majority of *their patients* would want to know ($P = 0.001$).[1] The study suggests that the physician needs to be attentive to cultural variance and must assess what each patient wants to know.

In a qualitative study carried out at London cancer clinics, it was noted that other factors modifying the extent of information patients wish to hear were linked to coping styles that were called 'faith, hope, and charity': *faith* when respect for physician expertise precluded need for details, *hope* when 'hope' entailed avoidance of detailed knowledge of unpleasant facts, and charity when bonding with fellow patients promoted recognition of the inevitable need to share both scarce resources and information, even when unfavourable.[2]

There is reason to question whether we are effective in assessing our patients' desire to participate in treatment decision-making. Indeed, even after a lengthy clinic interview, highly trained palliative care physicians were able to assess correctly the degree to which their patients wished to be actively involved in decisions about their own care in only a minority of cases (38–45 per cent, depending on the manner of data analysis).[3] Once again the need for a specific prospective assessment of patient wishes is suggested.

The significance of inadequate patient assessment during physician–patient communications is underscored by a study examining the ability of 143 UK cancer physicians to assess the psychiatric needs of 2297 oncology patients. Using self-report questionnaires, an impressive 36.4 per cent of the patients scored themselves in a manner indicating psychiatric morbidity. The misclassification rate by physicians was 34.7 per cent. The authors conclude: 'These data show that much of the probable psychiatric morbidity of cancer patients goes unrecognized and therefore untreated'.[4]

In reviewing the oncology communications literature, Maguire[5] noted that the number and severity of patients' concerns are predictive of later psychological distress, anxiety, and depression. Nevertheless, only a minority of patient concerns are elicited in clinical practice and patient-centred interviewing behaviours are used infrequently. Physicians also often fail to acknowledge patient distress and do not probe psychological and social issues. They tend to use a 'one shoe fits all' standard approach to communication that has been acquired during clinical practice without specific training. Furthermore, the communication problems of senior physicians working in cancer medicine are not resolved by time and clinical experience.[6]

A further problem is that the information we provide while communicating bad news is also likely to be incomplete. In an Australian study of audiotaped conversations in which 118 incurable cancer patients were informed of their prognosis by tertiary care oncologists, the physicians checked their patients' understanding of what they had been told in only 10.2 per cent of cases. While the majority were told about the aim of anticancer therapy (84.7 per cent), incurable status (74.6 per cent), and life expectance (57.6 per cent), only 36.4 per cent were told how anticancer treatment would affect their quality of life and only 29.7 per cent were offered a management choice.[7]

Giving the patient an audiotape recording of their doctor's comments or a written summary of the salient points covered,[8] or both written summary and tape recording,[9] improves patients' overall recall of the information provided and results in greater patient satisfaction.

Question 2. Given the documented deficiencies in giving bad news, what strategies might we use to assist us in these challenging discussions?

Many clinicians have found the mnemonic **SPIKES** to be a helpful aide-memoire.[10–13] Robert Buckman reminds us that 'bad news' is 'any news that adversely and seriously affects an individual's view of his or her future'. By extension, he suggests two guiding principles:[14]

- How 'bad' the news is can be thought of as the gap between the patient's expectations of the situation and the medical reality.
- Ascertaining how they perceive their situation is a precursor to understanding how 'bad' the news is from their perspective. Hence, a valuable rule is: 'Before you tell, ask.'

The **SPIKES** mnemonic suggests a strategy for approaching the communication of sensitive information.

Step 1 Setting. Ensure privacy; minimize distractions; involve significant others as desired by the patient; sit down (eye contact on the same level conveys your interest and concern—full attention; high priority; discussion will seem longer and feel less rushed); look attentive and calm; use active listening techniques (silence, repetition of patient's words, nodding, smiling, saying 'Hmmmm'); ensure availability (shut off mobile phone, avoid other interruptions).

Step 2 Perception. How does the patient perceive his or her medical condition and its seriousness? ('Before you tell, ask'.) '*What did you think when you coughed up the blood? What have you been told about all this so far?*' Adopt the vocabulary used by the patient in your response.

Step 3 Invitation. Inviting input about how much the patient wants to know respects autonomy. '*Are you the kind of person who wants to know all the details about what is going on? How much information would you like to have about your diagnosis and treatment?*'

Step 4 Knowledge: Before delivering the bad news, give some warning. '*The test results are back Anne, and I'm concerned about them.*' Use patient's language; avoid technical terms; give information in small packages, checking understanding after each. '*Any questions about all this so far?*' Integrating bad news is a process, not an event. Adjust the rate of providing information to the needs and resources of each patient.

Step 5 Empathy. Listen for, identify, acknowledge, and address the patient's emotions as they arise. '*These results are not what you were expecting, are they?*'—offering a box of tissues to your silently tearful patient—'*Hearing all this is a shock, I'm sure. It's not what either of us wanted to hear.*' Validate their feelings. '*It's not easy.*'

Step 6 Summary and strategy. Summarize information (with opportunities for the patient to respond and question) and set out a clear plan for further action, including tests, consultation referrals, treatment options, follow-up appointments. The message is that you remain ready to accompany them in a spirit of realistic optimism born out of a readiness to take advantage of all that is still possible.

Question 3. What are your goals for the communication that is about to occur?

It may be helpful to keep two questions in the forefront of your thinking when communications become complicated: '*What is going on here—for the patient and for me?*' '*What are my goals for this conversation?*' On bad days, asking 'What is going on here?' may help to avoid being reactive. Mr G. has been symptomatic for more than 6 months without a diagnosis, despite having consulted a health care professional without delay. While his frustration is understandable, his outburst underscores the significance of several issues. What life crises has he faced in the past? How did he cope? What are his current support systems?

Communication goals

The goals of patient–physician communication include the following.

Develop insight into 'who the person is' in each domain of personhood

It is whole persons, not bodies, who experience suffering. Relevant areas of concern include: the person's personality and character, past; family, cultural background, roles, relationship with self, political being, actions, the unconscious, physical body, secret life, perceived future, and transcendent dimension.[15]

Understand the nature of his illness or complaint

This is important both in terms of the pathophysiology of disease and how the patient experiences his infirmity, the *meaning* it has for him. We do not know the meaning or impact of the illness as experienced by the patient or family member unless we ask; if we do not ask, we will continually make assumptions based on our own projections.

Examine the nature of his suffering

Suffering occurs when there is a perceived threat to the integrity or continued existence of the person. It is individual in its origins and expression. It is intensely private.[16]

Foster coping and integration of reality

Uncertainty breeds anxiety and anxiety can paralyse coping mechanisms. Uncertainty is diminished when the goals of therapy are clarified. The three general goals of therapy are to cure, to prolong life, and to improve quality of life. In each of these settings it is important and usually possible to establish realistic positive goals based on the priorities of the individual. To identify and express a fear is to diminish it and render it more manageable. The unknown is less fearsome when we are accompanied by a skilled and compassionate health care provider.

Support ability to find meaning

Quality of life depends on a sense of meaning. Meaning is found in things we have accomplished or created; things loved—persons, places, music, ideas, books, films; things left as a legacy; things believed in. Paradoxically, meaning may also be found in suffering.[17] We can assist in the recognition of meaning by inquiring about these areas.

Support healing

Finding a sense of meaning promotes healing. Healing, in the broad sense that embraces human wholeness, is a psychosocial spiritual process which involves reconciliation with self, others, the Other, however defined. It is possible to die healed. Healing generally involves recognition of personal need; acceptance of self (which entails owning responsibility and accepting forgiveness—from self and others); transcendence of egoism, the preoccupation with self that inhibits relating; and entry into dialogue or other-centredness. In illness, transcendence and entry into dialogue are often expressed simply through acceptance of increasing dependency.

Enhance the physician–patient relationship

While optimal care generally involves a multidisciplinary team and the patient may look to any team member for support, the relationship between patient and doctor is particularly coloured with significance and offers a rich opportunity for the patient to feel supported, thereby aiding in the realization of the above goals.

Models of communication

Traditionally, in medical teaching, the physician–patient relationship has been conceptualized as existing within a continuum that extends from *subjective, empathic identification* at one extreme to *objective depersonalization* and *distancing* at the other. Both have rightfully been rejected, leaving the practitioner who opts for this model to claim a midpoint on the continuum, one that appropriately blends the two extremes. One is then caught between identification and depersonalization, the twin risks that can so easily compromise effectiveness.

On examination, two central weaknesses in this model of relating become evident. Is it not revealing that in our teaching we describe the patient–physician relationship in terms of ourselves? For in the above model, it is the physician who is being subjective, empathic, and identifying or objective, depersonalizing, and distancing. Our model betrays our preoccupation with self, how *I* am relating. Furthermore, it betrays a second bias, for there is a *relator* (the physician) and *one related to* (the patient), an active and a passive agent, and a resultant power differential between the two. The problem is that where a power differential exists, it stands in the way of trust, disclosure, and true dialogue.

There is a better model. Our relating will be enhanced if we abandon the traditional continuum altogether and adopt another perspective, one that arises out of recognition of two realities—the uniqueness of each individual and the shared vulnerability of the human condition. When viewed in the light of these perceptions the patient–physician relationship occurs between equals. Power is neutralized. It becomes easier to move beyond preoccupation with self; to focus on both the uniqueness and the otherness of the one related to. When the focus is on patient *uniqueness*, depersonalization is erased.

When our shared vulnerability is recognized, illusions of power are dispelled. In our insecurity it is easy to fall into the trap of feeling that our effectiveness is linked, in part, to the power differential intrinsic to the physician's role. We may look to the 'MDeity' persona as a placebo adjunct in therapeutics. Paradoxically, to hide in the power differential of our professional role is to diminish our effectiveness, since our success as healers is tied to our capacity to understand the other's experience of illness, and such an understanding is fed by openness in dialogue and, at best, that deep honesty of interaction referred to by Martin Buber as 'I–thou' relating.[18]

General principles of palliative care communication[19]

Dialogue between caregivers and the terminally ill is like no other form of communication. It can properly involve a degree of self-disclosure not appropriate in other forms of clinical discourse.[20] We communicate using plain language, symbolic language, and non-verbal communication.[21] Most communication is non-verbal. How aware are we of the non-verbal communication from our patients, from their families, from ourselves?

Most communication between people is impersonal, relating to the other as an object *(I–it relating)*. However, it is possible for contact, even when brief, to be person to person at the deepest level *(I–thou relating)*, thus calling forth a sense of identity, self-worth, meaning, and healing in the other.[18]

Effective communication demands attention to the circumstances and setting. It is enhanced when there is privacy, quiet, an absence of glaring lighting, and eye contact at the same level, as when both persons are sitting. Optimal communication demands *active* listening, which is an acquired skill. Am I really listening to what he is saying? Am I listening to what is being left unsaid? Am I listening to his body language and to my own? Am I watching for and neutralizing the power differential between us as caregiver and patient or family member? Do I recognize when the request is for accompaniment rather than for answers to unanswerable questions?

Question 4. How would you respond to Mr G.'s comments? What further information would be helpful to you? What are your goals for the communication that is about to occur?

You respond to M G. by saying that you will need the results of the biopsy in order to answer his questions fully, but that the shadow in the region of the pancreas may well be the reason why he has been having the back pain. He explodes, 'Well if it's cancer I'm going to sue the chiropractor and Dr X.' (the first doctor he had seen). You respond, 'I can appreciate your frustration, but you know Mr G., the problem in making the diagnosis that your doctor experienced is pretty typical for problems in the pancreas. They are often very difficult to diagnose because they tend to cause back pain that at first seems to be due to ordinary back strain. But before we jump to any conclusions why don't we get the tests we need and then I'll have some clear answers for you.'

Before ending the visit you scan the details of the history you have just taken and comment, 'It's a worry to have these things crop up isn't it? From what you've told me it's not the first time you've had to cope with difficult challenges. You were telling me that you lost your youngest son in a car accident, and more recently your wife to cancer. Those must have been tough times. Tell me more about how you got through all that.'

Mr G. tells you with fresh feeling about the death of his son Bob 10 years earlier at the age of 26. As the story unfolds he confides that he had been unable to work for almost a year after that because of heavy drinking, a problem that resurfaced with his wife's illness and death 3 years ago. He now lives with his remaining son Gordon, his daughter-in-law Shirley, and their two children, aged 7 and 9. He states that he is now a member of Alcoholics Anonymous (AA) and drinking is no longer a problem. Mr G.'s only other family member, his daughter Anne, lives out of town but keeps in close contact by telephone.

Mr G. is admitted to hospital. Biopsy confirms pancreatic carcinoma. Findings suggestive of liver and coeliac lymph node metastases are noted on CT scan. During these investigations Gordon G. telephones to request that his father not be told the diagnosis if it should be malignant. The same afternoon Anne calls in a state of high agitation echoing her brother's demand and adding that she wants her father to be referred to a medical centre in her city for further assessment.

Question 5. How would you respond to these requests? What are the key factors influencing your approach?

You recognize that your primary responsibility is to your patient and you are also aware of the barriers to coping that the conspiracy of silence imposes. However, Mr G. has a past history of difficulty dealing with stressful situations, including alcohol abuse, and it is clear that his children have had a longstanding exposure to this problem.

In addition to these factors you recognize further danger signals suggesting troubled communications in this family. Patient, son, and daughter have each in turn reacted precipitately, without discussion involving other family members. You respond to Gordon by suggesting a meeting in which you can discuss his concerns in person. On hearing from Anne, your recommendation becomes a family meeting.

Question 6. Who should be present at this meeting? What are your specific goals?

Family meetings can be a highly effective and powerful tool for achieving several important ends in the shortest possible time. They provide an opportunity to assess the family system, observe family dynamics, and arrive at a shared understanding of diagnosis, prognosis, and management goals. They provide a forum for ventilation of feelings and the establishment of the foundations of trust on which future communications will depend. For both the patient and family, they may enhance reconciliation in relationships and promote a sense of control through participation in decision-making. A designated family spokesperson can be named and mutually acceptable norms for further communication established, including the fact that questioning and open dialogue are welcomed; often, particularly with a large family, this is most effectively accomplished through a designated person.

Who should attend? Ideally, the family should be represented by all those directly affected by the changes in the family system produced by the illness. Err on the side of over-inclusiveness. In addition to the physician, the caregiving team should be represented by such key figures as the primary care nurse, social worker, or psychologist. In our experience the caregiver side of the equation should be limited to two or three persons. More than this may inhibit easy discussion. Multidisciplinary representation and anticipated involvement with this particular family are the selection criteria.

It may be helpful to tape-record family meetings, particularly if some family members are unable to be present. Mutual agreement and consent to record the session should be obtained at the outset once the staff facilitator has explained the rationale.

Family system assessment

A number of issues are important to consider in the family meeting or assessment.

- **Who** is included in the nuclear family, extended family, social network? Anne is single. It turns out that there are no other family members, few friends, and no extended network that could be counted on to assist with home care or family support.
- **What** are the family system characteristics?
    - *Life-cycle-related issues.* In the G. family the presence of the patient and two grandchildren in crowded living quarters is complicated by the fact that Gordon is out of work.
    - *Relationships.* Are they enmeshed or disengaged? You later learn that Anne and her younger brother Gordon have always found their relationship difficult, characterized by competition and mutual resentment. Are there dyads, triads, or coalitions? Anne and her mother had always seen themselves as presenting a unified wall of reason in the face of male instability in the G. family. With the death of her mother Anne has felt isolated and has an even greater need to 'take charge'.
    - *Past ability to cope with crisis.* In addition to Mr G.'s known problems in dealing with crises, his son Gordon has a history of intermittent alcohol abuse, Shirley has a history of depression, and Anne has bouts of anxiety and considerable unpredictability, particularly since her mother's death.
    - *Response to current illness.* Changing roles and relationships are clearly to be watched for in this family with minimal internal resources and significant stressors at the time of diagnosis.
    - *Physical, emotional and financial resources.* These are very limited, as noted above.
    - *Immediate and long-term needs.* Without additional support, care in the home will be difficult as Mr G. becomes weaker.
    - *Risk of troubled bereavement.* Heightened risk of difficult grief resolution occurs with: parental grief reaction following the death of a child, social isolation, an ambivalent relationship with the deceased, presence of concurrent life crises, a short preparation time as with a sudden death, evident pining and clinging to the dying person, cultural or family repression of the expression of grief, and disenfranchised grief, as with a gay lover, mistress, or ex-spouse.[22–24] The G. family have ambivalent relationships and concurrent life crises as indicators that there is a high risk of problems during bereavement.

The family conference, which involved Gordon, Shirley, Anne, you as attending physician, and the primary care nurse, was convened later that week. It revealed the details outlined above and established a basis for future communications. Agreement was reached that Gordon would act as the family representative in discussions with the physician and would keep Anne informed.

In a lengthy discussion Gordon and Anne disclosed their fears that their father would go on a drinking binge and 'give up completely' if told the diagnosis. In response you explained that their father had a right to know about his own health status. You also reassured them that the details they had provided concerning their father's past coping problems were very useful. This led to the establishment of a plan to involve a social worker and to recommend to Mr G. that he maintain close contact with AA from the outset. When you had explained the test results and their father's palliative status in detail and offered to facilitate any further consultations they might wish, Anne agreed that there was no reason to carry through with her request for a second opinion at this time.

You then met alone with Mr G. and told him his diagnosis. The discussion occurred in private in a ward interview room. In response to his questioning you informed him that surgery would not be helpful, but that both standard chemotherapy and chemotherapy research protocols were available for consideration. Following further discussion, both of these options were declined by Mr G. You then explained that your goal would be to work with him to ensure that he was comfortable and able to live as fully as possible. You then reviewed in detail your management plans for his pain, insomnia, anorexia, and nausea.

Having established clear goals, you mentioned to Mr G. that you have great respect for all he has been through in recent years and wondered whether it might not be wise for him to contact his friends in AA so that they could offer their support through this difficult time. He agreed. In leaving, you mentioned that the social worker would be in to see him.

The next day you drop in to see Mr G. prior to his discharge from hospital. He greets you and thanks you warmly for your helpful chat the day before. He then adds, 'I'm glad it isn't serious. And say, I would prefer that you didn't say anything to the kids about any of this'.

Question 7. What is your interpretation of these unexpected comments? How will you respond?

Integration of news concerning a hard reality is a process, not an event. It requires time. Frequently, when the facts are overwhelming, it is possible to hear and deal with them only if they are presented slowly in small packages, one fact at a time. With his thanks and comment about it not being serious, Mr G. is expressing appreciation for the honesty and ground of trust that has been established in your relationship. He has also made it abundantly clear that he will need to move forward slowly as he grapples with all that you have discussed.

Denial

Does Mr. G.'s response represent denial? It seems important to recognize that there are at least two types of 'denial'. *Global denial* represents a total paralysis of coping. It constitutes a need to deny reality and hold on to illusion in the face of overwhelming fear. It is seen in the person who protests in the face of a 25 kg weight loss that the doctors have made a mistake in reading the pathology slides. Great skill and support are needed in dealing with this uncommon situation. In general, it calls for gentle but persistent confrontation to replace illusion with a gradually clearing picture of the reality at hand.

More frequently, as in the case of Mr G., we see *adaptive denial*. Such a strategy represents a creative response to a challenging reality. It chooses to focus on the positive; to filter in only those elements that the psyche can tolerate. Over time it generally leads to a deepening ability to integrate a conscious awareness of those parts of the situation that are necessary to ensure functioning.

Question 8. How should one respond to Mr G.'s admonition not to tell his family about his illness?

Clearly, having already discussed diagnosis and prognosis with his children, you find yourself in an awkward situation. Legally it is the patient's right to inform the family concerning diagnosis and prognosis, yet in the course of the family meeting it had seemed important to inform them fully in order to bring them on side and attain their trust. Thus you have already gone against his wishes and you recall only too well his earlier threat of litigation.

You recognize two options: either you tell him that you have already informed them, with an explanation concerning how this happened, or you say nothing about the family at this time, with the intent of telling them about his request and advising them to say nothing until the natural course of events leads him to speak to them about his condition.

Question 9. What would you do?

Frequently circumstances appear to support disclosure to family members about the diagnosis and prognosis prior to, or in lieu of, discussion with the patient. The current dilemma is a reminder that such a course of action is generally unwise. The physician's mandate is with the patient. However, when circumstances dictate preliminary disclosure to the family, the patient should be advised. To do otherwise is to invite further complications in communication and a lessening of trust.

When circumstances appear to necessitate disclosure of diagnosis or prognosis in the absence of the patient, it may be important respectfully to inform the family that this is rather unusual, and that you hope to involve the patient in subsequent family meetings.

'...I'm glad it isn't serious. And say, I would prefer that you didn't say anything to the kids about any of this.'

You pause before responding to Mr G., intentionally slowing the pace of the conversation while you assess the feelings that lie behind his words. In responding, your goal is to build on the deepening level of trust that you sense exists between you. You speak slowly, thoughtfully, and directly, addressing the part of Mr G. that has become linked to you in trust. 'Well, it's interesting you should say that. You need to know that both Gordon and Anne said the same thing to me the other day. They wanted to protect you in the same way that you now want to protect them. They were insistent that I not tell you about your condition because they were afraid that it would be difficult for you to deal with.'

'In listening to their concerns I felt it was important to discuss your medical condition with them. I hope that was all right. I do believe that they found our chat helpful. It seemed to make it easier for Gordon and Anne to plan together how they can be most helpful when you go home. You know, Mr G., maybe it would be a good idea for us all to have a chat together. Sometimes that sort of thing helps to clear the air. I'd be happy to help with that if you like.'

During the conversation that followed, Mr G. avoided further reference to his diagnosis and yet managed to acknowledge his willingness to accept assistance in discussing these sensitive issues with his children.

Question 10. Are you surprised by how that conversation went?

As is usually the case, a simple, direct, and honest approach that respects both the reality of the situation and the patient's wishes, in this case not to talk further at this time about prognosis, led not to confrontation but to a deepening ability to communicate. Many people, especially men, find it difficult to talk about feelings and charged personal issues. The offer of a supportive presence to facilitate difficult family discussions often relieves anxiety and permits a lessening of pervasive tensions for all involved.

Mr G.'s return home was facilitated by a further meeting with Gordon and Shirley. In the interest of airing issues that they might find difficult to discuss in their father's presence, it was held in the absence of Mr G. During this meeting they were supported in expressing their concerns about the crowded conditions in their home, the risk of Mr G. resorting to alcohol again, Gordon's loss of his job, their related financial worries, and Anne's involvement as 'out-of-town supervisor'. Arrangements were made to involve the family physician, a social worker, a home help nurse, and a palliative care nurse, and to discuss these plans, as well as the need for AA involvement, with Mr G. A meeting with Gordon, Shirley, and Mr G. followed. It was successful in establishing a shared plan of action that enabled discharge from hospital.

Mr G. returned home and remained there for 3 months with gradually progressive loss of weight and strength. During a visit by the palliative care nurse near the end of this period Mr G. commented, 'I'm a lot weaker then I was a week ago. How long do I have?'

Question 11. Who should answer this question? Should the nurse comment or refer this inquiry to the family doctor, or to you as the doctor who was involved in his inpatient care and in the previous discussions regarding prognosis? How would you respond to this question?

The fact that Mr G. asked the nurse suggests his sense of trust in their relationship and underscores the importance of team discussions concerning key issues of communication and family dynamics. The nurse in question had established good communications with the family physician from the outset. Also, she felt that it was not easy for Mr G. to ask such an intimate question and that it arose out of the bonds they had forged in their many chats. Thus she felt comfortable entering into a discussion with Mr G. that conveyed to him that his remaining time was probably limited, while avoiding any precise estimate of length of survival.

She concluded by saying, 'While I can't say with certainty how long you or any of my other patients will live, I can tell you that how ever long it may be, we will continue to be closely involved and we'll work with you to ensure that you are comfortable'. She informed the family doctor and the others involved in his care about the details of this discussion.

Discussing prognosis

Communication regarding prognosis is as integral a part of the care plan as pain control. The patient is most able to choose the person he or she feels most comfortable with in discussing such an intimate matter as dying. Generally, such discussions do not, as anxious family members fear, take away hope. Instead, if handled with sensitivity and support, they tend to bring the reassurance and increased ability to cope that is associated with diminished uncertainty. Patients near death are generally aware of their reality. Their hope often has more to do with the need for assurance of sustained symptom control, and accompaniment by family and health care team, than length of survival.

Hope and wishing are not the same things. For the dying, there is an important difference. Hope bespeaks a perspective on reality, a point of view. It is a child of the human spirit. It arises out of an experience of personal meaning and thus reflects a degree of inner peace. Wishing, in contrast, arises from a sense of need, dissatisfaction, and unrest. It reflects a sense of incompleteness. Hope is the product of adversity transcended, wishing of adversity denied. Hope is found in acceptance, the conscious attitude that accompanies integration. The one who accepts is freed to act, respond, and take control in new ways.

Question 12. What other issues might be raised at this time?

A number of issues should be kept in mind and opportunities to discuss them identified. Has Mr G. written a will? Have a Living Will and Enduring Power of Attorney been discussed? Are there particular symptoms or events that the patient or family fear may occur in dying? These should be discussed and reassurance given concerning the treatment for each.

What does Mr G. think comes after death? This may seem difficult to talk about, but it is an issue that is a concern for those who are dying and often looms as a taboo topic for family members, leaving the patient isolated with his thoughts, hopes, and fears. Has Mr G. any thoughts about a funeral or memorial service following his death? Would he like to suggest content that he feels would be particularly meaningful?

The goal in all these discussions is to enable coping by providing reassurance, diminishing uncertainty, naming fears, and promoting autonomy. It is important to keep the discussion of charged issues simple, low key, and supportive. The physician should adopt a tone that is respectful but which de-dramatizes and lends reassurance through evident comfort in chatting about these questions.

Several days later, because of mounting difficulties in contending with children, home, and his extensive needs, Mr G. was admitted to the palliative care unit. It seemed evident that he had days, at most, to live. He had mild confusion and a level of consciousness that seemed to wax and wane. He was no longer able to respond reliably to your questioning. He was tachypnoeic, had a tachycardia, and was profoundly weak but appeared, despite all that, to be comfortable.

Hours after his admission Anne arrived from out of town and demanded to see 'the doctor in charge'. As you arrive at the unit she meets you in the hall. She is highly agitated and obviously angry.

'Have you seen my father? What are you going to do for him? He is suffering greatly. This is unacceptable. You promised he wouldn't suffer. I should never have left him with Gordon. I should have brought him with me [to her city]. I have asked the nurse to give him something, but nobody does anything!'

Question 13. Discuss in detail how you would respond?

Your response will depend on what you *hear* in her outburst. What are the origins of her anguish? Is he suffering? Is the suffering mainly her own, her projections, amplified by years of ambivalence in their relationship? How can you be most helpful?

It is common for health care professionals to have a high need to serve and, as a result, to experience difficulty in setting limits. Many are all too ready to assume that they should be able to do more—to 'make it all better'. At the same time, it is common for people to assume that dying must be associated with suffering. Thus the death-bed scenario is frequently fraught with expectations concerning suffering on the part of both family and caregivers. The fact is that you have already assessed Mr G., reviewed his medications, and know that he is comfortable. Furthermore, you recall the nature of Anne's highly charged relationship with her father and suspect that ambivalence and guilt are fuelling her anger—a classic precursor to high-risk bereavement.

Rather than either reacting to Anne's impressive anger, or reassuring her there in the middle of the hallway that her father is not suffering, you once again pause before responding, both to provide the space needed for you to assess the likely origins of her anguish and in a deliberate effort to slow down and calm the situation. You then speak to her in a calm and quiet voice.

'Anne, hello! Glad you're here. When did you get in?'

'Look maybe you didn't hear me. Dad is suffering and I can't get any action around here. What does a person have to do?'

'Anne, I heard you loud and clear. And I think I can help. I'm here now, and so are you. You know that you and I share the same goal, that is, your Dad's comfort. I'm sure we can achieve that. Let's go in his room and see what the problem is.'

Without waiting for a response you turn and she follows you down the hall and into Mr G.'s semi-private room. You draw the curtains around the bed, speak quietly to the family of Mr G.'s roommate, informing them, by way of excusing the drawn curtains, that you will be having an important and private conversation and would appreciate privacy and silence, and gather two chairs which you bring to the bedside. Selecting the one closest to the head of the bed for yourself and motioning for Anne to take the one closest to the foot, you both sit down, Anne with evident reluctance and residual irritation.

Without speaking to Anne you calmly and silently watch Mr G. breathe for several minutes, time his respirations, and finally take his pulse. Still without comment, you examine his mouth, moisten his lips using the sponge and water on the bedside table, and put on a relaxation tape of soft instrumental music in the bedside cassette player and adjust the volume. At least 3 to 5 minutes have passed. It seems much longer. There has been no comment from either of you since entering the room.

'Now then Anne. What do you see as the greatest problem just now?'

'His pain! This is ridiculous! The man is in pain.'

'Well Anne, let's look at that more closely. If you watch, you will see that the moaning sounds he is making are timed to his expirations—when he breathes out. See ... There, again ... They represent a form of sighing that comes with relaxation. If they were due to pain they would be at other times as well and would be associated with tensing his muscles. Although he appears to be sleeping and not in contact with us, indeed your father is aware and benefits from family presence. Watch. If I take his hand and speak quietly to him, he will respond.' Taking his hand and slowly stroking his arm with your other hand, in time with his respirations, you speak softly but clearly near his ear, 'Mr G., Anne is here.' He stirs, attempts to open his eyes, and seems to say something, although it is inaudible.

During the conversation that follows Anne progressively relaxes. You answer her questions one by one and deal specifically with issues of hydration, nutrition, his ability to hear and be aware of touch, the need for a clean moist mouth, and the healing calming impact of music. The inappropriateness of CPR is touched on in a simple de-dramatizing manner that reassures: 'CPR has nothing to offer your Dad at this point. It would not significantly prolong his life and I'm sure you wouldn't want to add to his suffering.' The simple goals of good palliative care are gently articulated and the particular needs of this family reflected on.

You sit together for a while in what is now a peaceful silence, and then comment quietly, 'It's not easy, is it?' After a further silence of several moments you realize without turning that

Continued

Anne has started to cry. You offer her a tissue but do not touch her or take her hand, out of respect for her autonomy, her need to be in control, and the freshness of her expression of grief. It will all take some time.

Without speaking, you stand and motion for her to take your chair at the head of the bed. Before leaving the room, you clean and moisten his mouth once again and comment, 'Glad you're here Anne. I'm sure it means a lot to your Dad. You know, this is a good time to say anything that you want to tell him. He will hear you. If you need anything just press the bell. And by the way, when the tape gets to the end, just turn it over. The volunteers and nurses will be glad to help and can get you anything you need.'

Over the ensuing week Mr G.'s level of consciousness improved and, though weak, he was able once again to talk with family members and take fluids by mouth with assistance. Anne, Gordon, and Shirley visited regularly. They appeared tired and were irritable in relating to each other.

Question 14. Are there other interventions that you can suggest at this time or other topics that would be helpful to discuss in preparing the family for Mr G.'s impending decline?

Most families experience a heightening of interpersonal stresses when a family member is dying. It is often helpful to acknowledge this and to suggest strategies for coping. '*You know folks, it might be a good idea for you to draw up a schedule that takes into consideration when it is convenient for each of you to be here. There is no need for there to be more than one of you here at a time while your Dad is stable like this, and that way it will be possible for you to get some rest and deal with the other things that always seem to need doing.*'

Watch for decathexis, the normal separating off seen in many dying animals and a significant minority (perhaps 20 per cent) of palliative care patients, as death approaches. Reassure the family that this is not depression or anger.

Anticipate and explain 'death rattle'. Reassure the family that these sounds are due to upper airway secretions and are expected in a person who is this sick; they are not a problem for the patient, who is not aware of them.

Ask about Gordon and Shirley's children, their relationship with their grandfather, and their understanding of the seriousness of his illness. Suggest that they come to see him and offer assistance in talking to them about his condition. Children of all ages can be included with great benefit in the family experience of loss and grieving around death if the adults present are supportive.

Mr G.'s nurse notes that his respirations are irregular and his limbs and lips increasingly cyanotic. She feels that he is dying.

Question 15. What steps would you take, and why, both at this point and following Mr G.'s death?

At death

Ensure that Mr G. does not die alone. Sitting with him, in the absence of a family member, should be seen as a priority meriting the undivided attention of a caregiver, either volunteer or staff member. Dying alone is one of the most common fears of those who are terminally ill. A policy of accompaniment communicates clearly to the patient and family, to other patients and their family members present on the ward, and to caregivers alike, that it is 'safe to die here';

the individual is valued, and the time of dying is respected. Such a policy also enables the team to provide absent family members with a factual account of the death and reassurance that the patient was comfortable and not alone.

Encourage the family, including children, to be present as an important factor in facilitating subsequent grief work, and be attentive to their needs. Most are uncomfortable in the presence of death. The support of a team member who is able to gauge the need for caregiver presence or absence as a means of assuring support or privacy is very comforting.

Notify the priest, rabbi, or other representative of the relevant religion if that would be supportive for the patient or family.

When Mr G. dies, straighten the body and encourage absent family members to come in. Allow adequate time for this important gathering, and provide a generous supply of tissues, tea, and time for the therapeutic experience of shared acute grief to occur in a facilitating environment. At some point unobtrusively touch the body, thus signifying that it is natural to do so.

Consider whether it is important to let the family collect the deceased's personal effects. This may be particularly important following the death of a child. In this setting also consider whether a memento, such as a lock of hair or picture taken at the time of death, may facilitate future grief work.

Discuss having an autopsy as a step that may resolve subsequent doubts and questions during bereavement.

After death

As noted above, Gordon and Anne have an increased risk for troubled bereavement. Support programmes involving community-based self-help groups, a social worker, or pastoral care person have had a favourable impact on the morbidity and mortality associated with bereavement. Consider referral.

Consider attending the funeral as a means of: assisting the family in reviewing the illness, expressing respect for the family and patient, and addressing one's own personal feelings.[25]

References

1. **Bruera, E., Neumann, C.M., Mazzocato, C., Stiefel, F., and Sala, R.** (2000) Attitudes and beliefs of palliative care physicians regarding communication with terminally ill patients. *Palliat Med*, **14**, 287–98.
2. **Leydon, G.M., Boulton, M., Moynihan, C., *et al.*** (2000) Faith, hope and charity: an in-depth interview study of cancer patients' information needs and information-seeking behavior. *West J Med*, **173**, 26–31.
3. **Bruera, E., Sweeney, C., Calder, K., Palmer, L., and Benisch-Tolley, S.** (2001) Patient preferences versus physician perceptions of treatment decisions in cancer care. *J Clin Oncol*, **19**, 2883–5.
4. **Fallowfield, L., Ratcliff, D., Jenkins, V., and Saul, J.** (2001) Psychological morbidity and its recognition by doctors in patients with cancer. *Br J Cancer*, **84**, 1011–15.
5. **Maguire, P.** (1999) Improving communication with cancer patients. *Eur J Cancer*, **35**, 2058–65.
6. **Fallowfield, L., Jenkins, V., Farewell, V., Saul, J., Duffy, A., and Eves, B.** (2002) Efficacy of a Cancer Research UK communication skills training model for oncologists: a randomised controlled trial. *Lancet*, **359**, 650–6.
7. **Gattellari, M., Voigt, K.J., Butow, P.N., and Tattersall, M.H.** (2002) When the treatment goal is not cure: are cancer patients equipped to make informed decisions? *J Clin Oncol*, **20**, 503–13.
8. **Scott, J.T., Harmsen, M., Prictor, M.J., Entwistle, V.A., Sowden, A.J., and Watt, I.** (2003) Recordings or summaries of consultations for people with cancer. In: *Cochrane Library*, Issue 3. Oxford: Update Software.

9. **Bruera, E., Pituskin, E., Calder, K., Neumann, C.M., and Hanson, J.** (1999) The addition of an audiocassette recording of a consultation to written recommendations for patients with advanced cancer: a randomized, controlled trial. *Cancer,* **86**, 2420–5.
10. **Baile, W.F., Buckman, R., Lenzi, R., Glober, G., Beale, E.A., and Kudelka, A.P.** (2000) SPIKES—a six-step protocol for delivering bad news: application to the patient with cancer. *Oncologist,* **5**, 302–11.
11. **Buckman, R.** (1992) *Breaking Bad News: A Guide for Health Care Professionals.* Baltimore, MD: Johns Hopkins University Press.
12. **Buckman, R., and Baile, W.F.** (eds) (2001) *A Practical Guide to Communication Skills in Cancer Care* (CD-ROM or video set). Toronto: Medical Audio-Visual Communications.
13. **Buckman, R., Korsch, B., and Baile, W.F.** (1998) Part 2: Dealing with feelings. In: Buckman R, Baile WF (eds) *A Practical Guide to Communication Skills in Cancer Care,* (CD-ROM or video set). Toronto: Medical Audio-Visual Communications.
14. **Buckman, R.** (2003) The S-P-I-K-E-S strategy for breaking bad news. In: *Oncology Rounds from Princess Margaret Hospital.* Toronto: Princess Margaret Hospital University Hospital Health Network.
15. **Cassell, E.J.** (1991) *The Nature of Suffering and the Goals of Medicine.* Oxford: Oxford University Press, 37–43.
16. **Cassell, E.J.** (1991) *The Nature of Suffering and the Goals of Medicine.* Oxford: Oxford University Press, 30–47.
17. **Frankl, V.** (1963) *Man's Search for Meaning* (trans J Lasch). Boston, MA: Beacon Press.
18. **Buber, M.** (1973) *I and Thou* (trans RG Smith). Edinburgh: T. and T. Clark.
19. **Mount, B.** (1995) Managing genitourinary cancer: supporting the cancer patient: hospice care. In: Vogelzang NJ, Scardino PT, Shipley WW, Coffey DS (eds) *Comprehensive Textbook of Genitourinary Oncology.* Baltimore, MD: Williams and Wilkins.
20. **Feigenberg, L., and Shneidman, E.S.** (1979) Clinical thanatology and psychotherapy: some reflections on caring for the dying person. *Omega,* **10**, 1–8.
21. **Kubler-Ross, E.** (1969) *On Death and Dying.* New York: Macmillan.
22. **Worden, J.W.** (2001) *Grief Counselling and Grief Therapy: A Handbook for the Mental Health Professional.* New York: Springer.
23. **Parkes, C.M., and Weiss, R.S.** (1983) *Recovery from Bereavement.* New York: Basic Books.
24. **Institute of Medicine Committee for the Study of Health Consequences of the Stress of Bereavement.** Bereavement (1984) In: Osterweis M, Solomon F, Green M (eds) *Reactions, Consequences and Care.* Washington, DC: National Academy Press.
25. **Irvine, P.** (1985) The attending at the funeral. *N Engl J Med,* **312**, 1704–5.

Chapter 2

Managing pain in palliative patients

Mike Harlos and Leah MacDonald

Attitude

To enable each student to:

- Appreciate that pain is a subjective experience.
- Recognize that pain makes up only a portion of the cancer patient's 'total suffering'.
- Appreciate the importance of empowering the patient and/or the family to participate effectively in their pain management.

Skill

To enable each student to:

- Take an effective pain history.
- Consider appropriate investigations in evaluating pain.
- Formulate a pain management strategy using pharmacological and non-pharmacological intervention.
- Be able to prescribe opioids and non-opioid adjuvant medications appropriately.
- Anticipate and attempt to prevent common opioid side effects.
- Be aware of the potential role for interventional analgesia (e.g. spinal analgesia).

Knowledge

To enable each student to:

- Understand the basics of pain pathophysiology, specifically with regard to referred and neuropathic pain.
- Understand the basics of opioid pharmacology and the pharmacology of other agents used in pain control.

Mrs A.M. is a 56-year-old woman who has been a long-term patient at your family practice clinic. She was diagnosed 6 months ago with stage IIIB adenocarcinoma of the right lung. You have not seen her recently, as she temporarily relocated to a larger centre where her son lives and where radiation treatments were available. Her treatment included combined chemotherapy and radiation. While she had some initial response, a CT scan done 2 weeks ago showed an increase in tumour size of

Continued

the right lung primary tumour with some destruction of adjacent ribs, progression of mediastinal node involvement, and metastatic disease in the left lung. With no further chemotherapy or radiation therapy planned, Mrs A.M. has moved back to her own community. She comes to your office today, complaining of pain in her right chest.

Prior to her diagnosis of lung cancer, she has had no significant medical problems.

Mrs A.M. is married, and her 59-year-old husband is in good health. He has recently retired, and has been very supportive throughout the illness. Their son lives in another city, and they have a daughter who lives nearby.

Question 1. What information do you need to gather about Mrs A.M.'s pain in order to be able to help her?

Management of pain requires an understanding of its pathophysiology and classification, which will guide a comprehensive yet focused history, physical examination, and appropriate diagnostic tests.

Pathophysiology of pain

Pain originates through the activation of nociceptors by actual or potential tissue damage; these nociceptors can be stimulated in a variety of ways. Tumour bulk can initiate pain signals because of the mechanical pressure it puts on 'pressure receptors'. The inflammatory response induced by tumour growth and tissue damage leads to the release of numerous inflammatory mediators,[1] including leukotrienes, bradykinin, prostaglandins, substance P, and others, which also stimulate nociceptive neurons.

Afferent A-δ and C sensory nerve fibres carry signals from nociceptors to the dorsal horn laminae of the spinal column where they synapse with interneurons. The signal subsequently ascends primarily in the contralateral spinothalamic tract. This connection between the afferent nerves and the ascending pathways is modulated by a complex system of interneurons that can either inhibit or potentiate the pain signal. Axons in the ascending pathways then carry the nociceptive signal to the thalamus, where it is first perceived as pain. From there the signal is relayed to various areas of the cerebral cortex, leading to more complicated processing such as the ability to localize and remember pain or attach meaning and emotional responses to pain.

There are a number of descending pathways arising from the midbrain and brainstem which modulate the inhibitory neurons of the dorsal horn. Transmitters important in regulating this system include serotonin, norepinephrine, and the endorphin–enkephalin system (naturally occurring opioid-like substances). The analgesic effects of certain antidepressants probably relate to their effect on this system.

With chronic exposure to pain, the nervous system can undergo maladaptive structural and modulatory changes. Particularly in cases where there is damage to peripheral nerves or to the central nervous system (CNS) itself, a chronic state of abnormal excitability in neurons can develop, leading to persistent pain which is often difficult to treat. Activation of the *N*-methyl-D-aspartate (NMDA) receptor has been shown to play an important role in this phenomenon. NMDA receptor antagonists, such as ketamine and methadone, have been found to have an effect in both preventing and treating this type of pain condition. More information on these topics will be found in Chapter 3 on neuropathic pain.

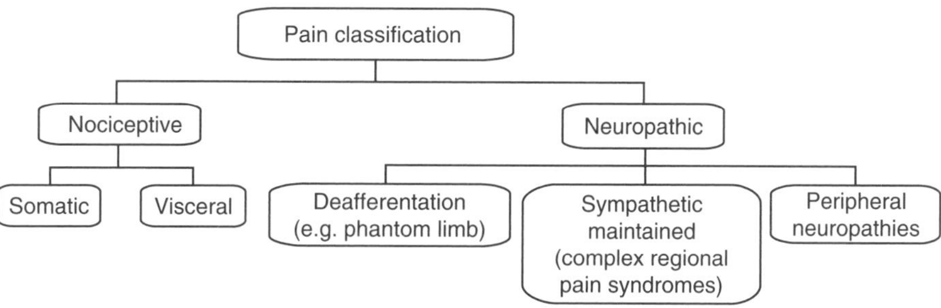

Fig. 2.1 Pain classification.

Pain classification

The two main mechanisms of pain are **nociceptive** and **neuropathic** (Fig. 2.1).

Nociceptive pain can be categorized as **somatic**, if it involves stimulation of nociceptors in the skin, muscle, bone, joints, and ligaments, or **visceral**, if it involves stimulation of nociceptors in the viscera, peritoneum, and pleural cavity.

Somatic pain tends to be well localized, aching, and often reproducible with local pressure in the affected area.

Visceral pain is generally diffuse and often described as 'pressure', 'squeezing', or 'crampy' pain. It is also more likely to be associated with autonomic stimulation, resulting in symptoms such as nausea and diaphoresis. Some patients will describe pain of visceral origin as discomfort rather than pain. Visceral pain can on occasion be referred to (experienced at) a remote superficial site of the body, owing to sharing of secondary neurons between the damaged viscera and the superficial site. An example of this is seen when liver irritation leads to right shoulder pain.

Neuropathic pain is caused by damage to the peripheral nervous system or the CNS. When peripheral nerves are injured they can become increasingly sensitive to stimulation, or may spontaneously fire. Common descriptors of the steady ongoing discomfort of neuropathic pain include burning, stinging, tingling, squeezing, prickly, crawling, and occasionally itching. The sudden discomfort of neuralgic pain, presumably caused by a spontaneous depolarization, may be described as stabbing, lancinating, shock-like, or ' like a lightning bolt'. Referred pain is also common in neuropathic pain, with discomfort experienced in the distribution of the nerve involved.

Clinical terms for the sensory disturbances associated with neuropathic pain include the following.[2]

- Dysesthesia: an unpleasant abnormal sensation, whether spontaneous or evoked.
- Allodynia: pain due to a stimulus which does not normally provoke pain, such as a light touch to the skin.
- Hyperalgesia: an increased response to a stimulus which is normally painful.
- Hyperaesthesia: increased sensitivity to stimulation, excluding the special senses.

Hyperaesthesia includes both allodynia and hyperalgesia, but the more specific terms should be used wherever they are applicable.

Brief episodic pain which occurs despite control of baseline pain is commonly termed 'breakthrough pain'. This reflects that fact that the pain stimulus has 'broken through' the analgesic regimen. This can occur because of an increase in pain stimulus from changes in the underlying illness such as tumour progression, or because of the development of tolerance to the analgesics.

One setting of breakthrough pain is pain that occurs only with activity, termed 'incident pain'. The possible triggering 'incidents' are numerous, and include dressing changes, mobilizing, breathing or coughing, bathing, and so on.

The pain experience

Pain is a complex phenomenon, an experience very much influenced by the emotional, socio-cultural, and spiritual context of the individual. The potential contribution of these factors must be considered in any palliative patient, for whom pain may hold an additional meaning related to death and dying that is not shared by those experiencing pain due to non life-threatening illness. The experience of suffering reflects the combined contribution of these factors. This has been described as 'total pain' (a term coined by Dame Cicely Saunders[3]) or 'total suffering'.[4]

Effective approaches to mitigate suffering associated with illness recognize that the suffering is *total suffering*; our approach to pain assessment and treatment should include sensitivity to the potential impact of non-physical influences.

The language of pain

Some patients may be more comfortable using physical pain terminology to describe their suffering, even if there are substantial emotional or spiritual components involved. They may lack insight into the complexity of their experience, or not wish to explore such issues. Sometimes the term 'anguish' would more accurately describe their suffering; however, some find it difficult to go beyond the language of physical pain. It is very important to believe patients when they describe pain, and to tease out the potential subtexts behind the statement 'it hurts', especially if the pain is not responding as expected to analgesic interventions.

Pain assessment

A thorough evaluation of pain involves:

- a comprehensive pain history
- an evaluation of the psychological state of the patient
- a physical examination, focused on identifying the source of pain if possible
- appropriate diagnostic tests if the source of pain is in doubt or if management plans would change according to the results.

The pain history

The pain history is essential for constructing an effective analgesic strategy. Pain characteristics and examples of how one might inquire about them are listed in Table 2.1. The general rule for history taking is to start with open-ended questions (*'Could you tell me about your pain?'*) and then add more specific questions as necessary. Patients often find pain difficult to describe and may be helped by providing potential descriptors.

As a routine, patients should be taught to quantify the pain intensity, for example with a numbered scale from zero to 10 (Fig. 2.2) such as on the Edmonton Symptom Assessment Scale.[5] This enables description of intensity in a language that has clear meaning to caregivers throughout the spectrum of possible care settings, and facilitates monitoring of changes in pain status.

Table 2.1 Pain assessment

Quality	Questions the interviewer might ask
Location	Where is the pain? Can you point right to it? Can you cause it by pressing there? Does it radiate anywhere?
Temporal pattern	When did it start? Is the pain constant/intermittent? If intermittent, are there sudden, stabbing pains? Crampy pains? Is it worse at certain times of the day? Is it getting worse/better?
Intensity	On a scale of zero to 10 (where zero is no pain and 10 is the worst pain you can imagine), how would you rate the pain you have right now...on average during the day...after activity?
Quality	How would you describe the pain? (Provide examples if necessary, e.g. dull, aching, burning, sharp, stabbing, squeezing, crawling, tingling etc.) Is the skin extremely sensitive, even to light touch such as clothing, shower spray?
Alleviating/ aggravating factors	Does anything make the pain better/worse? Is the pain connected to activity, such as moving, dressing changes, taking deep breaths, eating, bowel movements, etc.?
Effect of medications	What medications have you tried for the pain? How helpful are they?
Impact on lifestyle	What effect has the pain had on your daily activities? Is the pain interrupting your sleep?
Meaning	Are there specific concerns that you have about what is causing this pain, and what it might mean about your illness?
Previous history	Have you ever experienced similar pain in the past? If so, what was it caused by? Were there tests and treatments done... what were they, and what were the results?

The most accurate and meaningful assessment of pain intensity will come directly from the patient. Studies have shown that professional care providers underestimate the pain of the their patients,[6,7] especially in the elderly,[8,9] in children,[10] and in cases of chronic pain where facial features and physiological indicators of acute pain are missing. Similarly, family caregivers may under- or overestimate the amount of pain present.[11]

The clinician must keep in mind the uniqueness of each person's experience and description of pain, and that the complexities of the pain experience are not easily captured in a simple numerical scale.[12] While several pain scales have been found to be valid, reliable, and reproducible, some patients may rate their pain with a low number, trying to be stoic and avoid being alarmist or complaining. Others will consistently score in the 9–10 range, even though

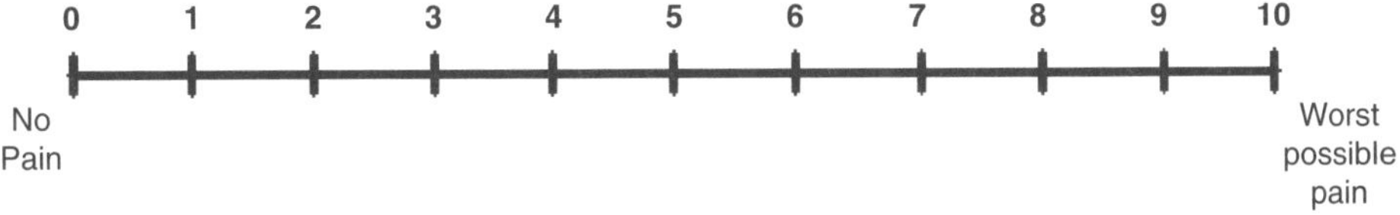

Fig. 2.2 Example of a numbered pain scale.

they may not appear to be in such severe discomfort; in such patients, the concept of *total pain* is often particularly relevant.

Physical examination

Physical examination of the pain patient should be guided by the clinical impression from the pain history. Whether specific systems (such as cardiovascular or respiratory) are examined in more detail will depend on clinical indications. However, there are some important general principles that should be considered in all pain evaluations.

Inspection/observation

'You can observe a lot just by watching'. (Yogi Berra).

- What is your overall impression—the 'gestalt'? Simply observing the patient during the history will provide extremely valuable information.
- Facial expression: grimacing, furrowed brow, appears anxious, flat affect.
- Body position and spontaneous movement: there may be positioning to protect painful areas, limited movement due to pain.
- Diaphoresis: can be caused by pain.
- Areas of redness, swelling.
- Atrophied muscles.
- Gait.
- Myoclonus: possibly indicating opioid-induced neurotoxicity (see below).

Palpation

- Localized tenderness to pressure or percussion.
- Fullness/mass.
- Induration/warmth.

Neurological examination A thorough neurological examination is important in evaluating pain because of the possibility of spinal cord compression and nerve root or peripheral nerve lesions.

- Sensory examination:
  - areas of numbness/decreased sensation
  - areas of increased sensitivity, such as allodynia or hyperalgesia.
- Motor examination: assessment of muscle strength
  (**Note:** Use caution in applying resistance to the extremities during motor testing if bone metastases exist or are suspected; it is possible to cause a pathological fracture including the humerus or femur.)
- Deep tendon reflexes (intensity, symmetry):
  - hyperreflexia and clonus point to an upper motor neuron lesion, such as spinal cord compression or cerebral metastases
  - hyoporeflexia: diminished or absent reflexes may indicate lower motor neuron impairment including lesions of the cauda equina of the spinal cord or leptomeningeal metastases.
- Sacral reflexes: diminished rectal tone may indicate cauda equina involvement of tumour.

Other Further areas of focus of the physical examination are determined by the clinical presentation. For example, evaluation of pleuritic chest pain would involve a detailed respiratory and chest wall examination.

Diagnostic investigations

After a history and physical examination it may or may not be necessary to order investigations to elucidate further the cause of a patient's pain. It is important to keep in mind the potential burden of an investigation, particularly in palliative patients, and realistically consider how the results might change the management. Such deliberations are undertaken in collaboration with the patient and family.

The main goals of diagnostic interventions for pain are as follows:

1. Confirm or rule out suspected causes of pain.
2. Define the anatomy of the area of concern, to guide possible therapeutic interventions such as radiation therapy, surgery, nerve blocks, or spinal analgesia.
3. Assess the extent of disease. This may be helpful in deciding the appropriateness of further investigations and interventions.

Which specific tests to consider will depend on the clinical situation at hand. The following are some common investigations and their potential roles.

Plain radiography

- Plain radiographs are specific in defining primary or metastatic tumour involvement of bone; however, small lesions may be missed (limited sensitivity).
- In evaluating chest pain, chest films may reveal rib destruction or intrathoracic tumour. A pleural effusion can be associated with a pressure sensation or aching discomfort.
- In evaluating abdominal pain, plain radiographs can demonstrate constipation, bowel obstruction, or free air (indicative of perforated abdominal viscus).

Radioisotope bone scans

- About 95 per cent sensitivity for bone metastases.
- May be difficult to distinguish from inflammatory or traumatic lesions (specificity not as high as plain radiographs).
- Typically do not demonstrate abnormality (false negative) in multiple myeloma or other tumours with primarily osteolytic features; plain radiographs are more accurate for such lesions.

Computed tomography (CT)

- Can produce high resolution images with very effective imaging of bone.

Magnetic resonance imaging (MRI) scans

- Particularly effective in producing high-resolution soft tissue images.
- The investigation of choice for possible spinal cord compression; availability may be a limiting issue.

Other Specific investigations may be appropriate for the presenting clinical scenario.

With guidance from you, Mrs A.M. tells you that her pain is an almost constant aching pain in her right chest that has been steadily increasing over the last few months. She describes it as 5 to 10 in intensity, increasing to 6 or 7 to 10 in the evening. It is not made worse with breathing. She has no areas of numbness or increased skin sensitivity of the chest wall, and no lancinating or stabbing pains. The pain does not radiate elsewhere. The pain covers a broad area, larger than what can be covered by her own hand on the chest wall.

She had been given tablets consisting of acetaminophen 325 mg with codeine 30 mg, of which she takes one or two as needed. She has been reluctant to use them because of the severe constipation they cause, and she finds them minimally helpful in reducing her pain when she does take them. Nonetheless, she is taking six to eight tablets daily.

Since you have not seen Mrs A.M. for some time, you explore a little further how she is coping with her terminal diagnosis. After some discussion, you conclude that depression or anxiety are not significantly exacerbating her pain.

On examination, Mrs A.M. is moderately cachectic. Her mood and range of affect seem normal. There is no chest-wall tenderness, and no areas of diminished sensation or hyperalgesia. Chest auscultation is unremarkable.

You do not order any investigations at this point; the pain that Mrs A.M. is describing is consistent with the progression of her lung tumour and you have a recent CT scan showing the extent of her disease.

Question 2. How would you classify Mrs A.M.'s pain?

Mrs A.M.'s pain is consistent with nociceptive somatic pain related to her right lung tumour invading local bone and soft tissues. The difficulty in reproducing the pain on physical examination (absence of tenderness) and the broad area where the pain is experienced could also be consistent with visceral pain. Although she is at risk for neuropathic pain from potential involvement of intercostal nerves, this does not seem to be a significant component of her current pain presentation. Based on the clinical and CT scan findings, you conclude that she probably has mixed pain, both somatic and visceral.

Question 3. How will you treat Mrs A.M.'s pain?

Basic principles of pain pharmacotherapy in palliative care

While each person and each clinical presentation of pain management presents a unique situation, there are basic principles of pain pharmacotherapy that can guide the construction of an analgesic strategy.

1. If the pain has been consistently present and is expected to remain so, it should be treated proactively rather than reactively. This means that regular doses of analgesics should be used (the 'by the clock' principle described by the World Health Organization [WHO]), titrated as needed for comfort.
2. Choose medications that are appropriate for the type of pain experienced by the patient, based on a detailed pain assessment. The WHO has developed a model for the pharmacological treatment of pain in the palliative patient that includes opioid and non-opioid analgesics, as well as adjuvant therapies (Fig. 2.3). Non-pharmacological treatment and interventional anaesthetic techniques are other potential tools in the management plan.

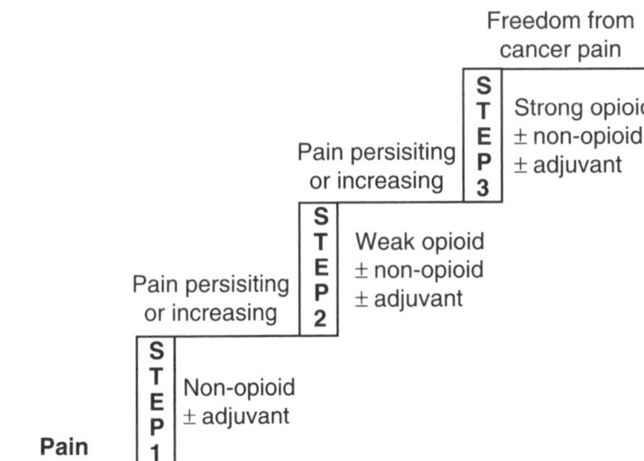

Fig. 2.3 WHO analgesic ladder. Modified from *Cancer Pain Relief* Geneva: World Health Organization.

3. Use short-acting (immediate-release) opioids for titration in poorly controlled pain. This facilitates a rapid response to changing opioid needs, and a more prompt achievement of therapeutic levels than with long-acting (sustained-release) opioids.
4. Simplify the route of administration, using the least invasive route capable of achieving acceptable analgesia; in most circumstances that is the oral route. While intravenous and subcutaneous routes have a faster onset, the oral route is just as effective in cases of stable pain when swallowing and absorption are not compromised. The large majority of cancer patients can achieve good control of even severe pain with oral opioids.
5. Always start a laxative when starting an opioid analgesic. Constipation will occur with all opioids, and it is much less difficult and burdensome for the patient to prevent constipation than to treat it once it becomes severe. **Concern about potential constipation should almost never be a reason to withhold the appropriate use of opioids for symptom control.** With a proactive approach, opioid-induced constipation can be managed. A stool softener such as docusate is often given concomitantly with a sennoside stimulant to begin with, and if needed more potent laxatives such as lactulose can be given. Avoid bulk-forming laxatives such as bran and psyllium products in frail patients with poor fluid intake, as they can cause obstipation. More information on constipation can be found in Chapter 18.
6. Since the majority of cancer pain patients with evenly controlled baseline pain will also experience daily episodes of breakthrough pain, always provide a breakthrough analgesic. Patients should feel confident that their breakthrough (or 'rescue') analgesic doses are reliably effective; they must feel empowered to address increases in pain should they occur. Important principles of managing breakthrough pain include the following.
    - Do not use long-acting opioids for breakthrough doses (except for methadone). The pharmacokinetics of long-acting drugs can result in delayed onset of action and potential for accumulation if used with a short dosing interval.
    - The breakthrough opioid dose must be proportionate to the total daily opioid dose: generally 50–100 per cent of the regular four-hourly dose, or 10–20 per cent of the total daily dose if long-acting opioids are being used as the regular opioid analgesic. As opioids are titrated, the breakthrough dose must also be adjusted accordingly.
    - Patients should be encouraged to take their breakthrough opioid as often as every 1–2 h, if needed. Oral opioids generally have a peak effect within approximately 60 min; patients

should not have to wait longer than this to repeat a breakthrough dose if necessary. It is extremely unlikely that an opioid-tolerant patient would develop respiratory depression from an aggressive approach to oral breakthrough analgesia, as the ability to ingest repeated doses will generally be limited by sedation before respiratory compromise develops.

- Anticipate the need for breakthrough doses and use them pre-emptively. For example, if there is a pattern of incident pain and an outing is planned that is likely to result in an increase in pain, then a breakthrough dose of opioid should be taken about an hour in advance.
- Repeated and consistent need for breakthrough doses (more than two or three a day) should prompt a re-evaluation of the pain and consideration of increasing the regular opioid dose. It could be that the patient does not have breakthrough pain but instead has poorly controlled baseline pain that is being managed with breakthrough pain doses to supplement the baseline opioid.

Specific medications

Non-opioid analgesics

Non-opioid analgesics include acetaminophen (paracetamol) and non-steroidal anti-inflammatory drugs (NSAIDs). These medications have a ceiling effect, beyond which increases in dose do not yield increased analgesia. The WHO analgesic ladder suggests a trial of these medications in cases of milder pain. If the pain is not well controlled, an opioid should replace or be added to the non-opioid analgesic.

Acetaminophen

Acetaminophen can be effective in different types of pain and, in view of its low incidence of adverse effects when used in appropriate doses, is a reasonable option in mild pain. Anecdotally, it can be surprisingly effective in headache due to increased intracranial pressure, bone pain, neuropathic pain, or other specific pains, even if opioids have been unhelpful. The maximum recommended daily dose of acetaminophen in adults is 4000 mg. However, if pre-existing liver disease is present, consider more conservative dosing or perhaps an alternative analgesic.

NSAIDs

NSAIDs act through inhibition of the enzyme cyclo-oxygenase (COX), which is involved in prostaglandin synthesis and contains subtypes COX-1 and COX-2. The COX-1 subtype is ubiquitous, and is involved in protection of the gastric mucosa and in platelet aggregation. COX-2 is involved in modulation of the complex inflammatory response. It is found in the brain and the kidney, and can be induced at sites of inflammation. COX-2 is not present in platelets.

It is believed that NSAIDs produce analgesia through a reduction in activation and sensitization of nociceptors caused by inflammatory mediators such as prostaglandins. Newer agents (rofecoxib, celecoxib) selectively inhibit the COX-2 subtype and do not impair platelet aggregation. They may cause fewer gastrointestinal mucosal lesions than non-selective NSAIDS. However, recent concerns regarding the cardiovascular safety of selective COX-2 inhibitors has led to the voluntary withdrawal of rofecoxib from the market, and to increased scrutiny of this group of medications as a whole.

When using NSAIDs, the prescriber should always keep in mind the potential renal and gastrointestinal toxicities, regardless of the NSAID chosen.

The lack of effect of selective COX-2 inhibitors on platelet aggregation should favour their use over non-selective NSAIDs in patients who have existing risk of bleeding or who have bleeding from solid tumours such as lung, kidney, or colorectal carcinomas.

Among the non-selective NSAIDs, the most commonly used classes include the following:

- salicylates such as ASA and choline magnesium trisalicylate
- acetates such as diclofenac, indomethacin, and sulindac
- proprionates including ibuprofen, ketoprofen, and naproxen.

There are no data indicating that one medication or class of NSAIDs is more effective than another. It is worth being familiar with one or two drugs from each class, as some patients who do not respond to one NSAID may respond to another from a different class. There is evidence that selective COX-2 inhibitors have an overall incidence of serious adverse events, including thrombosis, congestive heart failure, and high blood pressure, that is similar to or higher than that encountered with non-specific NSAIDs. Individualized assessment of each patient who is prescribed an NSAID is a useful approach to monitoring for the presence of these toxicities.

Opioid analgesics

Opioid analgesics include natural derivatives of the opium poppy, as well as synthetic and semisynthetic drugs which produce their effects through combining with opiate receptors and are blocked by naloxone.[13] The μ (mu) opiate receptor is the main site of action for the commonly used opioid analgesics.

Opioids are commonly considered as being either 'weak' (such as codeine), used for mild to moderate pain, or 'strong' (such as morphine and others), used for moderate to severe pain.

Potential adverse effects of opioid analgesics are listed in Table 2.2. Note that probably all opioids can have neuroexcitatory effects as can many of their metabolites.

Codeine Codeine is a naturally occurring opium alkaloid and is a pro-drug of morphine. Individuals who lack the cytochrome P-450 enzyme necessary for transformation of codeine to morphine may experience little analgesia from codeine; this may be as much as 7–10 per cent of the Caucasian population.[14] If this is suspected in a patient who is not responding as expected to codeine, an alternative opioid should be used.

Codeine may be used alone; however, it is commonly combined with a non-opioid analgesic such as acetaminophen. There is a ceiling effect to codeine that appears to be reached at approximately 60 mg parenterally, which limits its use to situations of mild to moderate pain. However, the data are inconsistent regarding the maximum effective dose.

Morphine Morphine is the prototypical strong opioid analgesic, and is the opioid recommended by WHO to be available worldwide. It is a naturally occurring opium derivative, and in Canada is available in oral (long-acting tablets, long-acting granules in capsules, and short-acting tablets and elixir), rectal (long- and short-acting suppositories), and injectable formulations. Morphine is predominantly metabolized by the liver into morphine-3-glucuronide (M3G) and morphine-6-glucuronide (M6G), which are excreted by the kidneys.[15] M6G is an active metabolite which binds to opioid receptors and has analgesic effects. M3G does not appear to have analgesic effects; however, it may play a significant role in the neurotoxic adverse effects of morphine. Morphine should be used cautiously in patients with renal insufficiency, or an alternative opioid should be selected if patients develop evidence of toxicity.

Table 2.2 Possible opioid side effects

Side effect	Cause	Potential action to take
Constipation	Activation of μ receptors in gut leading to decreased intestinal mobility	Proactively add laxative, stool softener Avoid bulking agents Patients do not develop tolerance to this side effect See constipation (Chapter 18)
Nausea/vomiting	Direct stimulation of the chemoreceptor trigger zone in the medulla GI motility and delayed gastric emptying Vestibular effects	If mild, reassure patient that tolerance will probably build (3–5 days) Use antinauseants such as metoclopramide, domperidone, haloperidol, or dimenhydrinate as needed
Sedation	Central effect	If mild, tolerance usually develops in 2–3 days May need to change (rotate) opioids Interventional analgesia Decrease opioid requirements through use of adjuvants, radiation therapy, or chemotherapy. Consider adding CNS stimulant such as methylphenidate
Urinary retention	Increase in bladder sphincter tone Relaxation of detrusor muscle	Consider decreasing opioid dose or trial of alternative opioid When possible, avoid concomitant administration of anticholinergics Consider pro-cholinergic medication
Pruritus	Release of histamine	Consider switching to a more synthetic opioid such as oxycodone, fentanyl, or methadone Antihistamines (co-administration of both H_1 and H_2 blockers) For itch related to spinal opioids, adding bupivacaine spinally may help; also consider parenteral ondansetron
Opioid-induced neurotoxicity (also see later in this chapter) Sedation, confusion Myoclonus Hyperalgesia Seizures	Opioids, their metabolities, or both Exacerbated by renal failure	Opioid rotation or dose reduction Hydration Benzodiazepine
Respiratory depression (Note: serious but uncommon in opioid-tolerant patients)	Central (brainstem) inhibition of respiratory drive	Administer oxygen Discontinue opioids If mild (patient easily roused, respiratory rate ≥ 8 bpm), observe If patient not rousable and respiratory rate <8 bpm, consider administering titrated doses of 0.04–0.08 mg of naloxone (1–2 ml of 1:10 dilution of the commercial 0.4 mg/ml preparation) subcutaneously or intravenously

Often, close monitoring for toxicity is all that is needed. The only opioid which is known not to accumulate either parent drug or metabolites in renal failure is methadone; it is metabolized in the liver and undergoes predominantly faecal excretion. Others are either known to accumulate or have been observed clinically to behave as if they accumulate in renal impairment.

Hydromorphone Hydromorphone is a semisynthetic morphine derivative with approximately five times the potency of morphine. In Canada, it is available in oral (long- and short-acting), rectal, and injectable formulations.

Hydromorphone is predominantly metabolized to hydomorphone-3-glucuronide, a potent neuroexcitant[16] that is renally excreted.[17]

Oxycodone Oxycodone is a semisynthetic morphine congener with short and long-acting oral formulations, and is a reasonable Step 2 drug on the WHO analgesic ladder (Fig. 3) in preparations combined with non-opioid analgesics such as acetaminophen/paracetamol. In formulations alone, it can be used in severe pain. Although reported as clinically inactive 18, its metabolite oxymorphone has analgesic properties and accumulates in renal failure 19, as does oxycodone, warranting caution in such circumstances.

Transdermal fentanyl Fentanyl is a highly potent synthetic μ agonist, approximately 100 times as potent as morphine. The transdermal patch formulation (Duragesic®) is a useful option in the management in moderate to severe pain. The patch is changed every 3 days, although there are individuals for whom a 2-day interval seems most effective. A subcutaneous depot is created beneath the patch, from which the opioid is absorbed systemically.

The onset of action is gradual after first applied, being close to peak levels within about 24 h. Similarly, the decline in serum drug level following patch removal is gradual, falling by 50 per cent in the first 17 h.[20] Because of the slow change in serum levels after dose changes, if there is unstable or severe pain opioids of more rapid onset should be used to stabilize pain control prior to use of the transdermal fentanyl patch.

There are no known active metabolites of fentanyl but further study is needed.

There is some evidence that transdermal fentanyl may be less constipating than other oral opioids.[21]

Specific circumstances in which transdermal fentanyl should be considered include the following.

- Compromised oral route:
  - dysphagia in head and neck cancers
  - oesophageal, gastric outlet, or bowel obstruction
  - decreased or variable level of consciousness.
- Poor compliance with oral medications.
- Preoccupation with medication regimen; anxiety about schedule.
- Adverse effects of other opioids.

In general, the dosing recommendation from the manufacturer should be followed for dose equivalences to morphine. Breakthrough doses are given with a short-acting opioid such as morphine or hydromorphone, and are generally calculated as 10–20 per cent of the total daily morphine equivalence of the transdermal fentanyl.

For example, a transdermal fentanyl patch of 100 μg/h is approximately equivalent to 315–404 mg/day of oral morphine, according to the manufacturer's conversion table. For breakthrough analgesia, one could prescribe 30–40 mg of oral morphine per dose.

If hydromorphone is chosen as a breakthrough opioid, the dose would be approximately one-fifth of the morphine dose, which would be 6–8 mg hydromorphone. This could be given every 1–2 h as needed.

Use caution when administering transdermal fentanyl to the frail elderly or those of small body weight. In particular, do not increase the dose more frequently than every few days, as drug accumulation may occur 1–2 weeks into the regimen, resulting in opioid overdose.

Methadone Methadone is a synthetic opioid developed in the 1940s that is having an increasing role in pain management. As described above, it has no known active metabolites, which makes it an attractive choice in renal insufficiency. With its structural difference from morphine, it can be considered for use in the rare patient who is truly allergic to morphine, or in those who develop pruritus from histamine release due to morphine and its congeners. Methadone is very inexpensive when prepared from powder form.

Methadone also has antagonism activity toward the NMDA receptor, which is implicated in the development of opioid tolerance, opioid-induced neurotoxicity, and neuropathic pain. There is some anecdotal evidence to support the effectiveness of methadone in these circumstances, but this is an area currently under investigation.

There are significant cautions that must be observed in the use of methadone. Its half-life varies from 13 to >100 h, although most people require dose intervals of 8–12 h. This difference between half-life and duration of effect can result in potentially dangerous drug accumulation over time,[13] which must be watched for, particularly in the dose titration phase.

Equivalent dosing between methadone and other opioids has been shown to depend on the existing opioid tolerance as reflected in the total daily opioid dose. Methadone's relative potency increases substantially in circumstances of high opioid dosing (Table 2.3), requiring close attention and clinical caution when converting.

There is recent evidence associating high doses of methadone with the potentially fatal ventricular arrhythmia torsade de pointes.[22] The clinical implications of this in palliative patients is not clear. However, in a recent publication a panel of experts did not recommend routine electrocardiograms in patients taking methadone.[23]

Meperidine pethidine Meperidine has a neurotoxic metabolite (normeperidine), which can accumulate in chronic use and cause potentially fatal seizures. Meperidine should not be used in palliative pain management except in unusual circumstances.

Converting between opioids: equivalent dosing Most studies looking at opioid equivalences have been undertaken using single doses in acute pain situations in patients who were not opioid tolerant. Tolerance develops with repeated dosing of a given opioid; however, this tolerance is not fully expressed when switching over to other opioids. This phenomenon is called 'incomplete cross-tolerance', and can result in opioid overdose if standard equianalgesic conversion tables are followed in patients on chronic opioid therapy. In order to account for incomplete cross-tolerance when converting from one opioid to another, the calculated conversion dose should be reduced by 30–50 per cent and titrated upwards as needed.

In situations of very high dosing, and most particularly in opioid-induced neurotoxicity, incomplete cross-tolerance may be very significant, and it may be best to undertake a gradual conversion to the new opioid over several days. Alternatively, one could abruptly stop the first opioid and use generous as-needed dosing of the alternative opioid until an effective dose is found. In such circumstances, consultation with experts in pain management should be considered.

Table 2.3 highlights current conversion ratios for selected opioids.

Table 2.3 Opioid dose equivalence ratios

Drug	Approximate equipotency with oral morphine (morphine:drug)
Hydromorphone	5:1
Oxycodone[24]	1.5:1 to 2:1
Codeine[1]	1:12
Methadone[25]	
Daily morphine dose (mg)	
30–90	3.7:1
90–300	7.75:1
>300	12.75:1
Transdermal fentanyl[26]	100:1

Special note on management of incident pain

Incident pain is particularly challenging to manage, as there may be severe pain with increased physical activity but little or no pain otherwise. Breakthrough dosing with high dosages of short-acting morphine or hydromorphone may result in sedation during periods of inactivity.

One approach is to use sublingual or intranasal doses of ultra-rapid onset short-acting opioids such as fentanyl or sufentanil[27–32] administered in anticipation of the 'incident' or activity. These medications generally have a duration of activity of approximately 1 h, resulting in less drowsiness between activities. A protocol for the use of fentanyl and sufentanil for the management of incident pain can be found at http://palliative.info/IncidentPain.htm

Adjuvant medications

Adjuvant pain control medications were first developed for non-analgesic indications, and were subsequently found to have analgesic activity in specific pain scenarios. They are often added to a treatment plan in cases of pain which is poorly responsive to opioids (such as neuropathic pain) or with the intention of lowering the total opioid dose and thereby mitigating opioid side effects.

Table 2.4 outlines examples of adjuvant medications and their potential indications.

Table 2.4 Examples of adjuvant analgesics

Type of medication	Examples	Proposed mechanism of action	Pain indication
Corticosteroids	Prednisone, dexamethasone	Inhibits inflammatory response to tissue damage Decreases peritumour oedema reduce spontaneous discharge in injured nerves	Multiple indications including spinal cord compression, headache from raised intracranial pressure, neuropathic pain
Alpha-2 adrenergic agonists	Clonidine	Decrease sympathetic transmitter release Pre- and post-synaptic inhibition	Refractory neuropathic pain

Continued

Table 2.4 Examples of adjuvant analgesics—*cont'd*

Type of medication	Examples	Proposed mechanism of action	Pain indication
Neuroleptics	Methotrimeprazine (levomepromazine)	?Antagonism of dopamine receptors in pain pathways	Limited role; pain with significant anxiety or concomitant delirium
Anticonvulsants	Gabapentin	Reduction of spontaneous nerve discharge ?Effect on voltage-dependent Ca^{2+} channel currents at post-synaptic dorsal horn neurons[33]	Neuropathic pain
Tricyclic antidepressants	Desipramine, nortriptyline, amitriptyline	Increase in monoamine activity in descending pain-modulating pathways	Neuropathic pain, particularly continuous dysaesthesia
NMDA receptor antagonists	Ketamine, dextromethorphan	Agent in intracellular events involved in opioid tolerance, opioid-induced neurotoxicity, and neuropathic pain	Neuropathic pain Opioid-induced neurotoxicity ?Situations of high opioid tolerance
Bisphosphonates	Pamidronate, clodronate, zoledronate	Inhibit osteoclast activity	Bone pain
Calcitonin		Osteoclast inhibition Uncertain mechanism in pain other than bone	Bone pain Sympathetically mediated pain Acute phantom pain

Mrs A.M. is describing moderate pain that has not responded well to a weak opioid (codeine) combined with acetaminophen. In view of the progression of her disease and severity of her current pain, a strong opioid will be needed.

You suggest that she start regular dosing of oral shorting-acting morphine, beginning with 10 mg every 4 h, with a breakthrough dose of 5 mg every hour as needed. You also provide her with a recommendation for starting docusate every morning and a sennoside laxative every evening, and you stress to her the importance of having regular bowel movements while on opioids.

Because of potential nausea when starting opioids, you supply her with a prescription for metoclopramide 10 mg tablets, to fill if needed, which can be taken up to every 4 h as required. You encourage her by telling her that should nausea occur, it is usually a side effect to which patients develop tolerance within a few days.

Question 4. Besides prescribing an opioid, are there any other interventions that might be helpful in achieving pain control?

In view of the rib destruction noted on the CT scan, it is worth exploring whether radiation therapy might help her pain. Even when chemotherapy and radiation are no longer possible as curative or life-prolonging treatments, they may palliate symptoms. An opinion from an appropriate consultant should be sought with regard to options, particularly in cases where a patient has not been seen recently by an oncologist.

> You contact Mrs A.M's radiation oncologist, who informs you that she has already had the maximum allowable dose of radiation to her right chest wall.

Interventional analgesia

Potential considerations include nerve block (such as an intercostal block for Mrs A.M.'s chest wall pain) and spinal analgesia (epidural or intrathecal administration of opioids, local anaesthetics, and other drugs). Generally, these interventions are considered when the systemic side effects of opioids (such as sedation) limit dosing. In-dwelling catheters can be tunnelled for long-term use, and the patient can be mobile with a portable pump.

Clinicians should consider referral to palliative medicine or pain consultants with experience in interventional analgesia for review of such options in challenging pain management situations.

> Mrs A.M. mentions that a friend of hers at the cancer clinic was taking a long-acting form of morphine. 'Couldn't I take those instead?' she asks.

Question 5. What is the role of long-acting opioid analgesics in pain management?

Long-acting opioid formulations are more convenient and are associated with improved compliance in management of chronic baseline cancer pain. However, they should not be used in uncontrolled pain, as their lengthy half-lives make titration difficult. Once the pain has been controlled, the dose of short-acting opioid can be converted to a long-acting formulation, simply by adding up the total daily dose and dividing it according to the recommended dosing schedule of the long-acting drug. For example, if a patient is taking morphine 20 mg every 4 h, that would be the equivalent of 60 mg of the long-acting morphine formulation every 12 h.

> 'Until your pain is well controlled it would be better for you to stay with short-acting morphine.'
>
> As promised, you call Mrs A.M. at home 3 days after your initial visit to inquire how she is doing with the morphine. You are disappointed to hear that she is still describing significant pain. On further questioning you learn that, despite your discussions, Mrs A.M.'s daughter has discouraged her from taking the morphine regularly and instead wants her to take it 'only as needed' to avoid 'getting addicted'. She is also worried about her mother driving while on opioids.
>
> You speak to Mrs A.M.'s daughter to explain that if she takes the analgesic only for pain control, the overwhelming likelihood is that she will never become addicted.

Common myths and misconceptions about opioids

1. Addiction (psychological dependence) is extremely uncommon when opioids are appropriately used for pain in palliative circumstances. Clinicians should be familiar with the distinction between the following.[34]

- Tolerance: a physiological state characterized by a decrease in the effects of a drug (e.g. analgesia, nausea or sedation) with chronic administration
- Physical dependence: the development of physical withdrawal symptoms when opioids are discontinued, when the dose is reduced abruptly, or when an antagonist (e.g. naloxone) or an agonist–antagonist (e.g. pentazocine) is administered
- Psychological dependence ('addiction' in former terminology): compulsive use of drugs for non-medical reasons characterized by a craving for mood-altering drug effects, not pain relief.

2. A common concern is that if opioids are started 'too early' in the illness, they will not be effective later. There is no basis for this belief; opioids have no ceiling effect and can be titrated as needed. There is some evidence that patients who have better control of chronic cancer pain will actually live longer.
3. Many people mistakenly believe that driving is not allowed while on opioids. This is not the case. In Canada and many other countries, administration of opioids is not a specific contraindication to non-commercial driving. People who are on stable doses and who are not drowsy are allowed to drive; the decision is left to the judgement of the driver. Immediately after a dose change, there may be 2–3 days of drowsiness, during which it may be safest to avoid driving.

Mrs A.M. and her daughter return to your office two weeks later, during which time you have been out of town. Mrs A.M.'s pain had increased, and your colleague has gradually increased her morphine to 40 mg every 4 h. She has been taking three 25-mg breakthrough doses daily. Her daughter is concerned about some mild confusion and 'twitching' that has developed. Mrs A.M. had been experiencing increased right chest pain, but now complains of being uncomfortable 'all over'.

Question 6. What is the probable cause of Mrs A.M.'s new symptoms? What would be an appropriate plan of action at this time?

Mrs A.M. is probably demonstrating early signs of opioid-induced neurotoxicity. This is addressed in detail in Chapter 6, but will be briefly reviewed here.

As clinicians are becoming more familiar and comfortable with prescribing opioids for pain in life-limiting illness, adverse effects related to neurotoxicity are being seen more often. Fortunately, these can often be managed through simple measures when recognized early.

Opioid-induced neurotoxicity (OIN) refers to a spectrum of effects seen during opioid therapy that can include delirium, hyperalgesia, allodynia, myoclonus, and seizures. These have been attributed to the opioid metabolites of meperidine (its metabolite normeperidine), and in particular to the 3-glucuronide metabolites of morphine and hydromorphone (M3G, H3G).[16] These metabolites are renally excreted, and are particularly prone to accumulate in conditions of dehydration or compromised renal function. There have also been reports of OIN associated with opioids with no known active metabolites, such as methadone[35,36] and fentanyl.[37,38] Therefore any opioid can be associated with OIN.

The cellular events implicated in OIN (raised intracellular calcium, cyclic AMP formation, phosphinoside hydrolysis[39]) appear to involve the NMDA receptor.[40]

Early signs of OIN include sedation and delirium. Myoclonic jerking is often first noted when patients are drifting off to sleep. These sudden muscular contractions can startle the patient awake and they may call out in distress, particularly if delirium is present.

If hyperalgesia is present as well, it can be challenging to distinguish between OIN and an increase in tumour-related pain. The distinction is critical, however, as the latter calls for an increase in opioid while the former requires dose reduction or a change in opioids.

Generally, opioid-induced hyperalgesia occurs along with other features of OIN, such as myoclonus and CNS side effects (lethargy or delirium). The pain tends to be generalized, and is not consistent with the known underlying disease; hyperalgesic patients develop pain everywhere, while previously their pain was related to areas of known disease. They will often call out in pain when moved, even if the activity appears unlikely to cause discomfort.

It may appear to those at the bedside that the patient is in uncontrolled pain, for which the offending opioid may then be increased. This can lead to a vicious circle in which the opioid is increased in order to address problems that it is actually causing (Fig. 2.4). A clue to this clinical scenario is a rapid escalation in opioid dose over a few days.

Managing opioid-induced neurotoxicity

Prevention

- Demonstrate caution in prescribing opioids with known active metabolites to patients with impaired renal function, such as pre-existing renal disease or volume depletion, and the frail elderly.
- Where clinically appropriate, maintain adequate hydration in patients on opioids. Decision-making around the question of hydration in the terminally ill is a complex issue. However, OIN is one indication for attention to hydration status.

Vigilance

- Watch closely for early signs of opioid metabolite accumulation and neurotoxicity such as sedation, delirium, myoclonus, and hyperalgesia.

Treating mild to moderate opioid-induced neurotoxicity

- Hydration to facilitate renal clearing of opioids and metabolites. Oral or parenteral hydration is usually appropriate, depending on clinical circumstances.

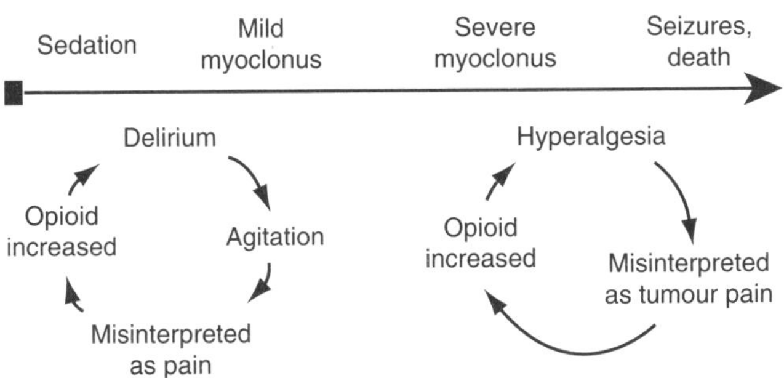

Fig. 2.4 Cycle of opioid toxicity.

- Decrease or change (rotate) the prescribed opioid. In mild OIN, once hydration is addressed it may be possible to continue with the current opioid. Using non-opioid interventions such as adjuvant drugs for neuropathic pain, radiation therapy, or nerve blocks may help decrease the opioid requirements. Changing to spinal analgesia permits a decrease in total opioid administered, and is an option. In moderate OIN, with frequent myoclonic jerks and more prominent CNS effects, it is unlikely that the offending opioid can be continued. Rotation to an alternative opioid will probably be necessary. In calculating conversions, be particularly cautious about incomplete cross-tolerance. Divide the calculated dose of the new opioid by **at least** 50 per cent. This is because in situations of OIN, the offending opioid may have been increased in an attempt to treat its own adverse effects, and the true opioid requirements may be substantially smaller.
- Consider adding a benzodiazepine such as lorazepam or clonazepam to help with the myoclonus.

Treating severe opioid-induced neurotoxicity

- Severe OIN is a life-threatening situation, manifest by continuous myoclonus, hypoactive delirium or unresponsiveness, and ultimately seizures and death.
- The offending opioid must be stopped. **Do not give naloxone**, unless clinically significant respiratory depression exists (uncommon in OIN because of the high tolerance of such patients); naloxone can actually worsen the neurotoxicity.
- Aggressive hydration is critical: intravenous hydration starting with a 500 ml bolus followed by normal saline 250 ml/h is one approach. Consider adding furosemide 20–40 mg i.v. every 6 h once volume status is repleted. Electrolytes should be monitored. Consider inserting a catheter in the bladder if there is uncertainty about the patient's ability to control bladder function. This will have the dual benefit of allowing close monitoring of urine output and ensuring that there is no risk of bladder distention.
- As-needed doses of an alternative (preferably structurally dissimilar) opioid can be given intravenously or subcutaneously when indicated by pain. These doses must be conservative, and cannot be estimated from the current dose of the offending opioid because of the hyperalgesia. For example, fentanyl 25–50 μg i.v. as needed may be a sufficient starting dose, regardless of the previous opioid administered (of course, if the OIN was due to fentanyl, a different opioid should be chosen). The pain should be seen to be present upon reassessment in order to reduce the risk that a transient self-limited episode of pain is needlessly managed with opioids.
- Benzodiazepines such as lorazepam or midazolam can be given parenterally if necessary; they may help the myoclonus, and are indicated if seizures develop.
- With the above approach, the manifestations of severe OIN usually diminish over several hours but may take days to fully resolve.
- Ongoing specific dosing with an alternative opioid is empirical, depending on the clinical circumstances.

Future trends and promising research

Areas of research and development in pain control that have potential for impact on palliative care include the following:

- the development of new NMDA antagonists and exploration of their role in managing tolerance, neuropathic pain, and opioid-induced hyperalgesia

- peripheral opioid μ-receptor antagonists such as methylnaltrexone and ADL 8–2698 for managing and perhaps preventing opioid-induced bowel dysfunction
- the role of cannabinoids in the management of pain,[41] including alternative drug delivery models and the development of cannabinoids with improved side-effect profiles
- expanding the role of interventional analgesia techniques, including portable in-dwelling infusion devices such as intrathecal catheters
- the role of intracellular messengers such as cyclic AMP and nitric oxide in pain modulation.

References

1. **Twycross, R.** (1994) *Pain Relief in Advanced Cancer.* New York: Churchill Livingstone.
2. **International Association for the Study of Pain® Task Force on Taxonomy** (1994) *IASP Pain Terminology* Available online at: http://www.iasp-pain.org/terms-p.html
3. **Clark, D.** (1999) 'Total pain', disciplinary power and the body in the work of Cicely Saunders, 1958–1967. *Soc Sci Med,* **49**, 727–36.
4. **Woodruff, R.** (1999) *Palliative Medicine–Symptomatic and Supportive Care for Patients with Advanced Cancer and AIDS* (3rd edn). Oxford: Oxford University Press.
5. **Bruera, E., Kuehn, N., Miller, MJ., Selmser, P., and Macmillan, K.** (1991) The Edmonton Symptom Assessment System (ESAS): a simple method for the assessment of palliative care patients. *J Palliat Care,* **7**, 6–9.
6. **Nekolaichuk, C.L., Bruera, E., Spachynski, K., MacEachern, T., Hanson, J., and Maguire, T.O.** (1999) A comparison of patient and proxy symptom assessments in advanced cancer patients. *Palliat Med,* **13**, 311–23.
7. **Guru, V., and Dubinsky, I.** (2000) The patient vs. caregiver perception of acute pain in the emergency department. *J Emerg Med,* **18**, 7–12.
8. **Cleeland, C.S., Gonin, R., Hatfield, A.K., *et al.*** (1994) Pain and its treatment in outpatients with metastatic cancer [see comments]. *N Engl J Med,* **330**, 592–6.
9. **Reynolds, K., Henderson, M., Schulman, A., and Hanson, L.C.** (2002) Needs of the dying in nursing homes. *J Palliat Med,* **5**, 895–901.
10. **Zarbock, S.F.** (2000) Pediatric pain assessment. *Home Care Provid,* 5, 181–4.
11. **McMillan, S.C., and Moody, L.E.** (2003) Hospice patient and caregiver congruence in reporting patients'symptom intensity. *Cancer Nurs,* **26**, 113–18.
12. **Collins, S.L., Moore, R.A., and McQuay, H.J.** (1997) The visual analogue pain intensity scale: what is moderate pain in millimetres? *Pain,* **72**, 95–7.
13. **Hanks, G., Cherny, N. and Fallon, M** (2004) Opioid analgesic therapy. In: Doyle D, Hanks GWC, Cherny N, Calman K (eds) *Oxford Textbook of Palliative Medicine.* Oxford: Oxford University Press, 316
14. **Eckhardt, K., Li. S., Ammon, S., Schanzle, G., Mikus, G., and Eichelbaum, M.** (1998) Same incidence of adverse drug events after codeine administration irrespective of the genetically determined differences in morphine formation. *Pain,* **76**, 27–33.
15. **Osborne, R., Joel, S., Grebenik, K., Trew, D., and Slevin, M.** (1993) The pharmacokinetics of morphine and morphine glucuronides in kidney failure [see comments]. *Clin Pharmacol Ther,* **54**, 158–67.
16. **Smith, M.T.** (2000) Neuroexcitatory effects of morphine and hydromorphone: evidence implicating the 3-glucuronide metabolites. *Clin Exp Pharmacol Physiol,* **27**, 524–8.
17. **Babul, N., Darke, A.C., and Hagen, N.** (1995) Hydromorphone metabolite accumulation in renal failure. *J Pain Symptom Manage,* **10**, 184–6.
18. **Levy, M.H.** (2001) Advancement of opioid analgesia with controlled-release oxycodone. *Eur J Pain,* **5** (Suppl A), 113–16.

19. **Kirvela, M., Lindgren, L., Seppala, T., and Olkkola, K.T.** (1996) The pharmacokinetics of oxycodone in uremic patients undergoing renal transplantation. *J Clin Anesth*, **8**, 13–18.
20. **Portenoy, R.K., Southam, M.A., Gupta S.K., *et al.*** (1993) Transdermal fentanyl for cancer pain. Repeated dose pharmacokinetics. *Anesthesiology*, **78**, 36–43.
21. **Radbruch, L., Sabatowski, R., Loick, G., *et al.*** (2000) Constipation and the use of laxatives: a comparison between transdermal fentanyl and oral morphine. *Palliat Med*, **14**, 111–19.
22. **Krantz, M.J., Lewkowiez, L., Hays, H., Woodroffe, M.A., Robertson, A.D., and Mehler, P.S.** (2002) Torsade de pointes associated with very-high-dose methadone. *Ann Intern Med*, **137**, 501–4.
23. **Al Khatib, S.M., LaPointe, N.M., Kramer, J.M., and Califf, R.M.** (2003) What clinicians should know about the QT interval. *JAMA*, **289**, 2120–7.
24. **Pereira, J., Lawlor, P., Vigano, A., Dorgan, M., and Bruera, E.** (2001) Equianalgesic dose ratios for opioids. a critical review and proposals for long-term dosing. *J Pain Symptom Manage*, **22**, 672–87.
25. **Ripamonti, C., Groff, L., Brunelli, C., Polastri, D., Stavrakis, A., and De Conno, F.** (1998) Switching from morphine to oral methadone in treating cancer pain: what is the equianalgesic dose ratio? *J Clin Oncol*, **16**, 3216–21.
26. **Donner, B., Zenz, M., Tryba, M., and Strumpf, M.** (1996) Direct conversion from oral morphine to transdermal fentanyl: a multicenter study in patients with cancer pain. *Pain* **64**, 527–34.
27. **Gardner-Nix, J.S.** (2001) Oral transmucosal fentanyl and sufentanil for incident pain. *J Pain Symptom Manage*, **22**, 627–30.
28. **Kunz, K.M., Theisen, J.A., and Schroeder, M.E.** (1993) Severe episodic pain: management with sublingual sufentanil. *J Pain Symptom Manage*, **8**, 189–90.
29. **Striebel, H.W., Wessel, A., Rieger, A., and Boerger, N.** (1993) Intranasal fentanyl for breakthrough cancer pain or incident pain. *Br J Anaesth*, **70** (Suppl 1), 109.
30. **Zeppetella, G.** (2000) An assessment of the safety, efficacy, and acceptability of intranasal fentanyl citrate in the management of cancer-related breakthrough pain. A pilot study. *J Pain Symptom Manage*, **20**, 253–8.
31. **Zeppetella, G.** (2001) Sublingual fentanyl citrate for cancer-related breakthrough pain: a pilot study. *Palliat Med*, **15**, 323–8.
32. **Jackson, K., Ashby, M., and Keech, J.** (2002) Pilot dose finding study of intranasal sufentanil for breakthrough and incident cancer-associated pain. *J Pain Symptom Manage*, **23**, 450–2.
33. **Nicholson, B.** (2000) Gabapentin use in neuropathic pain syndromes. *Acta Neurol Scand*, **101**, 359–71.
34. **Joranson, D.E., and Colleau, S.M.** (1998) Tolerance, physical dependence and addiction: Definitions, clinical relevance and misconceptions. In: Colleau SM (ed). *Cancer Pain Release 11*. Geneva: World Health Organization.
35. **Sarhill, N., Davis, M.P., Walsh, D., and Nouneh, C.** (2001) Methadone-induced myoclonus in advanced cancer. *Am J Hosp Palliat Care*, **18**, 51–3.
36. **Doverty, M., White, J.M., Somogyi, A.A., Bochner, F., Ali, R., and Ling, W.** (2001) Hyperalgesic responses in methadone maintenance patients. *Pain*, **90**, 91–6.
37. **Bruera, E., and Pereira, J.** (1997) Acute neuropsychiatric findings in a patient receiving fentanyl for cancer pain. *Pain*, **69**, 199–201.
38. **Adair, J.C., el Nachef, A., and Cutler, P.** (1996) Fentanyl neurotoxicity. *Ann Emerg Med*, **27**, 791–2.
39. **Harrison, C., Smart, D., and Lambert, D.G.** (1998) Stimulatory effects of opioids. *Br J Anaesth*, **81**, 20–8.
40. **Mao, J., Sung, B., Ji, R.R., and Lim, G.** (2002) Neuronal apoptosis associated with morphine tolerance: evidence for an opioid-induced neurotoxic mechanism. *J Neurosci*, **22**, 7650–61.
41. **Walker, J.M., Strangman, N.M., and Huang, S.M.** (2001) Cannabinoids and pain. *Pain Res Manage*, **6**, 74–9.

Chapter 3

Neuropathic pain

Dwight Moulin

Mrs. M.B. is a 58-year-old woman who presented with right shoulder girdle pain of 3 months' duration. Plain radiographs revealed erosion of the first and second ribs and a CT scan of the chest showed a right apical lung mass. Fine-needle aspiration biopsy established a diagnosis of adenocarcinoma of the lung. Treatment consisted of chemotherapy, local radiation therapy, and analgesic management. She had an excellent response, with tumour reduction for 4 months, and required only ibuprofen for pain related to right arm activity. She now presents with recurrent aching right shoulder pain associated with escalating burning pain radiating down the medial aspect of the upper arm and forearm into the fourth and fifth digits. She describes superimposed shock-like pain in the same distribution and sensitivity to light touch involving the medial forearm and hand. She rates her overall pain intensity in the range of 7–10/10. Her right hand feels clumsy and weak.

Question 1. What is the information you wish to obtain from the history which will help to formulate a treatment strategy?

The patient describes a recurrence of aching right shoulder girdle pain probably related to locally progressive disease with further rib erosion. This pain is somatic in nature. In addition, she describes burning stabbing pain down the right arm which sounds neuropathic. The distribution of the pain and weakness provides important clues as to the segmental levels of nerve injury. Because there is a risk of tumour extension into the epidural space, one should also ask about lower extremity weakness, unsteadiness, bladder symptoms, or other evidence of early spinal cord compression.

Question 2. What are the important features associated with neuropathic pain that you will look for on physical examination in this patient?

Physical examination

The physical examination in this patient targets the head and neck, the shoulder girdle, and the upper extremity region. Is there cervical spine or chest wall tenderness as evidence of local tumour extension? Tenderness in the upper trapezius might indicate secondary muscle spasm. Is there axillary or supraclavicular lymphadenopathy? Assessment of range of movement in the neck and shoulder girdle is important. Provocative manoeuvres that reproduce the pain are valuable to identify the pain-sensitive structures involved and to further characterize the pain syndrome. A positive Spurling's manoeuvre with neck lateral flexion and lateral rotation suggests cervical root involvement.[1] Demonstration of Tinel's sign by tapping over Erb's point in the supraclavicular fossa just lateral to the sternomastoid muscle suggests pathology in the brachial plexus. Erb's point localizes the brachial plexus and tapping over this area may reproduce tingling shooting pain down the arm. Swelling and discoloration of the arm further suggest tumour infiltration of the neurovascular pedicle with venous and lymphatic obstruction.

A screening neurological examination is vital to determine the extent of disease. Horner's syndrome ipsilateral to the pain is a worrying sign because it can be associated with tumour extension medially to involve the stellate ganglion or the sympathetic fibres along the T1 nerve root; this can be a sign of impending epidural disease and requires evaluation for evidence of spinal cord compression. Weakness in the finger flexors and intrinsic hand muscles indicates dysfunction in C8–T1 distribution at either the root level or lower trunk of the brachial plexus. Similarly, sensory loss and touch-evoked pain (allodynia) along the medial aspect of the arm and hand also indicate C8–T1 involvement. The application of ice in this distribution with the aberrant perception of intense heat is pathognomonic of neuropathic pain. A depressed triceps jerk indicates that the reflex arc at C7 or C8 level is involved.

Question 3. What is neuropathic pain?

Pathophysiology

Neuropathic pain arises from injury to the peripheral or central nervous system.[2] In the setting of cancer, the pain can be due to tumour infiltration or it can be treatment related. Surgery (e.g. postmastectomy pain syndrome), radiation therapy (e.g. radiation fibrosis of the brachial plexus), and chemotherapy (e.g. cisplatin) can all produce nerve damage. Shingles and post-herpetic neuralgia are also common in elderly patients with cancer. Pain is generated by both peripheral and central mechanisms. Mechanical compression of the peripheral nerve may produce nerve sheath pain by irritating the small primary afferents (nervi nervorum) that innervate nerve trunks. Demyelination and axonal disruption can result in accumulation of sodium channels that are sites of ectopic impulse formation. Peripheral nerve injury can also generate secondary central pain at the spinal cord level due to sensitization of the dorsal horn. Neuronal discharges in the dorsal horn become autonomous and are responsible for aberrant sensory transmission. This accounts for allodynia, exaggerated responses such as hyperalgesia to pinprick, and the aberrant sensation of ice as intense heat. Central sensitization is mediated largely by the action of glutamate on its various receptors in the dorsal horn, in particular activation of the *N*-methyl-D-aspartate (NMDA) receptor.

Question 4. What are the clinical features of neuropathic pain in this patient?

Clinical features

Mrs. M.B. manifests all the cardinal features of neuropathic pain:

- continuous burning pain—sometimes described as intense tightness or an icy feeling
- superimposed paroxysmal pain—often described as lancinating, jabbing, or shooting
- allodynia or touch-evoked pain—the aberrant sensation of pain in response to what is normally an innocuous stimulus such as light touch, warmth, or coldness.

She does not have Horner's syndrome but does manifest weakness and wasting of the finger flexors and intrinsic hand muscles. The distribution of the pain, aberrant sensation, and weakness all point to injury in the C8–T1 distribution. The intensity of the pain, the rapid evolution of neurological signs, and the short interval from radiation therapy strongly suggests tumour infiltration rather than radiation fibrosis as the underlying cause. Clinically, it can be difficult to differentiate C8–T1 nerve root involvement from tumour infiltration of the lower trunk of the brachial plexus. An MRI scan, if available, provides the best evidence of localization and extent of disease. Figure 3.1 shows a coronal MRI scan of the upper chest with evidence of a right Pancoast tumour infiltrating the brachial plexus. The MRI also shows erosion of the T1 and T2 vertebral bodies adjacent to the apical lung mass. This patient's clinical presentation is common in cancer pain; patients often present with mixed pain syndromes such as neuropathic and nociceptive (bone) pain.

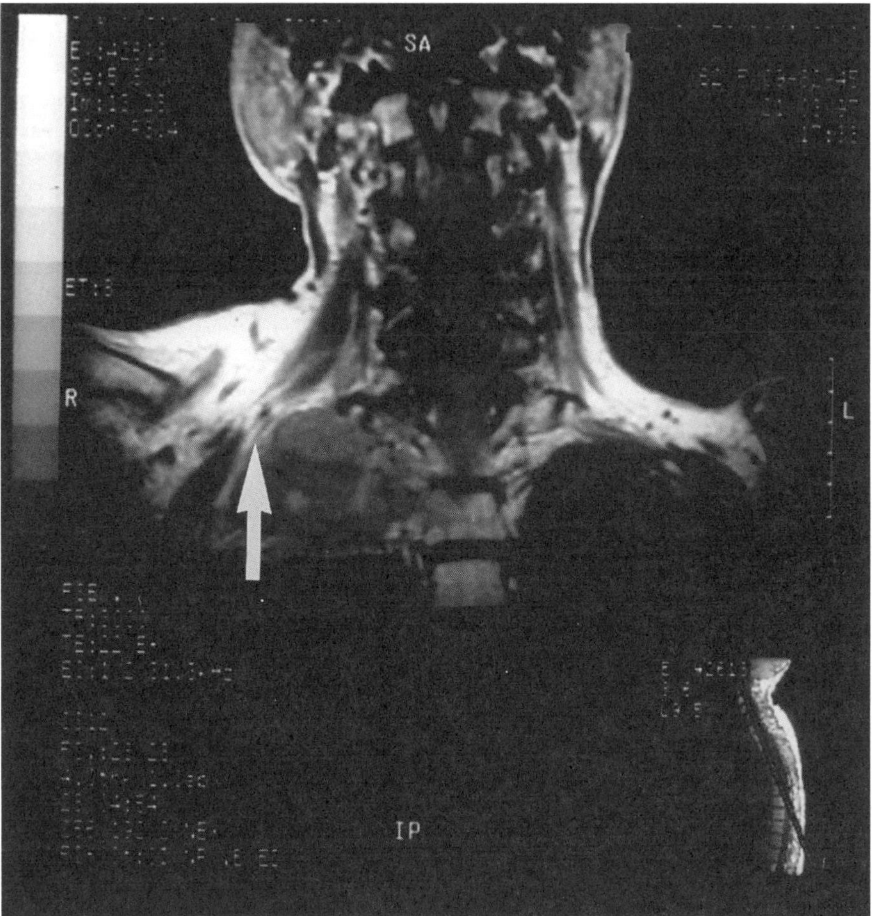

Fig 3.1 Coronal MRI of upper chest showing right Pancoast tumour adjacent to T1 and T2 vertebral bodies. The tumour invades the lower brachial plexus (arrow).

Question 5. What treatment would you recommend?

Treatment of neuropathic pain

Management of neuropathic cancer pain is based largely on survey data and extrapolation from randomized controlled trials of non-malignant neuropathic pain syndromes. However, a recent survey of 593 cancer patients treated by a pain service following World Health Organization (WHO) guidelines reported substantial pain relief in patients with nociceptive, neuropathic, and mixed pain syndromes.[3]

Table 3.1 lists the first- and second-line medications that have demonstrated efficacy in the management of neuropathic pain. First-line treatment involves the use of either a tricyclic antidepressant (TCA) or an anticonvulsant. TCAs relieve pain by blocking the reuptake of serotonin and norepinephrine at the spinal cord level. In addition, TCAs and anticonvulsants block sodium channels, a property which targets a major peripheral generator of neuropathic pain.

Systematic reviews show little evidence to guide selection between the various antidepressants and anticonvulsants.[4,5] Combined data from trials in painful diabetic neuropathy and post-herpetic neuralgia indicate that each class of agents provides at least 50 per cent pain relief in about one patient in three with no substantial differences in adverse effects. It is not certain that this response rate translates to neuropathic cancer pain. In addition, systematic reviews also suggest that the character of the pain does not predict response to any particular agent. For instance, there is no evidence that burning pain responds better to a TCA or that paroxysmal pain is better treated with an anticonvulsant.

Start with a preferred TCA or anticonvulsant and add an agent from the other class as required and tolerated. Amitriptyline is often considered to be the first-line TCA for neuropathic pain because it has sedative properties which sometimes allow patients to sleep with night-time dosing. However, anticholinergic side effects such as dry mouth and urinary hesitancy are sometimes intolerable, especially in older patients, and a switch to a more tolerable TCA such as desipramine or nortriptyline may be warranted. The usual starting dose is 10–25 mg at bedtime, with gradual increments every few days up to a total dose of 100–150 mg at bedtime. Do not use serotonin-specific reuptake inhibitors for neuropathic pain as they are much less likely to be analgesic.[6]

Gabapentin has become a first-line anticonvulsant for neuropathic pain, although there are no head-to-head trials to compare gabapentin with more conventional anticonvulsants such as

Table 3.1 Pharmacological treatment of neuropathic pain related to cancer

First-line drugs
Tricyclic antidepressants
Anticonvulsants
Topical lidocaine
Conventional opioid analgesics
Second-line drugs
NMDA antagonists
Methadone
Corticosteroids
Mexiletine
Continuous local anaesthetic infusion

carbamazepine and the former drug is much more expensive. The initial maintenance dose of gabapentin is 300–400 mg three times daily. However, some patients tolerate and benefit from gradually escalating doses up to 1600 mg three times daily. An open trial of gabapentin for neuropathic cancer pain suggests substantial benefit.[7] Carbamazepine remains a reasonable alternative. The initial maintenance dose of carbamazepine is 200 mg twice daily with increase of the dose as required and tolerated; trough blood levels can guide upward titration.

However, a recent randomized controlled trial of gabapentin for chemotherapy-induced painful peripheral neuropathy did not significantly improve the primary endpoints of pain intensity or sensory reuropathy.[8]

Topical local anesthetics are attractive for patients with localized neuropathic pain because they can provide significant pain relief with virtually no systemic side effects. This property is especially attractive in the elderly who are prone to post-herpetic neuralgia. Topical lidocaine 5 per cent applied as either a gel or a patch has been shown to be efficacious in the management of post-herpetic neuralgia with virtually no reports of side effects relative to placebo application.[9,10] Transcutaneous electrical nerve stimulation (TENS) may also be useful for localized neuropathic pain.

Opioid analgesics are useful in the management of neuropathic cancer pain, although the best evidence of efficacy comes from well-designed trials in non-cancer pain models.[11,12] If a patient presents with moderate to severe pain, a reasonable approach is to start a short-acting opioid analgesic such as oxycodone 5 mg with acetaminophen (paracetamol) 325 mg every 3–4 h as required for breakthrough pain while adjuvant analgesics are being initiated. The patient could then be switched to a controlled-release opioid such as morphine or oxycodone, if necessary, after or concurrent with trials of one or more adjuvant agents.

The patient has had inadequate relief from a combination of nortriptyline and gabapentin and has not tolerated controlled-release morphine or oxycodone because of sedation and hallucinations.

Question 6. What other treatment options would you suggest?

There is limited evidence that drugs with NMDA antagonist properties are useful in the management of neuropathic pain. Unfortunately, we do not have an NMDA antagonist available with proven efficacy and an acceptable side-effect profile. Ketamine is a commonly used i.v. anaesthetic with NMDA receptor blocking activity. Small double-blind placebo-controlled trials of i.v. ketamine have reported pain relief in post-herpetic neuralgia and a variety of chronic neuropathic pain syndromes, although psychomimetic side effects can be intolerable.[13] Small trials of low-dose oral ketamine suggest that this agent is beneficial and effective as an adjuvant analgesic in the management of intractable neuropathic pain in patients with advanced cancer.[14,15]

Dextromethorphan, a common cough suppressant, is another NMDA antagonist that has been studied in neuropathic pain states. Clinical trials involving dextromethorphan in chronic non-cancer pain have produced mixed results, whereas an open trial of dextromethorphan in cancer pain found that this drug was ineffective.[16]

Methadone is a synthetic opioid analgesic that has NMDA antagonist properties. Methadone is also attractive because it has excellent oral bioavailability, no known active metabolites, and availability at very low cost. However, it has a long and unpredictable half-life with increased potency in those patients who are already opioid tolerant. Although opioid rotation to methadone is more complex than with other opioids, uncontrolled trials of methadone suggest that this is a very useful drug in the management of neuropathic cancer pain.[17]

High-dose corticosteroids are extremely valuable in the short term in the management of a cancer pain crisis including neuropathic cancer pain. The mechanism of action of corticosteroids in producing analgesia is unknown, but may involve a reduction of peritumoral edema, a reduction of nociceptive cytokine production, and a direct oncolytic effect on neoplasms. Dexamethasone is the corticosteroid of choice because of its low mineralocorticoid effects. An initial dose of 100 mg tapered over 1–2 weeks have been used for episodes of severe acute pain associated with malignant plexopathy and epidural spinal cord compression.[18]

Lidocaine and mexiletine are local anaesthetic antiarrhythmic agents whose mechanism of action is sodium-channel blockade. Mexiletine is an oral congener of lidocaine. There is some evidence that mexiletine can relieve neuropathic pain in a diabetic neuropathy model.[19,20] The usual starting dose is 50 mg three times daily with dose titration up to 200 mg three times daily. Obtain an ECG prior to treatment to screen for a cardiac conduction disorder.

A continuous brachial plexus block using a local anaesthetic infusion can be salutary for severe intractable plexopathy pain and has the advantage of being an invasive and yet reversible technique.[21] Percutaneous cordotomy is a very useful technique for intractable unilateral cancer pain but works better for lumbosacral plexopathy than for brachial plexopathy.

> Mrs. M.B. was started on oral methadone and the dose was gradually escalated to 50 mg every 8 h. She had dramatic and sustained relief on methadone at this dose with minimal side effects until her death from progressive cancer 3 months later.

Future directions

NMDA receptor activation may play a key role as a central generator of neuropathic pain. Methadone may be a particularly useful opioid analgesic for neuropathic pain because of its NMDA antagonist properties, although this observation needs to be tested in randomized controlled trials. We also need novel analgesics that are more specific for NMDA receptors at the spinal cord level—this would provide selective analgesia with a side-effect profile that is far more favourable than any drug currently available for neuropathic pain. Other neural pathways are being actively studied as possible targets for pharmacotherapy as well as neuroablative and neurostimulatory interventions for neuropathic pain.

References

1. **Yeung, M.C., and Hagen, N.A.** (1993) Cervical disc herniation presenting with chest wall pain. *Can J Neurol Sci,* **20**, 59–61.
2. **Woolf, C.J., and Mannion, R.J.** (1999) Neuropathic pain: etiology, symptoms, mechanisms and management. *Lancet,* **353**, 1959–64.
3. **Grond, S., Radbruch, L., Meuser, T., Sabatowski, R., Loick, G., and Lehmann, K.A.** (1999) Assessment and treatment of neuropathic cancer pain following WHO guidelines. *Pain,* **79**, 15–20.
4. **McQuay, H.J., Tramer, M., Nye, B.A. *et al.*** (1996) A systematic review of antidepressants in neuropathic pain. *Pain,* **68**, 217–27.
5. **McQuay, H.J., Carroll, D., Jadad, A.R. *et al.*** (1995) Anticonvulsant drugs for management of pain: a systematic review. *BMJ,* **311**, 1047–52.

6. **Sindrup, S.H., and Jensen, T.S.** (1999) Efficacy of pharmacological treatments of neuropathic pain: an update and effect related to mechanism of drug action. *Pain,* **83**, 389–400.
7. **Caraceni, A., Zecca, E., Martini, C., and De Conno, F.** (1999) Gabapentin as an adjuvant to opioid analgesia for neuropathic cancer pain. *J Pain Symptom Manage,* **17**, 441–5.
8. Wong, G.Y., Michalak, J.C., Sloan, J.A., *et al* (2005). A phase III double blinded, placebo controlled, randomized trial of gabapentin in patients with chemotherapy-induced periphesal neuropathy: a North Central Cancer Treatment Group Study. American Society of Clinical Oncology Annual Meeting, abstract 8001.
9. **Rowbotham, M.C., Davies, P.S., and Fields, H.L.** (1995) Topical lidocaine gel relieves postherpetic neuralgia. *Ann Neurol,* **37**, 245–53.
10. **Rowbotham, M.C., Davies, P.S., Verkempinck, C., and Galer, B.S.** (1996) Lidocaine patch: double blind controlled study of a new treatment method for postherpetic neuralgia. *Pain,* **65**, 39–44.
11. **Watson, C.P.N., and Babul, N.** (1998) Efficacy of oxycodone in neuropathic pain. A randomized trial in postherpetic neuralgia. *Neurology,* **50**, 1837–41.
12. **Rowbotham, M.C., Twilling, L., Davies, P.S., Reisner, L., Taylor, K., and Mohr, D.** (2003) Oral opioid therapy for chronic peripheral and central neuropathic pain. *N Engl J Med,* **348**, 1223–32.
13. **Kingery, W.S.** (1997) A critical review of controlled clinical trials for peripheral neuropathic pain and complex regional pain syndromes. *Pain,* **73**, 123–139.
14. **Kannan, T.R., Saxena, A., Bhatnager, S., and Barry, A.** (2002) Oral ketamine as an adjuvant to oran morphine for neuropathic pain in cancer patients. *J Pain Symptom Manage,* **23**, 60–5.
15. **McQueen, A.L., and Baroletti, S.A.** (2002) Adjuvant ketamine analgesia for the management of cancer pain. *Ann Pharmacother,* **36**, 1614–19.
16. **Mercadante, S., Casuccio, A., and Genovese, G.** (1998) Ineffectiveness of dextromethorphan in cancer pain. *J Pain Symptom Manage,* **16**, 317–22.
17. **Bruera, E., and Sweeney, C.** (2002) Methadone use in cancer patients with pain: a review. *J Palliat Med,* **5**, 127–38.
18. **Hewitt, D.J., and Portenoy, R.K.** (1998) Adjuvant drugs for neuropathic cancer pain. In: Bruera E, Portenoy RK (eds) *Topics in Palliative Care,* Vol 2. New York: Oxford University Press, 41–62.
19. **Dejgard, A., Petersen, P., and Kastrup, J.** (1988) Mexiletine for treatment of chronic painful diabetic neuropathy. *Lancet,* **ii**, 9–11.
20. **Oskarssen, P., Lins, P.E., Ljunggren, J.G., and the Mexiletine Study Group** (1997) Efficacy and safety of mexiletine in the treatment of painful diabetic neuropathy. *Diabetes Care,* **20**, 1594–7.
21. **Vranken, J.H., Zuurmond, W.W., and de Lange, J.J.** (2000) Continuous brachial plexus block as treatment for the Pancoast syndrome. *Clin J Pain,* **16**, 327–33.

Chapter 4

Bone pain

Susan MacDonald and Jennifer Hall

Attitude

To enable the student to:

- Respect the negative impact of bone metastases on quality of life through pain, debility, the unwanted effects of analgesics, and other accompaniments of advanced disease.
- Recognize the value of patient and family input into the various options available to manage bone metastases.

Skill

To enable the student to:

- Prescribe long-acting and immediate release opioids to manage baseline bone pain and breakthrough (incident) pain.
- Select patients who are appropriate for referral to an orthopaedic surgeon and for treatment with focal radiation therapy, parenteral bisphosphonates, corticosteroids, hemibody radiation therapy, or radioisotope therapy.

Knowledge

To enable the student to:

- Describe the prevalence of bone metastases, the mechanism of pain, and common clinical features of pain from metastases to bone.
- Outline pharmacological and non-pharmacological interventions for bone pain.

Mr A.J. is a 68-year-old retired firefighter. Two years ago, he was found to have an elevated prostate-specific antigen (PSA). He underwent investigation and was determined to have advanced prostate cancer with metastases to the femurs and sternum. He elected to try hormonal therapy and did well for about 20 months. However, 3 months ago he began experiencing an ache in his right groin.

He is seen by his family physician, describing pain in his right groin and right hip. There is a general aching sensation at rest (3/10 on a pain scale) and the pain increases to '4–5/10'on walking more than a few blocks. He is using a cane. He indicates that he has tried acetaminophen (paracetamol) occasionally, and some of his neighbour's 'arthritis' pills, which helped a bit with the discomfort but also caused considerable epigastric pain. He has not tried any medication regularly, as he does not like taking pills.

On physical examination, he is noted to have lost approximately 2 kg since last seen. He has mild gynaecomastia. The range of motion of the right leg is normal but uncomfortable and reproduces the

Continued

pain that brought him to your office. Palpation of the leg reveals no obvious mass but is tender over the right greater trochanter. The neurological examination is normal.

Question 1. What are the possible diagnoses?

The most likely explanation of his pain is progressive bone metastases. Another possible diagnosis is osteoarthritis or muscle pain from some other mechanism. Fracture should be ruled out, but seems clinically unlikely given that the pain that is only moderately severe with walking. While cancer is not the only cause of new onset of bone pain in a patient with known metastatic disease, it is the most common cause. A history and physical examination should be carried out to rule out other causes which, if present, would prompt non-oncological interventions.

Question 2. Are bone metastases common? What is the pathogenesis?

Bone metastases are common in advanced cancer; about 60–80 per cent of patients will eventually encounter them.[1,2] Some malignancies have a particular predilection to spread to bone: breast, prostate, lung, kidney and thyroid cancers will account for approximately 80 per cent of all patients with metastatic bone disease.[3] The spread to bone is generally haematogenous. Bone metastases can be divided by radiological appearance into lytic, sclerotic, and mixed patterns.[4]

Lytic lesions are most commonly seen in multiple myeloma and breast and lung cancers, whereas sclerotic lesions are typically seen in prostate cancer. Multiple factors produced by tumours or the host modulate the occurrence and course of bone metastases. Known factors include parathyroid hormone-related factor (PTHrP) and a variety of inflammatory cytokines (both tumour and host produced). Working in variable combinations, they prepare the soil for tumour embedding and stimulate cycles of osteoclast–osteoblast activity. The overall effect imbalances the normal dynamic bone remodelling process between osteoclast-mediated bone resorption and osteoblast-mediated bone generation.

Sclerotic lesions are formed when new bone is deposited around tumour cells in the bone marrow. The mechanism is not fully elucidated, but many mediators are implicated including bone morphogenic proteins, fibroblast growth factors and endothelin-1.[4]

Question 3. What problems occur with bone metastases?

The development of bone metastases is an ominous occurrence, and the clinical complications for the patient can be significant. About 70 per cent of patients with bone metastases will develop pain, and it can be difficult to control. In addition, patients are at increased risk for hypercalcaemia, fracture, spinal cord compression, and bone marrow infiltration.[4] Some patients, particularly breast and prostate cancer patients, may live for many years with skeletal metastasis as the only site of metastases, and in this circumstance the morbidity of progressive bone metastases and its complications can be devastating.

Bone pain can have one or several different characteristics in any given patient. It may be a steady constant type of pain, or an intermittent pain that comes on with particular movements or positions. Pain can appear to migrate, with severe pain in one location for a few days which appears to shift to another, previously silent site with the earlier location no longer being so painful. It can significantly alter patients' ability to complete their activities of daily living.

Breakthrough pain is a major clinical feature of bone pain. Breakthrough pain can be defined as a transitory increase in pain to greater than moderate intensity that occurs on otherwise controlled baseline pain (i.e. of moderate intensity or less).[5] Breakthrough pain that occurs in a predictable manner with some kind of movement or procedure is called incident pain. Incident pain related to bone metastases carries a poor prognosis for satisfactory control, partly because incident pain commonly has a rapid onset and disappears quickly. Analgesic medications that would be able to manage such pain would need to have a very rapid onset but brief duration of effect. Traditionally, modest doses of immediate release opioid have been used on an as-needed basis for such pain. This approach can be helpful if breakthrough doses are taken prior to the onset of a predictable incident pain such as before taking a shower or going shopping. If incident pain is less predictable or lasts only a few minutes, oral opioids are less likely to be effective. Ultra-rapid onset opioids, such as sublingual fentanyl or sufentanil, or the oral transmucosal fentanyl citrate preparation, provide important alternatives to this difficult pain scenario.

Pain from bone metastasis can have many pathophysiological causes. There may be direct invasion into the bone matrix, causing microfracture. The periosteum can be pressurized by expanding tissue or by oedema. Nerves often travel through or near bone and can be compressed by contiguous tumour or bone collapse. Reflex muscle spasm can be a major component of bone-related cancer pain.[6] Chemical mediators contribute to nociception. For example, many inflammatory cytokines also enhance nociception.

Question 4. What investigations, if any, should be ordered for Mr J.?

Plain radiographs of the femur and acetabulum would be useful to rule out fracture and to assess the risk of possible fracture. Plain radiographs do not always identify metastatic disease, and for this reason the clinical picture should always be taken into account when there is a negative radiograph. A bone scan may also be helpful to document the overall burden of bone metastases and is much more sensitive at detecting metastatic deposits than plain radiographs. This outpatient procedure takes several hours; the patient is administered an i.v. injection of radiotracer and, later, lies on a table while being scanned. While this test can add valuable knowledge about the extent of metastatic bone deposits, it can be uncomfortable for patients with advanced disease.

> The family physician orders plain radiographs of the femurs and a bone scan. The radiographs demonstrate sclerotic lesions in the heads of both femurs, with mild cortical destruction on the right. The bone scan reveals multiple areas of uptake throughout the appendicular and axial skeleton, including the proximal femurs bilaterally.

Question 5. The patient asks you why only one of the areas of metastases is actually symptomatic. How would you respond?

The clinical scenario of multiple bone metastases has a number of features that are not fully explained. One is that only some metastatic lesions are painful, while others with very similar radiographic appearance are not. Why even some large metastases remain painless is not fully understood,[7] although one can speculate that the relative presence of nociceptive cytokines and other chemicals in the tumour milieu play a role.

Question 6. How should the patient's painful bone metastases be managed?

Occasionally treatment is begun before pain is felt, for example if specific radiological criteria for high risk of fracture are identified.[8,9] Potential interventions for painless metastases include radiotherapy to attempt to reduce the size of a large or dangerously placed metastasis, or orthopaedic surgery to stabilize a potential fracture.

Regardless of whether there is a potential treatment to reduce or eliminate further metastasis to the skeleton, the pain that the patient is experiencing must itself be managed.[10,11] Analgesic drugs are a mainstay for bone pain. As with any other cancer pain, the weakest analgesic that is effective is a reasonable goal. Following the recommendations of the World Health Organization (WHO), one should begin with a non-steroidal anti-inflammatory drug (NSAID) with or without a weak opioid.[12,13] If the pain is intermittent, the patient can be started on as-needed doses of opioid. If the patient requires more than a few doses of pain reliever every day, it is reasonable to introduce regular (scheduled) dosing. Once the patient is comfortable with the prescribed dose of opioid, long-acting formulations can be used to reduce the frequency of medication doses. Always allow the patient to have an appropriate amount of opioid available to use for rescue of breakthrough dosing. Use the number of breakthrough doses as a guide to determining whether the regular dose should be increased.

Question 7. How do NSAIDs work?

NSAIDs are effective as analgesics in pain and have been extensively studied in non-cancer pain. The WHO has recommended NSAIDs without opioids for the treatment of mild cancer pain and in combination with opioids in the treatment of moderate to severe pain. NSAIDs appear to have a dual mechanism of action. First, they inhibit peripheral prostaglandin synthesis, which attenuates the formation of oedema and reduces prostaglandin-induced pain sensitization. In addition, this class of drugs probably has a central mechanism of action that is independent of the prostaglandin synthesis inhibition. Although NSAIDs have been used extensively for the management of bone pain, analgesic superiority in treating this type of pain over other types of nociceptive pain has not been clearly demonstrated.[13,14]

Question 8. What side effects are you concerned about? How could you prevent some of them?

Unfortunately, a significant number of side effects are associated with NSAIDs. They include dyspepsia, allergic reactions, gastrointestinal bleeding, accelerated congestive failure, hypertension, and renal failure. The incidence of gastrointestinal bleeds is increased in patients with advanced age, prior complications with NSAIDs, co-morbid illnesses, or corticosteroid use. These factors may make it tempting for the clinician to discontinue the NSAID even if an analgesic benefit has been achieved. Instead, a more conservative approach would be to ensure that renal function is monitored from time to time in high-risk patients; and gastrointestinal cytoprotection in the form of misoprostol or a proton pump inhibitor are prescribed for patients with NSAID-related epigastric pain or other factors that would put them at particularly high risk for peptic ulcer.[15] Many cancer pain consultants do not routinely use ulcer prophylaxis in low-risk patients started on NSAIDS. Attention to adequate hydration may be required to ensure optimal renal function in patients taking this class of medication who have poor oral intake.

Question 9. What is the role of COX-2 inhibitors in bone pain?

A newer class of NSAIDs, COX-2 inhibitors, was primarily designed to reduce the gastrointestinal risks of non-selective NSAIDs. Unfortunately, they are also associated with a significant incidence of side effects and some COX-2 inhibitors have now been withdrawn from the market. The efficacy of these medications in the management of painfrom bone metastases compared with traditional NSAIDs is not yet well defined. The non-gastrointestinal side effects, including thrombosis, congestive heart failure, and high blood pressure, are probably worse with COX-2 inhibitors than with non-selective NSAIDs.[14]

If renal function precludes the use of NSAIDs, then corticosteroids once or twice daily will provide a similar or superior anti-inflammatory effect without renal toxicity. In general, they are used on a short-term basis (up to several weeks) in view of the long-term adverse effects of corticosteroids.

The role of anti-inflammatory drugs for bone pain remains incompletely evaluated. While clinicians often describe these agents as being particularly effective for bone pain, the evidence supporting this practice is modest at best.[14]

Acetaminophen in doses of up to 4 g/day can be administered alone or can add to the analgesic effect of opioids. Hepatic toxicity is described in acute poisoning with acetaminophen or in chronic administration in patients with pre-existing liver dysfunction, but is thought to be a very low risk in most clinical settings of chronic administration.

Question 10. Are there non-pharmacological analgesic interventions that should be offered?

Simple non-pharmacological methods of pain management should always be considered. Non-weight-bearing techniques, heat, ice, and sometimes gentle massage can help reduce pain. An assessment by both occupational and physical therapists can yield information to help reduce or prevent pain. Modification of the home or workplace with equipment such as walkers, wheelchairs, and grip bars can help. Many patients have better pain relief when a combination of medications and supportive therapies are employed.

Question 11. Mr J has indicated that his baseline pain worsens when he walks or bears weight. Is this an important problem to consider as you construct an overall analgesic strategy?

Bone pain carries a poor prognosis for control. One of the reasons for this is that incident pain, such as pain with movement, is commonly a significant component of the overall pain experience. Long-acting opioids can manage the baseline pain, but short-acting opioids may be too slow to be helpful in brief episodes of movement-related pain. Opioid neurotoxicity can occur if baseline opioids are increased to manage a relatively larger component of incident pain.

> Mr J. is started on immediate release hydromorphone (he had nausea when administered morphine several years ago) and is then switched to the same dose in a long-acting hydromorphone preparation once pain relief is obtained. He takes occasional acetaminophen for breakthrough. You advise him to return to see his medical oncologist, but he is not interested in chemotherapy or other oncological treatment at this time. You warn him that he will probably need further treatment in the future, and arrange that he continue to see you in follow-up monthly.

Question 12. Over the next few months, the pain progresses to the point where he finds it difficult to walk, particularly because of pain on the right hip region. What additional interventions could be offered?

He needs repeat radiographs of the pelvis and femurs to decide whether radiation therapy would be appropriate or whether there is a high risk for a fracture and need for a referral to an orthopaedic consultant. Radiation therapy in conjunction with analgesics has long been a standard treatment for painful bone metastasis. The goals of radiotherapy are to reduce pain, prevent fracture, and reduce the risk of contiguous tumour growth.[16]

Radiation can be administered to individual metastatic deposits in single fractions.[17] Single-fraction radiotherapy is often used in patients who cannot tolerate the process of receiving several fractions of radiotherapy, or in patients who live too far away to travel for several treatments. Single-fraction radiation therapy to isolated bone metastases (remote from radiation therapy sensitive tissues such as the spinal cord or colon) has the about the same analgesic effect as multifraction courses and is much less expensive. The radiotherapy treatment itself is generally painless, causes few or no side effects, and takes only a few minutes. Usually the primary cause of patient concern is the discomfort while lying on the table for treatment, or the discomfort in travelling to and from the treatments. Occasionally there will be a flare of bone pain shortly after the radiotherapy, but this usually subsides over the next few days. Management includes warning patients about this possibility and increasing the pain medication doses until the flare passes. Generally the area of treatment includes some normal tissue beyond the metastatic deposit. If the volume of the irradiated field is high, single-fraction treatment may not be possible and treatments may be divided into several sequential fractions.

There has recently been a Cochrane Review of the outcome of radiotherapy for painful bone metastases.[18] Localized radiation is only occasionally associated with long-term toxicity. The reviewers determined that 'one patient in four given radiotherapy will get complete relief at one month' and that one-third of patients would experience 50 per cent pain relief. The benefit of radiation can be experienced quickly; however, most patients require several weeks before they notice maximum improvement in their pain. It is advisable to mention to patients that as their analgesic requirements lessen, they may notice more of the somnolent side effects of these drugs. This would indicate the correct time to begin to reduce the amount of analgesic. Mr J. will need plain radiographs of the pelvis and femurs to evaluate the extent of bone disease, and whether radiotherapy or surgery should be considered.

The actual mechanism of analgesic action of radiation therapy is still not well understood. Since pain reduction is generally quick (days to weeks) it is likely that the initial analgesic effect is secondary to an alteration of the tumour–host milieu with reduction of locally produced chemical mediators.

Question 13. Can bone metastases be prevented?

There are strategies that can potentially reduce the risk of bone metastases occurring in the first place. In general, the aim of chemotherapy is to reduce further spread of the cancer and reduce or remove the primary tumour. Prevention of spread to the bones could also be included as a reasonable expectation of a successful chemotherapy regimen. Once bone metastases have developed, some malignancies, such as prostate or breast cancer, can be particularly sensitive to hormonal therapy. The goal of hormonal therapy includes prevention of further spread, as well as possible reduction of pain and reduction of the risk of skeletal events.[4] These options should be discussed with an oncologist, and will not be explored in detail in this text.

The use of bisphosphonates has been identified as an important oncological innovation during the last few years, for two primary indications: prevention of bone metastases and their complications; and control of acute cancer-related bone pain.[19] Bisphosphonates inhibit bone resorption through several mechanisms, and are a treatment of choice for hypercalcaemia of malignancy. They have been administered prophylactically in patients at risk for bone metastases, they are particularly well studied for breast cancer and myeloma, and found to be effective. Bisphosphonates can prevent or reduce the incidence of a variety of cancer-related skeletal events, including fractures, pain, the number and severity of future bone metastases, hypercalcaemia, spinal cord compression, and the need for orthopaedic surgery or radiation therapy.[20] Although bisphosphonates are used for hypercalcaemia of malignancy, a normal calcium value does not preclude their use for bone pain. The actual risk of causing clinically significant hypocalcaemia from bisphosphonates is very low and fear of this complication should not preclude their use.

Question 14. Would bisphosphonates be useful for Mr J.?

Chronic administration of oral bisphosphonates such as clodronate is useful for preventing bone metastases and reducing the risk of bone-related complications, but there is little evidence of the effectiveness of oral bisphosphonates in managing acute bone pain episodes. However, i.v. bisphosphonates such as clodronate, pamidronate, and zoledronate can relieve acute pain from bone metastases and are an important tool in the palliative management of painful bone metastases.[21] Clodronate can also be administered subcutaneously.[22] The American Society of Clinical Oncology Bisphosphonates Expert Panel has recently outlined guidelines for the use of bisphosphonates in breast cancer.[23] These guidelines will no doubt continue to evolve with further clinical experience and study in this area. Newer more potent bisphosphonates are now available, but there is need for direct comparative studies between them to be able to recommend one over another. Mr J. is currently a candidate for parenteral bisphosphonates as part of an overall analgesic strategy for his bone disease.

Question 15. Is there a role for calcitonin in patients with bone disease?

Another systemic intervention for painful bone metastases is salmon calcitonin. Administration of this hormone in pharmacological doses has been shown to reduce the amount of pain, particularly in osteoporotic fractures of the vertebrae. Physiologically, calcitonin is a peptide that is distributed widely in the human body. It modifies calcium and bone metabolism by a direct inhibitory effect on osteoclasts; the main effect is to produce a marked reduction in bone resorption. However, it also appears to exert at least some analgesic effect at the level of the central nervous system. Salmon calcitonin has been used in the pharmacological management of osteoporotic compression fractures as well as for Paget's disease, prevention of osteoporotic fractures, and hypercalcaemia. Although it has been shown to be of benefit in some patients with metastatic bone disease, the evidence for its efficacy in the relief of all types of bone pain is less clearly defined, particularly when used for a prolonged period of time.[24–27] Salmon calcitonin can be delivered by either subcutaneous injection or intranasal spray. The required dose is in the range 100–200 IU/day. Side effects are uncommon, and include allergy, hypocalcaemia, and nausea. Most patients who are going to experience relief of pain will see some benefit within 2 weeks. It is not known for how long administration should continue, but in responders one would generally administer salmon calcitonin for a few months. Some clinicians start both a bisphosphonate and calcitonin at the same time when a patient presents with a new vertebral fracture, although the practice needs further study to document its effectiveness.

Plain radiographs are obtained and reveal worrying results: there is >50 per cent erosion of the cortex of the neck of the right femur. A consultation with an orthopaedic surgeon is obtained. The right femur is found to be at high risk for fracture and the patient is advised to consider prophylactic pinning. The patient and his wife wish to know the risks of both not pinning the femur and of having the surgery before they make up their mind.

Question 16. Describe the role of an orthopaedic consultation for a patient with bone metastasis

Orthopaedic evaluation is needed to advise which lesions are best treated with surgical interventions, and which should not be operated upon. Most fractures are associated with large lytic lesions, particularly those that extend through the cortex of the bone. However, other types of lesions may require surgical repair. Some lesions (e.g. renal cell carcinoma) tend to be highly vascular, and surgery can carry a risk of severe haemorrhage. In general an orthopaedic opinion should be obtained earlier rather than later. An ideal arrangement is a multidisciplinary cancer pain clinic where orthopaedic surgeons are part of the team. When possible, closed intramedullary nailing is the preferred treatment, with the goal of unsupported use of the limb. The goal is to maintain weight bearing in the lower limbs and function of the upper limbs.[28] Pinning a weight-bearing bone usually reduces pain and improves function, and even patients with a life expectancy of only a few months can potentially be candidates for this procedure.[29]

Question 17. If Mr J. does not have the surgery, what other treatments could he have?

In patients for whom surgical pinning and further radiation therapy are not an option, the two goals are to prevent fracture of the limb and to control pain. This may be done through immobilization. The patient will require evaluation and treatment by occupational therapists and physiotherapists to reduce the risk of fracture and prevent complications of immobilization. If the bone fractures, treatment is aimed at reducing pain and disfigurement. Prevention of skin breakdown, control of pain, and improved quality of life are key goals of care for the patient who has experienced a pathological fracture of a weight-bearing bone.

Mr J. decides to have the surgery and is admitted several days later. The surgery goes well and there are no postoperative complications. He goes home 6 days after the surgery and feels relatively well. He is fully ambulatory, and interference of function by pain is greatly reduced. Over the subsequent several months, however, the left groin has become painful. On repeat radiological imaging, the left hip is found to have metastatic disease but is not at high risk for fracture and an orthopaedic intervention is not indicated.

Mr J. receives a brief course of radiation to the left pelvis region. He feels well again with good control of left groin pain within days of completing the radiation treatment. He is using long-acting opioids and requires two to three breakthrough doses daily with activities.

He notices over the next several months that he is becoming more fatigued. He now reports that his arms, shoulders, back and left ankle are also painful. A bone scan reveals multiple new sites of metastatic disease.

Question 18. Would further radiotherapy be of benefit?

If a limited number of specific sites were causing pain, localized radiotherapy would be a reasonable treatment. However, if there are many painful bony lesions, it may be beneficial to consider larger radiation fields. Hemibody radiation is an important palliative intervention, and can be given when several metastases are located within a generalized region such as the pelvis and hips. The radiation field would be enlarged to include as much of the lower body as possible. The larger the body area exposed to radiation, the higher is the risk of toxicity. The side effects of hemibody radiation correlate with the radiosensitive structures within the field of delivery. For example, hemibody radiation of the lower body can result in diarrhoea.[30] The real risk of toxicity is generally considered to be modest, given the short overall survival in patients with a high burden of tumour.

When the entire skeleton is afflicted with multiple sites of bone metastasis, consideration should be given to the use of radiopharmaceuticals.[31,32] The isotopes used in the treatment of bone metastasis are [^{32}P]chloride and [^{89}Sr]chloride.[30] These isotopes accumulate in active sites of bone turnover, such as metastatic deposits, and emit β radiation. The radioisotope is injected and the radiation goes directly to the entire skeleton with over half generally absorbed into the bone. Excess isotope is excreted in the urine. Studies have shown that this is an effective analgesic treatment, and results are similar regardless of which isotope is used. The exact mechanism by which the pain is reduced is uncertain. The main toxicity of note is myelosuppression; patients with renal failure may be at added risk as the agents are cleared through the kidney. Patients with urinary incontinence can present particular problems for possible skin or bed contamination by radiation.

Radiopharmaceuticals are less widely used than external beam radiation, probably because of their high cost. Because of their slow onset of action, patients should have a life expectancy of months or greater.

Mr J. receives wide-field radiation therapy to the pelvic region, and within 48 h describes improved comfort.

A month later he experiences rapidly progressive mid-thoracic back pain over the course of 3 days and comes in to the emergency department with numbness and weakness of the legs up to the mid-thoracic level. On examination he has spastic myelopathy and a palpable bladder. He is in severe pain, and there is tenderness over the mid-thoracic spine at about the T6 vertebral body with palpable paraspinal muscle spasm. You order a plain radiograph of the thoracic spine. There is collapse of the T6 vertebral body with destruction of the pedicles consistent with metastatic cancer.

Question 19. What is the diagnosis? What treatment should be considered?

Mr J. has epidural spinal cord compression due to extension of bone-based tumour into the epidural space. Epidural spinal cord compression is associated with contiguous bone metastasis about 95 per cent of the time, and for this reason plain spine radiographs are a useful screening tool. Collapse of a vertebral body due to tumour is a strong predictor of epidural cord compression. Definitive imaging of the thecal sac is warranted, as there may be other areas of silent epidural disease above and below the area of collapse seen on MRI; imaging the bones can identify patients who could be candidates for spinal surgery. In addition to imaging, Mr J. needs a catheter inserted in his bladder, parenteral opioids for the severe pain, and skin care.

Corticosteroids are used for the initial management of spinal cord compression prior to more definitive treatment with surgery or radiotherapy.[33] Prednisone, dexamethasone, or other corticosteroids can be used. The recommended dosages for spinal cord compression vary widely depending on the source, but most agree that higher doses in the order of ≥24–36 mg/day of dexamethasone or its equivalent are appropriate.

Surgical intervention, if required, may include vertebrectomy, decompression, and reconstruction with methyl methacrylate or another stabilizing technique.[34] These procedures can preserve function and reduce intractable pain from spinal metastases. Surgery can have a better outcome than external beam radiation therapy.[35] However, surgery is generally reserved for patients who have a prognosis measured in at least months and are medically able to tolerate it.

High-dose corticosteroids without radiation therapy or surgery can provide many weeks of palliation from pain from disseminated bone metastases and cord compression. It is an important palliative intervention that is frequently employed at the end of life or to help control pain until radiation therapy or other interventions have time to work.

Mr J. agrees to a course of high-dose steroids followed by 10 fractions of spinal radiation therapy. Within about 2 weeks of starting radiation therapy his mobility is improved, but he continues to have moderate weakness and bladder failure. He can walk with assistance. He is able to reduce the dose of steroids, and his appetite is improved. Over the next 8 weeks he develops progressive respiratory difficulty from lung metastases, and he dies peacefully from pneumonia with his family at his side.

Summary

Bone pain secondary to metastatic cancer can reduce patient function and quality of life. Early identification and rapid intervention with pharmacological and non-pharmacological treatments may improve functional status and quality of life. Although opioids are still the drugs of choice for management of this type of somatic pain, agents such as NSAIDs, bisphosphonates, calcitonin, and others, singly or in combination, can be effective. Radiotherapy and surgical interventions can reduce the risks of fracture, improve pain control, and therefore maintain function. The skills and knowledge of the interdisciplinary team are important in the management of bone pain.

Future directions

Despite considerable progress to date, patients with bone metastases often have pain and often experience complications such as cord compression and hypercalcaemia. Much further work is needed to understand the pathophysiology of bone metastasis and to develop more effective oncological interventions to prevent and manage this devastating scenario.

References

1. **Galasko, C.S.B.** (1986) Skeletal metastases. *Clin Orthoped,* **210**, 18–318.
2. **Periera, J.** (1998) Management of bone pain. In: Portenoy R, Bruera E(eds) *Topics in Palliative Care,* Vol 3. New York: Oxford University Press, 79–116.
3. **Lote. K., Walloe, A., and Bjersand, A.** (1986) Bone metastases, prognosis, diagnosis and treatment. *Acta Radiol Oncol,* **25**, 227–32.
4. **DeVita, V.T., Bellman, S., and Rosenberg, S.A.** (2001) *Cancer, Principles and Practices of Oncology* (6th edn). Philadelphia, PA: Lippincott–Williams and Wilkins, 2713–28.
5. **Portenoy, R.K., and Hagen, N.A.** (1990). Breakthrough pain, definition, prevalence and characteristics. *Pain,* **41**, 273–81.
6. **Hagen, N.A.** (1999) Reproducing a cancer patient's pain on physical examination: bedside provocative maneuvers. *J Pain Symptom Manage,* **18**, 406–11.
7. **Front, D., Schneck, S.O., Frankel, A., and Robinson, E.** (1979) Bone metastases and bone pain in breast cancer. Are they closely associated? *JAMA,* **242**, 1747–8.
8. **Frassica, F.J., Frassica, D.A., Lietman, S.A. *et al.*** (1998) Surgical palliation of malignant bone pain. In: Portenoy R, Bruera E (eds) *Topics in Palliative Care,* Vol 3. New York: Oxford University Press, 139–62.
9. **Fidler, M.** (1973) Prophylactic internal fixation of secondary neoplastic deposits in long bones. *BMJ,* **1**, 341–3.
10. **Mercadante, S.** (1997) Malignant bone pain: pathophysiology and treatment. *Pain* **69**, 1–18.
11. **Ripamonti, C., and Fulfaro, F.** (2000) Malignant bone pain: pathophysiology and treatments. *Curr Rev Pain,* **4**, 187–96.
12. **Joishy, S., and Walsh, D.** (1998) The opioid-sparing effects of intravenous ketorolac as an adjuvant analgesic in cancer pain: application in bone metastases and the opioid bowel syndrome. *Pain Symptom Manage,* **16**, 334–9.
13. **Mercadante, S., Casuccio, A., Agnello, A., Pumo, S., Kargar, J., and Garofalo, S.** (1999) Analgesic Effects of nonsteroidal anti-inflammatory drugs in cancer pain due to somatic or visceral mechanisms. *J Pain Symptom Manage,* **17**, 351–6.
14. **Wright, J.M.** (2002) The double-edged sword of COX-2 selective NSAIDs. *Can Med Assoc J,* **167**, 1131–7.
15. **Hunt, R.H., Barkun, A.N., Baron, D., *et al.*** (2002) Recommendations for the appropriate use of anti-inflammatory drugs in the era of coxibs: defining the role of gastroprotective agents. *Can J Gastroenterol,* **16**, 231–40.
16. **Saarto, T., Janes, R., Tenhunen, M., and Kouri, M.** (2002) Palliative radiotherapy in the treatment of skeletal metastasis. *Eur J Pain,* **6**, 323–30.
17. **Branislav, J.** (2001) Single fraction external beam radiation therapy in the treatment of localized metastatic bone pain. A review. *J Pain Symptom Manage,* **22**, 1048–58.
18. **McQuay, H.J., Collins, S.L., Carroll, D., and Moore, R.A.** (2002) Radiotherapy for the palliation of painful bone metastases (Cochrane Review) *Cochrane Library Issue,* **3**.
19. **Johnson, I.S.** (2001) Use of bisphosphonates for the treatment of metastatic bone pain. Survey of palliative physicians in the UK. *Palliat Med,* **15**, 141–7.

20. **Bruera, E.D., and Sweeny, C.** (2003) Bone pain. In: Bruera ED, Portenoy RK (eds) *Cancer Pain Assessment and Management.* New York: Cambridge University Press, 413–28.
21. **Fulfaro, F., Casuccio, A., Ticozzi, C., Ripamonti, C.** (1998) The role of bisphosphonates in the treatment of painful metastatic bone disease: a review of phase III trials. *Pain,* **78**, 157–69
22. **Roemer-Becuwe, C., Vigano, A., Romano, F.,** ***et al.*** (2003) Safety of subcutaneous clodronate and efficacy in hypercalcemia of malignancy: a novel route of administration *J Pain Symptom Manage,* **26**, 843–8.
23. **Hillner, B.E., Ingle, J.N., Berenson, J.R.,** ***et al.*** (2000) American Society of Clinical Oncology guideline on the role of bisphosphonates in breast cancer. American Society of Clinical Oncology Bisphosphonates Expert Panel. *J Clin Oncol,* **18**, 1378–91.
24. **Mystakidou, K., Befon, S., Hondros, K., Kouskouni, E., and Vlahos, L.** (1999) Continuous subcutaneous administration of high-dose salmon calcitonin in bone metastasis: pain control and beta-endorphin plasma levels. *J Pain Symptom Manage,* **18**, 323–30.
25. **Guay, D.** (2001) Adjunctive agents in the management of chronic pain. *Pharmacotherapy,* **21**, 1070–81.
26. **Schiraldi, G.F., Soresi, E., Locicero, S.,** ***et al.*** (1987) Salmon calcitonin in cancer pain; comparison between two different treatment schedules. *Int J Clin Pharmacol Ther Toxicol,* **25**, 229–32.
27. **Kreeger, L., and Hutton-Potts, J.** (1999) The use of calcitonin in the treatment of metastatic bone pain. *J Pain Symptom Manage,* **17**, 2–5.
28. **Galasko, C.S.B.** (2004) Orthopaedic principles and management. In: Doyle D, Hanks GWC, Cherny N, Calman K (eds) *Oxford Textbook of Palliative Medicine* (3rd edn). Oxford: Oxford University Press, 268.
29. **Janjan, N.** (2001) Bone metastasis: approaches to management. *Semin Oncol,* **28**, 28–34.
30. **Kantoff, P.W., Carroll, P.R., and D'Amico, A.V.** (2002) *Prostate Cancer: Principles and Practice.* Philadelphia, PA: Lippincott–Williams and Wilkins, 595–601.
31. **Lewington, V.J.** (2002) Symposium of Interventional Nuclear Medicine: a practical guide to targeted therapy for bone pain palliation. *Nucl Med Commun,* **23,** 833–6.
32. **Pons, F., and Fuster, D.,** (2002) Under-utilization of radionuclide therapy in metastatic bone palliation. *Nucl Med Commun,* **23**, 301–2.
33. **Twycross, R.** (1994) The risks and benefits of corticosteroids in advanced cancer. *Drug Saf* **11**, 163–78.
34. **Gokaslan, Z.L., York, J.E., Walsh, G.L.,** ***et al.*** (1998). Transthoracic vertebrectomy for metastatic spinal tumors. *J Neurosurg,* **89**, 599–609.
35. **Patchell, R., Tibbs, P.A., Regine, W.F.,** ***et al.*** (2003) A randomized trial of direct decompressive surgical resection in the treatment of spinal cord compression caused by metastasis. *J Clin Oncol,* **21**(Suppl), 237.

Chapter 5

Visceral pain

Raymond Viola and Pippa Hall

This chapter will build on the learning objectives listed in Chapter 2 and also enable each student to:

- Recognize the unique characteristics of visceral pain compared with somatic and neuropathic pain.
- Describe mechanisms of visceral pain production.
- Describe strategies for managing visceral pain.

> You are the family doctor for Mrs D.S., a 68-year-old housewife and widow with three adult children. Previously well, she presented with painless jaundice 3 months ago and was diagnosed with non-resectable adenocarcinoma of the head of the pancreas with liver metastases. A stent was placed to bypass the extrahepatic biliary obstruction. She was offered standard chemotherapy with gemcitabine, but she declined this treatment.
>
> After surgery, she returned to live alone in her own home, followed monthly by you. Today she comes to your office for her regular scheduled appointment, and reports that she has severe pain, worsening over the past 3 weeks. She is accompanied by her 30-year-old daughter.

Question 1. How would you obtain a complete and relevant pain history from Mrs S.?

A systematic approach to obtaining a pain history is outlined in Chapter 2. During the interview, you particularly observe Mrs S.'s behaviour because both verbal and non-verbal communication is important for the completion of a pain history.[1]

> With your guidance, Mrs S. reports to you that she has a constant, dull, and poorly localized upper abdominal ache, which she also feels in her mid-back area. On a pain measurement scale of 0–10, she says that the pain is 6 most of the time. If she lies flat on her back it increases to 8/10, but if she curls into a fetal position on her side it decreases to 4/10. She is having trouble sleeping because of the pain. She is using tablets of acetaminophen (paracetamol) 325 mg with codeine 30 mg to treat this pain, taking two at a time up to four times daily. She indicates that this does not help much and that she experiences nausea intermittently during the day, without any vomiting. She has a poor appetite and believes that she has lost 5 kg since her surgery. She has little energy. Her bowel movements have decreased from daily to every 3–5 days since the pain began. She takes magnesium hydroxide every few days to help stimulate a bowel movement, but these movements are associated with considerable straining and the stools are small and hard. She reports no urinary problems and no neurological symptoms.

Question 2. After the history, which aspects of the physical examination would you want to perform in order to assess Mrs S.'s condition further? Why?

The examination of Mrs S. should begin with a general physical examination, followed by a focused examination of her abdomen and back. The abdomen should be examined for the presence of palpable masses, areas of tenderness, hepatomegaly, signs of bowel obstruction, and signs of ascites (distension, fluid thrill, shifting dullness). She should be examined for areas of back tenderness. A rectal examination should be performed because of her constipation.

> On examination, she is not jaundiced, appears thinner than a month ago, and is in moderate distress, holding her abdomen while sitting in the chair. She moves slowly and is tearful at times. Examination of the abdomen shows no distension, but on palpation she has a vague fullness in the epigastric area which is tender to deep pressure. There is no evidence of gastric distension. The liver is not enlarged, there is no shifting dullness, and bowel sounds are present. There is no tenderness in her back and no restriction of spinal movement. Rectal examination reveals hard stool present in the rectum.

Provocative manoeuvres can elicit pain from cancer of the pancreas, and can suggest the presence of a retroperitoneal pain-sensitive structure.[2] To perform this manoeuvre, the patient is instructed to sit upright on the examining table with the legs extended horizontally and resting on the bed. A pillow is positioned beneath the lumbar spine and the patient is instructed to lie down; the positioning of the pillow results in extension of the thoracolumbar spine.

A positive provocative manoeuvre occurs if the patient's back, flank, or abdominal pain is reproduced by extension of the spine and is relieved promptly by sitting upright again. There should not be any tenderness of the spine on direct percussion.

> This manoeuvre clearly accentuates Mrs S.'s pain.

Question 3. What are the possible causes of Mrs S.'s abdominal pain? What is the most likely cause?

The positive retroperitoneal stretch manoeuvre indicates that the retroperitoneum is probably the site of the pain. Inflammatory processes, such as an abscess or pancreatitis, and cancer-related processes, such as metastatic tumour or primary pancreatic neoplasm, are common causes. The most probable cause of her pain is the primary pancreatic cancer. Other possible causes, such as hepatic capsular distension, bowel obstruction, ascites, and bone or soft tissue lesions of the back, are less likely based on the history and physical examination.[3] Constipation may be contributing to the abdominal pain. While many factors contribute to Mrs S.'s pain, you conclude that she has a visceral pain syndrome.

Question 4. What is visceral pain?

A viscus is an organ within a major body cavity and is innervated by the autonomic nervous system.[4] Visceral pain arises from disease in these internal structures. The association with the autonomic nervous system plus the generation of sensations from body areas whose activities are usually not consciously evident can produce confusing symptom patterns.

Question 5. What are the clinical features of visceral pain?

The clinical features of visceral pain differ from those of somatic pain. Although visceral pain perception may occur acutely, such as when a hollow viscus becomes obstructed, distended, and inflamed (e.g. malignant bowel obstruction; see Chapter 19), it often occurs late in the course of a disease because significant tissue destruction is usually required before such pain can be perceived. It is usually poorly localized by the patient and is difficult to describe, in contrast with somatic pain. More accurate localization occurs if adjacent somatic structures become involved with the disease process. Visceral pain syndromes are often associated with symptoms related to autonomic nervous system activation. These symptoms may include nausea, vomiting, weakness, sweating, and changes in heart rate and blood pressure, especially if the pain is acute. Visceral pain commonly produces referred pain, where pain and hyperalgesia are perceived at somatic sites distant from the stimulus.[5,6]

Question 6. What are the possible mechanisms of pain production in disease processes causing visceral pain? What mechanisms may be active in producing pain from pancreatic cancer?

Under experimental circumstances, the viscera are generally insensitive to some of the usual painful stimuli associated with somatic pain, such as cutting, tearing, or burning. However, this may not be true in clinical situations where inflammation is present.[5] Mechanisms of visceral pain include the following:[7]

- distension of a hollow viscus (e.g. bowel obstruction)
- abnormal contraction of a hollow viscus (e.g. urinary bladder spasms)
- stretching of the capsule of a solid viscus (e.g. liver capsular distension)
- ischaemia of visceral muscle (e.g. myocardial infarct)
- chemical stimulation of the serosa or mucosa (e.g. peritonitis)
- traction or torsion of mesentery (e.g. volvulus of the bowel)
- necrosis of a viscus.

The mechanism underlying referred pain remains unclear. It may be related to innervations of both visceral and somatic structures by the same sensory nerve (dual innervations) or to central nervous system convergence of sensory inputs.[5]

Pancreatic cancer pain may result from distension of the common bile duct or the pancreatic duct secondary to obstruction or release of pancreatic enzymes producing inflammation, both examples of visceral pain.[5] Other mechanisms of pancreatic cancer pain include stretching of retroperitoneal nerves, invasion of autonomic or somatic nerves, and peripancreatic neuritis. Back pain may be caused by retroperitoneal invasion by the malignancy.[3] Pancreatic cancer pain is primarily visceral in origin early in the disease, but can become mixed, with somatic and neuropathic components in addition to more than one mechanism of visceral pain, as the disease progresses.[8,9] Acknowledging the probable presence of multiple mechanisms is important when considering therapy.

Question 7. Would you recommend performing any investigations to help diagnose and manage Mrs S.'s pain? Why?

No further investigations are necessary at this point. The history and physical examination, if properly done, have diagnostic reliability[10] and, in the case of Mrs S., have provided a diagnosis which has a high probability of accuracy. Further diagnostic procedures will not affect the diagnosis or the treatment options that should be offered.

Question 8. Why does Mrs S. have anorexia, nausea, and constipation?

These symptoms have multiple possible causes in this patient. Anorexia and cachexia are common symptoms experienced by persons with advanced pancreatic cancer, but their pathophysiology is only partially understood (see Chapter 7). While severe pain alone can cause nausea and anorexia, visceral pain, such as that arising from the pancreas, is often associated with stimulation of autonomic reflexes which can produce nausea.[5] Gastroparesis is common in advanced cancer, partly because of autonomic dysfunction. This can result in several gastrointestinal symptoms including anorexia and nausea.[11] Opioid use may aggravate this motility problem, but may also produce nausea by direct stimulation of the chemoreceptor trigger zone and by vestibular stimulation. Constipation, caused by opioid use, decreased food and fluid intake, and possibly decreased mobility, may cause or aggravate anorexia and nausea. Anxiety may also cause or exacerbate nausea.

Question 9. What treatment options are available to manage Mrs S.'s pain?

> You explain to Mrs S. and, with her approval, to her daughter that you believe that her pain is coming from the pancreatic cancer, but that much can be done to control it. You also point out that she is constipated and that this may be aggravating the pain and other symptoms.

The principles of therapy for chronic cancer pain also apply to visceral pain. For moderate to severe visceral pain, oral morphine is the agent of choice. Non-opioid analgesics, such as non-steroidal anti-inflammatory drugs (NSAIDs) and acetaminophen, and adjuvant analgesics, such as corticosteroids, may contribute to pain control.[5] Antineoplastic therapies can provide symptom control benefits and should be considered when visceral pain is present. Radiotherapy can relieve pain caused by cancer of the pancreas, and the addition of the nucleotide analogue chemotherapy agent 5-fluorouracil may enhance the radiotherapy effect.[12] The chemotherapy agent gemcitabine improves symptoms related to pancreatic cancer, including pain, in about a quarter of patients.[13] Other systemic approaches for treating pancreatic cancer are being investigated, including new chemotherapeutic agents, somatostatin analogues,[14] and immunotherapy.[15] Patients can be offered the opportunity to participate in clinical trials of such innovative treatments.

Coeliac plexus block, a sympathetic neurolytic procedure, is safe and effective (in expert hands) in relieving visceral pain associated with pancreatic cancer early in the course of the disease.[9,16,17] It may be offered early in patients with severe pain, since a randomized controlled study has demonstrated that splanchnicectomy (coeliac plexus block) prevents pain from appearing, relieves or reduces pain that is present, and prolongs life.[18]

Non-pharmacological treatments can help to control pain and optimize quality of life. Physical modalities available include massage, transcutaneous nerve stimulation, and acupuncture.[19] Psychosocial interventions include distraction techniques, imagery, relaxation, hypnosis, and cognitive–behavioural therapy.[5] A physiotherapist, social worker, psychologist, or spiritual counsellor could be consulted to help administer some of these therapies.

Question 10. What other aspects of Mrs S.'s care need to be addressed and how would you address them?

Mrs S.'s anorexia, nausea, and constipation must be managed. Anorexia and nausea may respond to control of the pain and improvement in bowel function. In addition to specific nutritional advice, you can consider pharmacological management as outlined in Chapter 7.

Home care services, especially nursing, should be optimized with Mrs S.'s agreement. Psychosocial and spiritual issues will need to be addressed further once the physical symptoms are controlled.[20]

With Mrs S.'s agreement, discussion and planning of her care takes place with the participation of her daughter. They agree to inform the rest of the family about the plans. To assist with the monitoring and management of her pain and other symptoms, you request daily home care nursing visits. Since she is unable to manage her home and self-care adequately alone, she also agrees to accept home-making assistance. She wishes to remain in her own home for as long as possible, and believes that this plan will help her do so.

You recommend to Mrs S. that she start taking regular morphine. Referring to an opioid equianalgesic table, you prescribe morphine 5 mg orally every 4 h around the clock. You review with her the proven benefits of regular dosing for ideal management of constant pain, taking advantage of the 4-h duration of analgesia provided by oral morphine. You suggest that she set her alarm for the middle of the night to prevent missing that dose. Breakthrough pain will be managed with morphine 5 mg orally when needed, available at hourly intervals. The effect of this regimen will be reviewed by you by telephone or by a home care nurse in 24 h. If pain remains uncontrolled and side effects are minimal, the dose can be increased in 25–50 per cent increments, daily if necessary. Titration of the morphine dose will continue until the pain is adequately controlled, according to Mrs S., or intolerable side effects occur. Sustained-release morphine can be substituted once stable pain relief is achieved.

Potential side effects of opioid use are also discussed with Mrs S. Because she is already experiencing nausea, regular domperidone 10 mg orally four times daily is prescribed, plus 10 mg orally every hour if needed for breakthrough nausea. Prochlorperazine suppositories are also prescribed for breakthrough nausea in case vomiting prevents the oral use of anti-nauseants. Mrs S. is badly constipated; indeed, her rectum is blocked by hard stool. Disimpaction is gently carried out by the home care nurse, with follow-up daily enemas until the bowel is clear. At the same time, a senna laxative is prescribed and bisacodyl suppositories are made available for use every 2 days if no bowel movement has occurred. Close follow-up of her bowel function is planned, with escalation of the bowel regimen as necessary to ensure that a bowel movement occurs at least once every 3 days.

You discuss the use of NSAIDs and adjuvant analgesics, but Mrs S. prefers not to initiate more than two new agents at this time, especially in view of the nausea that she is already experiencing. You also recommend that she consider having a coeliac plexus block performed, but she declines, wishing to try systemic analgesics first. She states that she would consider a block or radiotherapy later, if necessary, but that she does not want to consider any chemotherapy. You indicate to her that if the above interventions prove ineffective or are not tried, a trial of a temporary epidural can be considered with a view to permanent placement if it is effective.

Research and future considerations

Cancer researchers continue to explore possible roles for new systemic therapies for pancreatic cancer.[21] Innovative methods of performing visceral sympathetic blocks have been described and studied, but their appropriate use remains to be determined.[22–24] Studies are revealing that different opiate receptors, such as the κ-receptor, may be specifically responsible for visceral pain. In the future, opioids targeted for specific receptors may be available, minimizing side effects.[25] During the past decade, clinicians have increased their use of methadone for managing patients with difficult chronic pain syndromes. Because it acts as an antagonist at the *N*-methyl-D-aspartate receptor, in addition to its opioid agonist effects, methadone is postulated as providing improved pain control when opioid analgesic tolerance has occurred or a significant component of the pain is neuropathic.[26,27] The role of methadone in the management of visceral pain remains to be determined. Finally, basic pain research continues to inform pharmaceutical companies and clinicians about the potential for developing new agents and about novel uses of existing drugs for managing visceral pain.[6]

Bibliography

Cervero, F., and Laird, J.M.A. (1999) Visceral Pain. *Lancet* **353,** 2145–8.

Portenoy, R.K., Forbes, K., Lussier, D., and Hanks, G. (2004) Difficult pain problems: an integrated approach. In: Doyle D, Hanks, GW, Cherny N, Calman K (eds) *Oxford Textbook of Palliative Medicine* (3rd edn). Oxford: Oxford University Press, 438–58.

References

1. **Weston, W.W., Brown, J.B., and Stewart, M.A.** (1989) Patient-centred interviewing. Part I: Understanding patients' experiences. *Can Fam Physician,* **35**, 147–51.
2. **Hagen, N.** (1999) Reproducing a cancer patient's pain on physical examination: bedside provocative maneuvers. *J Pain Symptom Manage,* **18(6),** 406–411.
3. **Patt, R.B.** (1993) Classification of cancer pain and cancer pain syndromes. In: Patt RB (ed) *Cancer Pain.* Philadelphia, PA: J.B. Lippincott, 16.
4. **Anonymous** (1989) Viscus. In: *Churchill's Illustrated Medical Dictionary.* New York: Churchill Livingstone, 2094.
5. **Portenoy, R.K., Forbes, K., Lussier, D., and Hanks, G.** (2004) Difficult pain problems: an integrated approach. In: Doyle D, Hanks, GW, Cherny N, Calman K (eds) *Oxford Textbook of Palliative Medicine* (3rd edn). Oxford: Oxford University Press, 438–58.
6. **Cervero, F., and Laird, J.M.A.** (1999) Visceral pain. *Lancet,* **353**, 2145–8.
7. **Patt, R.B.** (1993) Classification of cancer pain and cancer pain syndromes. In: Patt RB (ed) *Cancer Pain.* Philadelphia, PA: J.B. Lippincott, 6.
8. **Portenoy, R.K.** (1992) Cancer pain: pathophysiology and syndromes. *Lancet,* **339**, 1026–31.
9. **Ischia, S., Ischia, A., Polati, E., and Finco, G.** (1992) Three posterior percutaneous celiac plexus block techniques—a prospective, randomized study in 61 patients with pancreatic cancer pain. *Anesthesiology,* **76**, 534–40.

10. **Sackett, D.L., Haynes, R.B., Guyatt, G.H., and Tugwell, P.** (1991) *Clinical Epidemiology—A Basic Science for Clinical Medicine* (2nd edn). Boston, MA: Little, Brown, 19–21.
11. **Billings, J.A.** (1994) Anorexia. *J Palliat Care*, **10**, 51–3.
12. **Moertel, C.G., Frytak, S., Hahn, R.G., *et al.*** (1981) Therapy of locally unresectable pancreatic carcinoma: a randomized comparison of high dose (6000 rads) radiation alone, moderate dose radiation (4000 rads + 5-fluorouracil), and high dose radiation + 5-fluorouracil: The Gastrointestinal Tumor Study Group. *Cancer*, **48**, 1705–10.
13. **Burris, H.A., Moore, M.J., Andersen, J., *et al.*** (1997) Improvements in survival and clinical benefit with gemcitabine as first-line therapy for patients with advanced pancreas cancer: a randomized trial. *J Clin Oncol*, **15**, 2403–13.
14. **Hejna, M., Schmidinger, M., and Raderer, M.** (2002) The clinical role of somatostatin analogues as antineoplastic agents: much ado about nothing? *Ann Oncol*, **13**, 653–68.
15. **Kaufman H,L., Di Vito, J., and Horig, H.** (2002) Immunotherapy for pancreatic cancer: current concepts. *Hematol Oncol Clin North Am*, **16**, 159–97.
16. **Eisenberg, E., Carr, D.B., and Chalmers, T.C.** (1995) Neurolytic celiac plexus block for treatment of cancer pain: a meta-analysis. *Anesth Analg*, **80**, 290–5.
17. **Polati, E., Finco, G., Gottin, L., Bassi, C., Pederzoli, P., and Ischia, S.** (1998) Prospective randomized double-blind trial of neurolytic coeliac plexus block in patients with pancreatic cancer. *Br J Surg*, **85**, 199–201.
18. **Lillemoe, K.D., Cameron, J.L., Kaufman, H.S., Yeo, C.J., Pitt, H.A., and Sauter, P.K.** (1993) Chemical splanchnicectomy in patients with unresectable pancreatic cancer: a prospective randomized trial. *Ann Surg*, **217**, 447–57.
19. **Thompson, J.W., and Filshie, J.** (1998) Transcutaneous electrical nerve stimulation (TENS) and acupuncture. In: Doyle D, Hanks, GW, MacDonald N (eds) *Oxford Textbook of Palliative Medicine* (2nd edn). Oxford: Oxford University Press, 421–37.
20. **Doyle, D.** (1992) Have we looked beyond the physical and psychosocial? *J Pain Symptom Manage*, **7**, 302–11.
21. **Moore, M.J.** (2002) Pancreatic cancer: what the oncologist can offer for palliation. *Can J Gastroenterol*, **16**, 121–4.
22. **Leksowski, K.** (2001) Thoracoscopic splanchnicectomy for the relief of pain due to chronic pancreatitis. *Surg Endosc*, **15**, 592–6.
23. **Vranken, J.H., Zuurmond, W.W.A., and de Lange, J.J.** (2001) Increasing the efficacy of a celiac plexus block in patients with severe pancreatic cancer pain. *J Pain Symptom Manage*, **22**, 966–77.
24. **Mercadante, S., and La Rosa, S.** (2002) CT-guided neurolytic splanchnic nerve block by an anterior approach. *J Pain Symptom Manage*, **23**, 268–70.
25. **Gebhart, G.F., Su, X., Joshi, S., Ozaki, N., and Sengupta, J.N.** (2000) Peripheral opioid modulation of visceral pain. *Ann NY Acad Sci*, **909**, 41–50.
26. **Watanabe, S.** (2001) Methadone: the renaissance. *J Palliat Care*, **17**, 117–20.
27. **Bruera, E., and Sweeney, C.** (2002) Methadone use in cancer patients with pain: a review. *J Palliat Med*, **5**, 127–38.

Chapter 6

Neurological effects: opioids

Sharon Watanabe and Yoko Tarumi

Attitude

To enable each student to:

- Adopt a proactive approach to the management of opioid neurotoxicity.

Skill

To enable each student to:

- Recognize opioid neurotoxicity.
- Differentiate opioid neurotoxicity from other clinical syndromes.
- Identify risk factors for opioid neurotoxicity.
- Apply an appropriate management strategy for opioid neurotoxicity.
- Perform opioid rotation.

Knowledge

To enable each student to:

- Classify opioid adverse effects.
- Understand the pathophysiological basis of opioid adverse effects.

Mr. M. is a 62-year-old man who lives with his spouse. He was diagnosed with non-small-cell carcinoma of the lung 2 months ago, at which time he presented with progressively severe low back pain and right proximal thigh pain for which he had been taking ibuprofen 400 mg orally two to three times a day. Bone scan and accompanying plain radiographs revealed mixed osteolytic and osteoblastic abnormalities in the fourth and fifth lumbar vertebrae, the right sacro-iliac joint, and the neck of the right femur. He began a chemotherapy regimen together with palliative radiotherapy. He was started on immediate-release morphine 10 mg orally every 4 h round the clock, 5 mg orally every hour as needed for breakthrough pain, and a laxative regime. Two weeks ago, as Mr. M. had been taking three to four breakthroughs doses per day, his morphine was increased to 15 mg every 4 h round the clock.

Mr. and Mrs. M. now present to your office for follow-up. Since the increase in the morphine dose, they have noticed that his legs and arms occasionally jerk when he relaxes and watches television. It also wakes him up in the middle of the night.

Question 1. What is the probable diagnosis?

The patient has myoclonus, which is an opioid adverse effect (Table 6.1). Adverse effects of opioids can be categorized into those that typically occur upon initiation of therapy or with significant dose escalation, and those that generally develop with chronic administration.

Adverse effects that appear upon initiation or escalation of opioids are, in general, extensions of therapeutic effects. They include nausea, constipation, and drowsiness, sometimes associated with cognitive impairment. Tolerance to these effects usually develops within days, except for constipation. Respiratory depression is rare if the opioid dose is carefully titrated.

Adverse effects associated with chronic administration of opioids are manifestations of central nervous system hyperexcitability. These include myoclonus, delirium, hallucinations, and hyperalgesia. Myoclonus is a sudden brief shock-like involuntary movement caused by active muscular contractions that may involve a whole muscle or may be limited to a few muscle fibres.[1] Severe opioid-induced neurotoxicity may lead to generalized tonic–clonic seizures. Opioid-related hallucinations are most commonly visual or tactile.[2] Hallucinations may occur alone,[3] or in combination with cognitive failure and psychomotor agitation, i.e. hyperactive delirium.[4] Hyperalgesia is defined as an exaggerated nociceptive response to noxious stimulation, whereas allodynia is defined as a nociceptive response to innocuous stimulation.[5] Clinically, these phenomena present as worsening of the pre-existing pain syndrome and generalized pain with touch, respectively.

It is appropriate to screen proactively for adverse effects of opioids. Patients may not spontaneously report hallucinations and should be specifically queried regarding visual, auditory, and tactile hallucinations. The last of these refers to a benign and generally emotionally neutral experience of being touched, such as the sensation of having a hand resting on the shoulder.[3] Also, the presence of cognitive failure can be missed unless a screening tool such as the Folstein Mini-Mental State Examination is employed.[6,7]

> Mr. M. denies seeing or feeling things that are not really there. His Folstein Mini-Mental State Examination score is 29/30; the expected normal score for his age and educational level is 28/30.

Table 6.1 Classification of opioid adverse effects

Early phase
Nausea
Constipation
Sedation and cognitive impairment (hypoactive delirium)
Respiratory depression
Late phase
Myoclonus
Generalized tonic–clonic seizures
Hallucinations alone, or with agitation and cognitive impairment (hyperactive delirium)
Hyperalgesia or allodynia

Question 2. What is the differential diagnosis?

Myoclonus should be distinguished from tremor, asterixis, and focal seizures. Tremor is more continuous and rhythmic. Asterixis presents as a recurrent abrupt lapse in postural tone of the outstretched arms. Focal seizures tend to be confined to one area of the body, whereas myoclonus usually involves many different areas over time.

Generalized tonic–clonic seizures may be caused by brain metastases or metabolic derangements.

Hallucinations and cognitive failure may be manifestations of delirium from many other aetiologies (see Chapter 24).

Hyperalgesia may be misinterpreted as worsening nociception (tissue destruction by tumour or other causes). This may lead to an increase in opioid consumption, which may aggravate the toxicity. Allodynia may be a feature of neuropathic pain, in which case it is localized to one focal area of neurological dysfunction. Allodynia associated with opioid neurotoxicity tends to be generalized.

Question 3. How do opioids cause neurotoxicity?

While all opioids in high doses may have neurotoxic properties, adverse effects are thought to be mediated in large part via their active metabolites. The effects of opioid metabolites have been best described for morphine, which is metabolized mainly to 6- and 3-glucuronides.

Morphine-6-glucuronide binds to the μ opiate receptor and is a more potent analgesic than morphine. Accumulation of morphine-6-glucuronide has been associated with the development of respiratory depression, confusion, and nausea in humans.[8,9]

Morphine-3-glucuronide, on the other hand, has a low affinity for the μ opiate receptor. Its site of action is currently unknown, although there is evidence that it activates excitatory central nervous system pathways.[10] Experimental administration of morphine-3-glucuronide to animals produces neuroexcitatory effects such as hyperalgesia, allodynia, myoclonus, and seizures.[11] The evidence linking elevated morphine-3-glucuronide levels with neuroexcitatory toxicity in humans is limited.[12] Normorphine is another morphine metabolite that has been suggested to have neuroexcitatory effects.[13]

Neurotoxicity has also been attributed to metabolites of other opioids. In patients receiving meperidine, neurotoxicity has been correlated with levels of the metabolite normeperidine.[14] Hydromorphone-3-glucuronide has been shown to have neuroexcitatory effects in animals that reproduce a range of behaviours consistent with the spectrum of opioid neurotoxicity observed in humans.[15]

Question 4. What factors may contribute to the development of opioid neurotoxicity?

Renal failure has been well documented to cause accumulation of opioids and their metabolites,[16] and has been associated clinically with the development of opioid neurotoxicity.[12,16,17] Dehydration can also impair renal clearance of all renally excreted opioid or metabolite.

Some medications may precipitate opioid toxicity by interfering with renal function, for example non-steroidal anti-inflammatory drugs (NSAIDs)[18] and ACE inhibitors.[19] One study linked the occurrence of morphine neurotoxicity with the concomitant use of psychotropic agents and NSAIDs.[20]

Mr. M. has been drinking the equivalent of eight glasses of fluid per day and has normal renal function. He continues to use ibuprofen two to three times a day. His only other medications are laxatives.

Question 5. What is the management of opioid neurotoxicity?

If pain is well controlled, it is reasonable to try decreasing the dose of opioid by increments of at least 25 per cent. A number of retrospective studies[21,22] suggest that this strategy is effective in reducing opioid neurotoxicity.

If pain is not well controlled, the following options may be considered:[23]

1. Reduce the opioid dose while applying other analgesic interventions. These include the addition of non-opioid drugs, applying treatments to target the cause of pain, and using regional anaesthetic or neuroablative measure. While they may be useful in selected cases, all these approaches have potential limitations, such as polypharmacy, delayed onset of effect, and need for specialized resources.
2. Maintain the opioid dose and manage the neurotoxic effects symptomatically. This approach entails polypharmacy with the attendant risks of increased adverse effects, drug interactions, and diminished compliance.
3. Switch to a different opioid. This procedure, also known as opioid rotation or opioid substitution, may maintain analgesia while allowing the metabolites responsible for neurotoxicity to be cleared. A number of retrospective series and prospective uncontrolled studies suggest that this strategy is often effective.[24–28]

Mr. M. states that his pain is well controlled. He has not required any breakthrough morphine doses for the past week. Therefore you advise him to reduce the morphine dose to 10 mg every 4 h round the clock and 5 mg every hour as needed for breakthrough pain. You also suggest that he discontinues the ibuprofen. You reinforce the importance of drinking as much as possible to promote elimination of the morphine metabolites that are causing the myoclonus.

You call Mr. M. 2 days later, and he reports that the jerking has resolved and his pain remains under good control. He has required only one breakthrough morphine dose since his visit to your office. You decide to switch him to sustained release morphine 30 mg orally every 12 h.

Over the next 2 months, Mr. M.'s analgesic requirements gradually increase to sustained release morphine 60 mg every 12 h and immediate release morphine 10 mg every hour as needed for breakthrough pain. One day you receive a telephone call from Mrs. M. She reports that Mr. M. has been complaining of increased generalized pain during the past week. She gave him four breakthrough morphine doses 2 days ago, and at least five breakthrough doses yesterday. She has already given him three breakthrough doses today and has noticed that he is becoming drowsy and restless.

Upon further inquiry, Mrs. M. reports that Mr. M. has been disoriented at times, jerking, and picking at the air. Mrs. M. is also concerned that he has not taken anything by mouth except his pills since last night.

You ask Mrs. M. to bring Mr. M. to your office. However, Mrs. M. does not think that it is possible because of his restlessness and pain. You arrange to visit him at home later that day.

On arrival, you find Mr. M. to be drowsy and restless. Although complaining of pain, he gets up and down from the chair without difficulty. He scores 12/30 on the Folstein Mini-Mental State Examination. He appears dehydrated. He has frequent sudden brief shock-like involuntary movements of his extremities. He is generally sensitive to light touch. You do not find any localized bony tenderness.

Question 6. What is the diagnosis and what would you do?

Mr. M. has myoclonus, delirium, and allodynia, which suggest moderately severe neurotoxicity from morphine. Dehydration is probably an aggravating factor. Given the severity of the neurotoxicity, you decide to rotate the opioid.

Question 7. How do you perform an opioid rotation?

First, select an alternative opioid. There is little evidence on which to base the selection of an alternative opioid. It is best to switch to a short-acting opioid in order to be able to titrate the dose more rapidly during the initial dose-finding period. Morphine, hydromorphone, and oxycodone are widely available in short-acting formulation.

Fentanyl is most commonly used in a transdermal patch formulation, which is not usually changed more often than once every 72 h. The long titration interval limits the usefulness of fentanyl for outpatient opioid rotation in the setting of moderately severe opioid neurotoxicity. Fentanyl is also available in a parenteral formulation that can be administered by continuous subcutaneous or intravenous infusion. Although this technique allows for easier titration, it is cumbersome to apply in an outpatient setting unless there is considerable home care nursing support available.

Methadone does not have any known active metabolites and therefore may carry a lower risk of opioid neurotoxicity. However, its long and variable half-life, as well as the uncertainty of its equianalgesic ratio compared with other opioids, make it suitable for use only by experienced clinicians.

Tramadol is both an opioid receptor agonist and an inhibitor of norepinephrine and serotonin reuptake. As its analgesic efficacy is similar to that for codeine-like opioids, it is not a suitable option for opioid rotation.

Second, calculate the dose as described in Table 6.2.

You decide to use immediate release hydromorphone. Assuming that Mr. M. is using an average of four breakthrough doses per day, the total daily morphine dose is 160 mg. This converts into hydromorphone 32 mg/day. A 25 per cent dose reduction gives 24 mg/day, or 4 mg every 4 h round the clock with 2 mg every hour as needed for breakthrough pain.

Table 6.2 Calculation of new opioid dose for opioid rotation

1. Calculate the total daily dose of the current opioid, including round-the-clock and breakthrough opioid doses
2. Calculate the total daily dose of the new opioid using standard equianalgesic ratios (morphine:hydromorphone 5:1; morphine:oxycodone 1.5:1)
3. Decrease the total daily dose of the new opioid by 20–30%, in order to account for incomplete cross tolerance*
4. Divide the reduced total daily dose by 6 to calculate the four-hourly round-the-clock dose
5. Calculate the breakthrough dose as approximately 10% of the total daily dose

*Cross-tolerance refers to the fact that tolerance to one opioid can confer tolerance to another opioid. Incomplete cross-tolerance occurs when tolerance to the new opioid is less than tolerance to the previous opioid; in other words, there is greater sensitivity to the effects of the new opioid.

Question 8. What other supportive measures would you implement?

If hallucinations or agitation are present, a neuroleptic should be prescribed (see Chapter 24).

Myoclonus does not usually require treatment. However, if it is severe or if there is a concern that generalized seizures may occur, then there is limited evidence to support the use of baclofen, diazepam, clonazepam, midazolam, valproic acid, or dantrolene sodium.[23] However, these drugs may cause additional adverse effects, especially on cognition.

You prescribe haloperidol 1 mg orally twice a day around the clock and every hour as needed for agitation and hallucinations. As Mr. M.'s oral fluid intake is unreliable, you arrange for the home care nurse to start hydration by hypodermoclysis (normal saline 2 l/day). You also ask for blood to be drawn at home to exclude other causes of delirium. You include a complete blood count and differential urea, creatinine, electrolytes, calcium, and albumin.

The laboratory results return showing that the calcium is 2.86 µmol/l (normal range: 2.10–2.55 µmol/l) with an albumin of 30 g/l (normal range 35–50 g/l). Urea is 13.8 mmol/l (normal range 1.2–3.5 mmol/l) and creatinine is 118 µmol/l (normal range 62–115 µmol/l). The other results are unremarkable.

You decide to manage the hypercalcaemia with a subcutaneous infusion of clodronate 1500 mg in normal saline 500 ml over 4 h at home.

Two days later, you make a follow-up home visit to Mr. M. He is more alert, has no further hallucinations, and has only occasional myoclonus. He denies severe pain.

Future research directions

Clinical trials are needed to compare different strategies for the management of opioid neurotoxicity, such as opioid dose reduction and opioid rotation. Research to provide a rational basis for the selection of opioids for rotation is also required.

References

1. **Marsden, C.D., Hallet, M., and Fahns, S.** (1982) The nosology and pathophysiology of myoclonus. In: Marsden CD, Fahns S (eds) *Movement Disorders*. London: Butterworth, 196–248.
2. **Lawlor, P., Gagnon, B., Mancini, I., *et al.*** (2000) Occurrence, causes, and outcome of delirium in patients with advanced cancer. *Arch Int Med*, **160**, 786–94.
3. **Bruera, E., Schoeller, T., and Montejo, G.** (1992) Organic hallucinosis in patients receiving high doses of opiates for cancer pain. *Pain*, **48**, 397–9.
4. **Lawlor, P.** (2002) The panorama of opioid-related cognitive dysfunction in patients with cancer. *Cancer*, **94**, 1836–53
5. **Merskey, H., and Bogduk, N.** (eds) (1994) *Classification of Chronic Pain: Descriptions of Chronic Pain Syndromes and Definitions of Pain Terms* (2nd edn). Seattle, WA: IASP Press, 210–11.
6. **Folstein, M.F., Folstein, S., and McHugh, P.R.** (1975) 'Mini-Mental State': a practical method for grading the cognitive state of patients for the clinician. *J Psychiatr Res*, **12**, 189–98.
7. **Bruera, E., Miller, L., McCallion, J., Macmillan, K., Krefting, L., and Hanson, J.** (1992) Cognitive failure in patients with terminal cancer: a prospective study. *J Pain Symptom Manage*, **7**, 192–5.
8. **Osborne, R.J., Joel, SP., and Slevin, M.L.** (1986) Morphine intoxication in renal failure: the role of morphine-6-glucuronide. *BMJ*, **292**, 1548–9.

9. **Hagen, N.A., Foley, K.N., Cerbone, D.J., Portenoy, R.K., and Inturrisi, C.E.** (1991) Chronic nausea and morphine-6-glucuronide. *J Pain Symptom Manage*, **6**, 125–8.
10. **Bartlett, S.E., Dodd, P.R., and Smith, M.T.** (1994) Pharmacology of morphine and morphine-3-glucuronide at opioid, excitatory amino acid, GABA and glycine binding sites. *Pharmacol Toxicol*, **75**, 73–81.
11. **Sjogren, P.** (1997) Clinical implications of opioid metabolites. In: Portenoy RK, Bruera E (eds) *Topics in Palliative Care*, Vol. 1. New York: Oxford University Press, 163–75.
12. **Sjogren, P., Dragsted, L., and Christensen, C.B.** (1993) Myoclonic spasms during treatment with high doses of intravenous morphine in renal failure. *Acta Anaesthesiol Scand*, **37**, 780–2.
13. **Glare, P.A., Walsh, T.D., and Pippenger, C.E.** (1990) Normorphine, a neurotoxic metabolite? *Lancet*, **335**, 725–6.
14. **Kaiko, R.F., Foley, K.M., Grabinski, P.Y., Heidrich, G., Rogers, A.G., and Inturrisi, C.E.** (1983) Central nervous system excitatory effects of meperidine in cancer patients. *Ann Neurol*, **13**, 180–5.
15. **Wright, A.W.E., Mather, L.E., and Smith, M.T.** (2001) Hydromorphone-3-glucuronide: a more potent neuro-excitant than its structural analogue, morphine-3-glucuronide. *Life Sci*, **69**, 409–20.
16. **Ashby, M., Fleming, B., Wood, M., and Somogyi, A.** (1997) Plasma morphine glucuronide (M3G and M6G) concentrations in hospice inpatients. *J Pain Symptom Manage*, **14**, 157–67.
17. **Hagen, N., and Swanson, R.** (1997) Strychnine-like multifocal myoclonus and seizures in extremely high-dose opioid administration: treatment strategies. *J Pain Symptom Manage*, **14**, 51–8.
18. **Fainsinger, R.L., Miller, M.J., and Bruera, E.** (1992) Morphine intoxication during acute reversible renal insufficiency. *J Palliat Care*, **8**, 52–3.
19. **Fainsinger, R., Schoeller, T., Boiskin, M., and Bruera, E.** (1993) Cognitive failure and coma after renal failure in a patient receiving captopril and hydromorphone. *J Palliat Care*, **9**, 53–5.
20. **Potter, J.M., Reid, D.B., Shaw, R.J., Hackett, P., and Hickman, P.E.** (1989) Myoclonus associated with treatment with high doses of morphine: the role of supplemental drugs. *BMJ*, **299**, 150–3.
21. **Caraceni, A., Martini, C., De Conno, F., and Ventafridda, V.** (1994) Organic brain syndromes and opioid administration for cancer pain. *J Pain Symptom Manage*, **9**, 527–33.
22. **Hawley, P., Forbes, K., and Hanks, G.W.** (1997) Opioids, confusion and opioid rotation. *Palliat Med*, **11**, 63–4.
23. **Cherny, N., Ripamonti, C., Pereira, J., *et al.*** (2001) Strategies to manage the adverse effects of oral morphine: an evidence-based report. *J Clin Oncol*, **19**, 2542–54.
24. **de Stoutz, N.D., Bruera, E., and Suarez-Alamazor, M.** (1995) Opioid rotation for toxicity reduction in terminal cancer patients. *J Pain Symptom Manage*, **10**, 378–84.
25. **Ashby, M.A., Martin, P., and Jackson, K.A.** (1999) Opioid substitution to reduce adverse effects in cancer pain management. *Med J Aust*, **170**, 68–71.
26. **Maddocks, I., Somogyi, A., Abbott, F., Hayball, P., and Parker, D.** (1996) Attenuation of morphine-induced delirium in palliative care by substitution with infusion of oxycodone. *J Pain Symptom Manage*, **12**, 182–9.
27. **Mercadante, S., Casuccio, A., and Calderone, L.** (1999) Rapid switching from morphine to methadone in cancer patients with poor response to morphine. *J Clin Oncol*, **17**, 3307–12.
28. **Mercadante, S., Casuccio, A., Fulfaro, F., *et al.*** (2001) Switching from morphine to methadone to improve analgesia and tolerability in cancer patients: a prospective study. *J Clin Oncol*, **19**, 2829–904.

Chapter 7

Anorexia–cachexia syndrome

Paul Walker and Eduardo Bruera

Attitude

To enable each student to:

- Adopt a perspective on the limitations of enteral and parenteral nutrition.
- Understand the devastating effect of anorexia–cachexia on patients and their families.

Skill

To enable each student to:

- Identify the clinical problem of cachexia and describe simple techniques for assessing nutritional status.
- Apply a model dietary strategy designed to assist anorexic patients.
- Identify the clinical situations where hyperalimentation may be of value to patients with advanced illness.
- Recognize the symptoms commonly associated with cachexia.

Knowledge

To enable each student to:

- Describe the pathophysiology of cachexia and recognize that in advanced cancer patients it is not simply a direct result of anorexia and reduced food intake.
- Describe the possible cause of cachexia in cancer patients.
- State the relative value of agents that may be useful in relieving the symptoms and nutritional problems of cachexia.

You are asked to see a distressed patient and his family. Mr G. is a 62-year-old man, with a long smoking history, who was recently diagnosed with non-small-cell lung cancer in the right mainstem bronchus, adjacent to the carina. At the time of diagnosis widespread bony metastases were evident on the bone scan. Prior to Mr G.'s diagnosis he had gradually lost weight over 3–4 months. When he developed a cough productive of bloody sputum, he visited his family doctor and a subsequent work-up provided the diagnosis. He recently completed a course of palliative radiotherapy to the right hilar region.

Continued

On meeting this gentleman he greets you with a smile from the bed where he is lying and asks you to call him by his nickname, 'Slim'. However, his wife appears very concerned and immediately begins to enlist your help. Mrs G. is pleased that his coughing and production of bloody sputum have stopped since his radiation therapy, but she is concerned that he continues to have a very poor appetite, taking small amounts of food at mealtimes with no great desire for his favourite desserts. She shows you a family photograph and you can immediately see by comparison that 'Slim' is wasting. She also points to his trousers, pulling up his belt loop and revealing trousers that appear two sizes too large for him. Mrs G. states that a week ago they took Mr G. to the emergency department to have his weight loss of 15 kg assessed. A gastroscopy clinic was conveniently under way at that time and Mr G. underwent an endoscopy. Mrs G. was told that everything looked normal.

In talking to Mr G. you learn that he is almost bedridden with little energy, but otherwise does not feel too bad. He denies any pain or difficulty swallowing. In the remainder of your history you uncover no further pertinent information. He has no history or symptoms suggesting diabetes mellitus.

On physical examination, a very slender gentleman is evident; although he is communicative, he is obviously not energetic. His heart rate is 105 and regular, blood pressure is 100/60 mmHg, respiratory rate is 18 pm, and temperature is 36.6°C. Examination of the oral cavity is unremarkable except for the presence of dentures. Examination of the chest reveals a barrel chest with an increased anterior–posterior (AP) diameter. Breath sounds are normal but somewhat distant. His trachea is midline, and upon enquiry he denies any substernal discomfort. Examination of the cardiovascular system is unremarkable, except for tachycardia. Abdominal examination is normal; there are no masses, tenderness, or organomegaly. There is little else to be gleaned from the physical examination except that you are left with the distinct impression that he has lost a significant amount of weight, has little subcutaneous fat present, and marked diffuse muscle atrophy. He cannot rise from a chair without 'pushing off' with his arms.

Question 1. What is the clinical problem?

The clinical problem is that of cachexia. The term cachexia comes from the Greek *kakos*, signifying bad, and *hexis*, which implies a state of being. There are no strict diagnostic criteria, yet the syndrome is commonly recognized to include weight loss, anorexia, fatigue or weakness, chronic nausea, decreased performance status, and psychological distress from changes in body image.[1] Patents with this condition can have any number of these phenomena, of varying severity, in combination. This devastating syndrome increases in prevalence with advancing disease and occurs in more than 80 of cancer and AIDS patients before their death.[2,3] It results in increased morbidity and is correlated with a shortened survival time.[4] This wasting syndrome is estimated to account for 10–22 per cent of cancer deaths and for complications that may cause death, such as infection.[4]

Weight loss is more frequent in solid tumours than in haematological malignancies. An exception is breast cancer, where fatigue is more prominent than weight loss or anorexia.[5,6]

Question 2. What are the possible causes of weight loss in advanced cancer?

Many possible factors can contribute to weight loss in the cancer patient. However, the most common form of malnutrition is the **anorexia–cachexia syndrome**, sometimes termed **primary anorexia–cachexia.**[7] This is an incompletely understood condition. It was previously thought

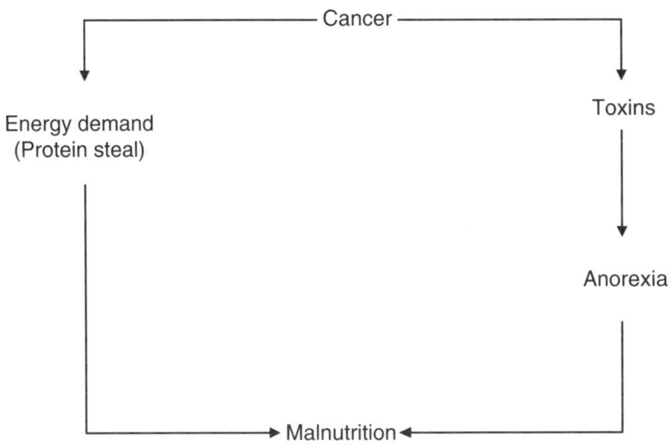

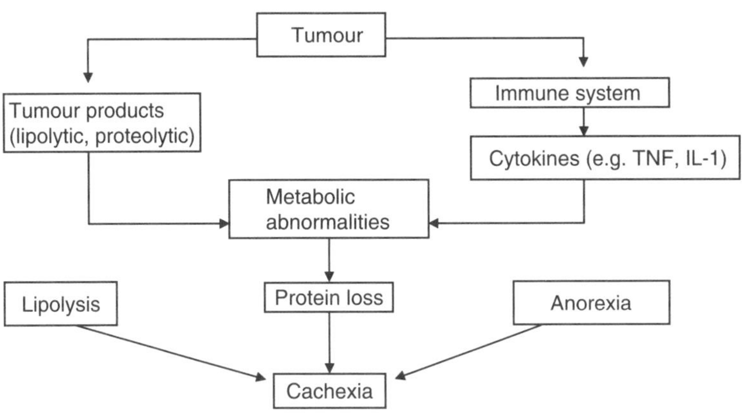

Fig. 7.1 Anorexia–cachexia syndrome.

to be caused by the extreme metabolic demands of the tumour, which would steal nutrients from the patient. The tumour was also believed to excrete 'toxins' which would produce anorexia and the resulting starvation component (Fig. 7.1). This old view has been replaced by an emerging model which, rather than viewing the tumour as a metabolic furnace, approaches the problem as a complex multifactorial process.

The old 'energy steal' and starvation theory is known to be false in primary cachexia. Metabolic response, as determined by resting energy expenditure, is found to be highly variable in cancer. Cancer patients have decreased, normal, or increased energy expenditure.[4] The old model also held that anorexia contributed significantly to weight loss. We now know that loss of fat and muscle tissue commonly precedes a decrease in calorie intake.[2] Studies performed with the goal of increasing nutritional status via parenteral nutrition have failed to provide benefit.[4,8,9]

It is clear that primary cancer cachexia involves more than a simple deficiency of calorie intake. Although anorexia is frequent and can aggravate the wasting syndrome by altering food intake, it is an associated factor rather than the cause of cachexia.

Weight loss that occurs in cancer patients differs from that found in starvation victims. In starvation there is preferential loss of body weight from fat, accounting for three-quarters of the of the weight loss, with only a small amount of weight loss occurring from loss of muscle. In contrast, cancer patients lose weight equally from muscle and fat, and do not have this muscle-sparing effect.[4,7] The concept of an energy steal is inconsistent with the findings that patients with a very large tumour burden may show no sign of cachexia, while others with a very low burden of tumour weight may have severe wasting. It has been shown that weight loss is not related to tumour burden, but rather to tumour type. Weight loss occurs in 90 per cent of patients with gastric or pancreatic cancer, but has a much lower frequency in breast cancer, and may occur in as few as 30 per cent of patients with non-Hodgkin's lymphoma.[3–5]

Although cachexia is commonly thought of as associated with cancer, AIDS, and chronic infections such as tuberculosis, it also occurs in patients with advanced chronic obstructive pulmonary disease, congestive heart failure, rheumatoid arthritis, endstage renal disease, and the frail elderly. Cachexia in these varied conditions is a consequence of a chronic systemic inflammatory response. What is known about cancer cachexia may apply, at least in part, to consideration of these other wasting disorders.[10]

Other conditions can occur that cause caloric deprivation and malnutrition. This is known as **secondary cachexia**. Examples include:[7]

- oesophageal and bowel obstruction
- stomatitis, dysphagia, odynophagia
- severe constipation
- vomiting
- severe pain
- dyspnoea
- depression
- delirium
- social or financial difficulties.

Conditions that cause impaired gastrointestinal absorption (short gut/dumping syndrome, exocrine pancreatic insufficiency, severe diarrhoea), significant loss of proteins (frequent drainage of ascites or pleural fluid, nephrotic syndrome), or loss of muscle mass (deconditioning, hypogonadism) may also cause secondary cachexia.[7] Many causes of secondary cachexia may respond to cause directed therapies. Therefore it is imperative that they be identified and treated as part of a comprehensive approach.

In primary anorexia–cachexia, the current view is that a combination of tumour by-products and host cytokine release combine to produce major metabolic alterations, changes in neuro-hormonal regulation, and autonomic failure.[7,11] Host cytokines produced in the presence of cancer have been shown to play a role in a wide variety of chronic diseases.[10] In cancer, tumour necrosis factor (TNF), interleukin 1 (IL-1) and IL-6, and interferon-α lead to anorexia, asthenia, loss of body weight, and metabolic changes such as increased lipolysis and decreased synthesis of protein and lipids.[8] In addition, the tumour may itself produce substances that can lead to cachexia. A proteolysis-inducing factor, which produces a reduction in body weight without production of anorexia, has been identified from animal tumours and the urine of cancer patients.[8] There is also evidence that tumours produce substances that result in lipolysis. In HIV and cancer cachexia, serum testosterone levels are decreased and associated with weight loss and disease progression.[7]

Question 3. Do you have enough information to state the likely cause of Mr G.'s weight loss?

The cause of this patient's malnutrition is almost certainly cancer-induced anorexia–cachexia syndrome. He exhibits the characteristic anorexia and weight loss, without any evidence of secondary cachexia. The patient's history and record of weight loss is sufficient to make the diagnosis.[12]

Question 4. Would laboratory investigations help with your diagnosis?

Although laboratory investigations are abnormal in cancer cachexia they are not definitive. Commonly, anaemia and low serum albumin (out of proportion to the degree of starvation) are evident. A high serum C-reactive protein level indicates active inflammation and correlates with cachexia and poor prognosis. Testing of C-reactive protein levels may help to identify patients whose decline in nutritional status is linked to inflammatory cytokines.[13,14] Indeed, a normal C-reactive protein in a cachectic patient should stimulate a particular review of the causes of secondary cachexia.

Question 5. Was the gastroscopy helpful? Was it required?

The normal gastroscopy ruled out extrinsic compression of the oesphagus by tumour or radiation oesophagitis. The stomach was also found to be free of ulcers and erosions, and presumably there was no duodenal ulcer. However, the necessity of this investigation is questionable as the patient exhibited no dysphagia or odynophagia.

> You are interrupted in your thoughts because the patient is beginning to vomit. Further questioning reveals that he has an almost continual low-grade nausea which he rates at 7/10 in severity. He may vomit two or three times a day. Mr G. has tried dimenhydrinate which he has obtained over the counter, but it has produced little relief. The nausea has been present for the last 4 days, gradually becoming worse.

Question 6. Why is this man chronically nauseated?

Nausea caused by gastroparesis as a result of autonomic dysfunction would be the presumed aetiology.[15] Autonomic dysfunction has been documented in cancer patients, especially if cachexia and poor performance status are present. This is reflected in gastrointestinal symptoms, such as chronic nausea, anorexia, and constipation. Cardiovascular phenomena such as tachycardia, postural hypotension, and syncope have also been documented. Mr G. exhibited both tachycardia and a low blood pressure. Other causes of chronic nausea such as bowel obstruction, antineoplastic therapy (chemotherapy or abdominal radiation therapy), raised intracranial pressure, metabolic abnormalities such as hypercalcaemia, and peptic ulcers do not appear likely in our patient. For completeness, determination of the serum calcium level would be useful. Opioid analgesics are a frequent cause of nausea,[16] and more than 80 per cent of patients with advanced cancer receive opioids before death. Chronic constipation can also be a cause of chronic nausea.

Question 7. What would you recommend to help manage his nausea?

Metoclopramide is a very useful agent in this setting.[16] Its dual action as a central dopamine and serotonin antagonist and its prokinetic effect on the stomach[7] may explain why it is an effective agent. It is typically used in 10 mg doses by mouth or subcutaneously every 4–8 h or as a continuous subcutaneous infusion (watch for akathisia and, although uncommon in long-term use, tardive dyskinesia).[16] Domperidone is another prokinetic agent that can be effective.

A dose of metoclopramide 10 mg is given subcutaneously. When you check on the patient an hour later his nausea has almost completely resolved. You write him a prescription for metoclopramide 10 mg tablets, one to be taken 30 min before meals and at bedtime. You obtain basic bloodwork to assess for anaemia and electrolyte imbalance secondary to vomiting and screen for hypercalcaemia. Arrangements are made to see Mr G. in a week.

A week has passed and you see Mr G. in clinic. His nausea is reduced to a low level which does not trouble him and he no longer vomits. Today, he expresses severe concern about his lack of appetite, stating that this has worsened such that he barely touches his food now. Mrs G. states that she has obtained cans of a high calorie nutrient drink which she feeds to Mr G. but he only manages to take 1½ cans per day. She is fearful that her husband will 'starve to death.' His son requests that he receives 'tube feeding or intravenous feeding'.

Your assessment reveals that Mr G. is further fatigued and that he feels that his quality of life has decreased since he is not able to partake in family meals. He has continued to be ambulatory in the home, although he takes long periods of rest through the day and required a wheelchair to come to clinic today. Physical examination reveals little change from when you saw him a week ago.

Question 8. How would you respond to Mrs G.'s concern that her husband's appetite is worsening and her fear that he will 'starve to death'?

Mr G. is experiencing severe anorexia, a hallmark of the cachexia syndrome. Families often feel that the lack of appetite is the cause of the problem, and that if their loved one could simply eat enough the malnutrition would be overcome. It is important to explain to the family that a metabolic abnormality underlies this problem, with the depressed appetite occurring secondarily. While decreased calorie intake secondary to this suppressed appetite does contribute to poor nutritional status, it must not be seen as the primary mechanism. As a physician you must also consider whether mechanisms of secondary cachexia are present which may benefit from nutritional intervention.[7]

Family members can sometimes make mealtimes a battle ground when they strenuously force food, with the best intentions, on their anorexic family member. Often it is useful to explain that the patient should only eat what he or she feels like eating, emphasizing that the body may not be able to use excessive nutrient intake to build muscle or fat because the cancer has caused an altered metabolism. The change in body image that occurs in cachexia related to cancer and AIDS can cause severe distress to patients and loved ones. Open discussion of this fact and how it reflects the seriousness of the patient's condition may be helpful.[17]

Question 9. How would you answer the son's question regarding enteral and parenteral nutrition?

In view of the underlying severe metabolic state there is a limited role for aggressive nutritional approaches. The current viewpoint is that the use of parenteral nutrition does not have a major role in advanced cancer care.[12] There is strong evidence from 70 prospective randomized controlled trials performed in the 1980s that using artificial nutrition for advanced cancer patients produced no improvement in patient survival, performance status, quality of life, strength, treatment toxicity, or psychological issues.[9] However, the following groups of patients may benefit from enteral or parenteral nutrition:

- patients with a starvation component (usually bowel obstruction), with a life expectancy from the cancer that would allow expected benefit[7,12]
- cachectic patients with potentially curable tumours requiring short-term nutritional support[12]
- surgical patients before tumour resection.[12]

When selectively considering parenteral nutrition the patient and family need to be made aware of the associated risks. Two meta-analyses of chemotherapy trials found that parenteral nutrition was associated with a fourfold increase in risk of infection, with resulting decrease in survival.[18,19] Other possible complications of intravenous catheter placement include pneumothorax and thromboembolism. Side effects of parenteral nutrition include electrolyte and fluid imbalance and hepatic dysfunction.[12]

Enteral nutrition through gastrostomy tubes has been used for patients with reduced oral intake due to dysphagia or obstruction (e.g. cancer of the oesophagus, head and neck cancers). Aspiration pneumonia, diarrhoea, nausea, abdominal cramps, and bloating are inherent risks of enteral nutrition. When a normal functioning bowel is present, there is no additional benefit from the use of a parenteral nutrition over enteral feeding.

Question 10. What treatment would you propose? How would you monitor the effect of your treatment?

It is important to discuss how the metabolic alterations in cachexia inhibit the effective use of nutrients. This poor nutritional utilization will limit the ability of nutritional repletion. Keeping this in mind, the following points for optimizing nutrition are helpful.

- A dietician may help in answering nutritional questions and giving advice on calorie and protein intake.
- Use of a whey protein source is often palatable. Alternatively meat, poultry, and fish are excellent protein sources.
- High-calorie foods may be added (e.g. margarine, cheese).
- Offer small helpings of food the patient desires at mealtimes and throughout the day.

- Avoid the mealtime battle. Emphasis should be placed on having a congenial social gathering at the family mealtime without excess concern regarding nutritional needs.
- Regarding food choices and mealtimes, it may help to experiment and 'go with what works'.

The progestational drugs megestrol acetate and medroxyprogesterone acetate have a significant effect in cachexia of advanced cancer and AIDS. Controlled trials have shown improvement in appetite, caloric intake, and nutritional status.[11,20–24]

Megestrol acetate has been the agent under most intense study. It has also shown beneficial effects on patients' sensations of well-being, fatigue, and reported quality of life.[11,23] Unfortunately, it has shown no effect on survival. A suggested starting dose is 320–480 mg/day. A higher dose may be required for some patients to respond, and the dose may be titrated up to 800 mg/day. Although the mechanism of action of these beneficial effects is unclear, an effective increase in the deposition of fat occurs.[25] The mechanism of action of megestrol acetate may be related to central appetite stimulation, anabolic effects, glucocorticoid activity, or cytokine modulation.[26] The main concern with these agents is their high cost and possible side effects, such as venous thrombosis, oedema, breakthrough vaginal bleeding, hypoglycaemia, hypertension, Cushing's syndrome, alopecia, adrenal suppression, and adrenal insufficiency if the drug is stopped abruptly.[7] Most commonly, patients who take megestrol acetate experience mild or no side effects, and about half (dependent on the daily dose) describe relief of symptoms from anorexia–cachexia. Treatment with megestrol acetate would be appropriate for Mr G. at this point. If available, it is appropriate to consider supportive counselling for both the patient and family, as severe stress is becoming apparent. This may also help to deal with issues regarding body image.

Continued attention should be paid to ongoing symptom control, particularly the avoidance of constipation. The use of a symptom assessment tool in a consistent fashion is advisable.

In the absence of significant ascites, pleural effusion, or oedema, monitoring the patient's weight, together with appetite evaluation, is the most appropriate way to determine if your treatment has an impact on malnutrition. These assessments should be supplemented by simple measures of function (activity at home) and muscle strength (rising from a chair and hand dynamometry if available). Subjective well-being is more important than objective measurement, as the patient's weight may stabilize or decrease more slowly, yet the patient feels better.

Question 11. Mr G.'s son asks about the use of marijuana and zinc to stimulate appetite. He also states that he has heard good things about something called 'hydrazine'. How will you respond?

Cannabinoids such as dronabinol showed improvement in mood and appetite but not in weight gain.[7] This class of substances has undesirable side effects such as impairment of cognition, memory, motor function, and perception. Dronabinol is not commonly used as it is less efficacious in cachexia then megestrol acetate and has a more adverse side-effect profile. Other drugs, such as cyprohepatadine, hydrazine sulphate, and pentoxyphylline, have not shown effectiveness in clinical trials. Taste alterations can occur with cancer cachexia. One study found that taste alterations were associated with decreased zinc levels and improved with zinc supplementation; further research is awaited.[27]

Following discussion with Mr G. and his family you write him a prescription for megestrol acetate 160 mg orally to be taken three times daily. Both the dietician and clinical psychologist have been notified and will be seeing the patient the same day and in follow-up. A symptom assessment scale is administered for the first time. A weight is obtained and a visiting home nurse is arranged for ongoing follow-up.

In the subsequent weeks your telephone discussions with the home care nurse reveal that Mr G. and his family are coping better. His severe anorexia has abated and he is able to participate in mealtimes. His weight has stabilized. Mr G.'s functional status has improved and he now accompanies his wife on short outings to go shopping.

Six weeks later Mr G. has been admitted to the hospital because of hemiplegia secondary to brain metastases. Extensive liver metastases are present and the lung tumour has increased in size. In discussions with Mr G., and also reflecting his symptom assessment scores, it is apparent that severe continuous nausea and anorexia are the most distressing symptoms. Dyspnoea and many of the other symptoms on the assessment are also poorly controlled. He has difficulty swallowing medications, and those that he does swallow are often regurgitated. He complains that his dentures hurt and that the food he attempts to eat does not taste right. He has mild bone pain in the lumbar spine and both femora. In talking to Mr G. you elicit that he is mildly confused. Looking at him, you notice that he has lost weight since you last saw him. He has little subcutaneous fat, his cheeks are drawn, his ribs are prominent, and bony prominences are evident over the greater trochanters and sacrum. A red area of skin is present over the coccyx. You note from the chart that he is on a continuous subcutaneous infusion of metoclopramide.

Question 12. What are the causes of the patient's symptoms?

This patient has multiple symptoms from his advanced disease. The severe anorexia and chronic nausea can be attributed to the anorexia–cachexia syndrome.

Bone pain from skeletal metastases explains the lumbar spine and femoral pains. Increased intrapulmonary tumour mass is probably responsible for the dyspnoea. Cachexia has placed him at risk for pressure ulcers (bed sores). The loss of subcutaneous fat and muscle leaves bony prominences evident and at risk of skin breakdown, which we can see over his coccyx. Weight loss can cause misalignment of dentures and subsequent pain. The alteration of taste is common in cancer patients; however, this occurs independent of the presence of weight loss. It is also worth noting that he is at high risk for dehydration and the subsequent problems that this may cause.

Question 13. Are there other treatments for anorexia–cachexia that could be considered?

Mr G.'s main distress continues to be related to chronic nausea, anorexia, and asthenia related to his cachexia. He is no longer able to swallow megestrol acetate tablets and, even if he could, it may be that there is a better agent in this setting of multiple symptoms and a limited life expectancy. Corticosteroids have been shown to improve anorexia and asthenia in cancer patients.[11,28–33] This effect appears to be subjective as no improvement in nutritional status can be proved.

The mechanism of action for this effect is unknown, but it is speculated that it could be related to the inhibition of substances secreted by the tumour or immune system. The main difference between corticosteroids and megestrol acetate is that the subjective improvement induced by corticosteroids is not consistently accompanied by increased food intake or improved nutrition and is probably of shorter duration, lasting 3–4 weeks.[29,31]

Dexamethasone, methylprednisolone, prednisone, and hydrocortisone have all been found to be effective. The optimum dose of the various corticosteroids is not established; in the individual patient, titrating doses over several days is reasonable. Corticosteroids have multiple beneficial symptomatic effects including analgesia, antiemetic effects, and amelioration of symptoms due to cerebral oedema (brain metastases), as well as spinal cord and nerve compression and dyspnoea due to lymphangitis carcinomatosis. The short-term complications of using these agents include glucose intolerance, delirium, and immune suppression resulting in oral candida infections. Common long-term complications are cushinoid habitus, osteoporosis, and steroid myopathy, more so with fluorinated corticosteroids such as dexamethasone. In patients with limited life expectancy a short course of corticosteroids may improve quality of life while having little impact on mortality.

At this point Mr G. would benefit from administration of a corticosteroid to improve symptoms of chronic nausea, anorexia, and asthenia caused by his cachexia. Symptoms referable to cerebral oedema from brain metastases will probably improve and this alone may relieve the patient's hemiplegia. The additional analgesic effect of corticosteroids would add to the relief of bone pain. Mr G. has extensive liver metastases and, although he does not yet have right upper quadrant pain from liver capsule distension, the addition of a corticosteroid, for the above reasons, may also prevent this problem from developing. It may be possible that Mr G.'s dyspnoea would be improved by this drug; however, this remains speculative.

You decide that it would be wise to give most drugs parenterally at this point. You continue with the continuous subcutaneous metoclopramide and decide to add dexamethasone 10 mg subcutaneously in the morning. Your rationale for using this dose is to see if the beneficial effect can be achieved quickly, with the drug then rapidly tapered to the minimum dose that achieves satisfactory symptom control. You elect to discontinue any further use of megestrol acetate. Nursing attention is directed towards mouth care, with the provision of ice chips and cold beverages as desired. Physiotherapy and occupational therapy are requested to optimize function and comfort and to discourage the development of pressure ulcers and joint contractures. The patient is assessed for dehydration and the advisability of hypodermoclysis. The patient's multiple problems of brain metastases, bone pain, and dyspnoea are appropriately assessed and treated. Psychological and spiritual support may need to be increased as this gentleman nears his death.

As a result of your interventions you note that Mr G.'s level of distress is markedly reduced within 2 days. Although he still takes little by mouth, his nausea is better controlled. The symptom assessment scores show that the patient's rating of his appetite and energy has improved. The hemiplegia has improved since starting the dexamethasone. In the following days his functional status improves to the point that he can sit in a chair for short periods. This improvement continues for a week, after which Mr G. becomes progressively bed-bound and unresponsive, and dies.

Summary

The anorexia–cachexia syndrome is the result of abnormal metabolism secondary to substances released from the cancer and the immune system. Anorexia, weight loss, asthenia, and chronic nausea often result. Because of the severe catabolic state, nutrients are not effectively utilized, which explains why aggressive nutritional treatment has failed to be of benefit. Continuing and optimizing oral nutrition is a cardinal point of management. The priority should be to improve patient comfort by managing troublesome symptoms. To this end three classes of drugs have been proved to be beneficial. Prokinetic drugs, such as metoclopramide and domperidone, are helpful for relief of chronic nausea and early satiety. These symptoms are thought to be partly related to gastroparesis secondary to autonomic dysfunction caused by malnutrition. Progestational agents, of which megestrol acetate has been most intensively studied, improve appetite and the overall sensation of well-being, as well as promoting weight gain through an increase in fat deposition. These agents are considered appropriate in the setting of a slowly progressive illness for which the expected survival is of the order of several weeks to months. Corticosteroids, such as dexamethasone, improve both anorexia and asthenia for a limited period of time with no benefit seen in nutritional status. Several symptoms, in addition to those caused by cachexia, can be relieved with corticosteroids. However, the side effects of corticosteroids can be a problem. Severely ill patients with a shorter expected survival and multiple symptom problems may benefit from corticosteroids.

Future directions

Research in this field is leading to increasing optimism that the processes involved in producing the anorexia–cachexia syndrome are being elucidated. This new knowledge leads to new strategies proposed to lessen this destructive syndrome (Table 7.1). Some strategies (e.g. exercise, nutraceuticals) await initial clinical testing, while others (e.g. fish oil) have controversial results that are hotly debated.

Clinicians now recognize that patients with cachexia suffer physically, emotionally, and socially, as do their caregivers. Together with supportive counselling, drug therapies and nutritional interventions are now recognized as effective treatments that reduce this cause of suffering. The study of anorexia–cachexia has resulted in expanding the focus from assessment of appetite and weight alone to outcomes that directly benefit patients such as increased muscle mass and improvement in function. Associated with this is the hope that patients will also have improved therapeutic tolerance to beneficial interventions such as chemotherapy or surgery.

The anorexia–cachexia syndrome is a complex problem that requires an active interdisciplinary team for effective management. This includes, but is not limited to, nurses, nutritionists, physicians, and rehabilitation experts.

Table 7.1 Areas of future research

Thalidomide[34]
Melatonin[35]
Non-steroidal anti-inflammatory drugs[36]
Anabolic and androgenic anabolic steroids[37,38]
β_2 mimetics[39]
Immunonutrition[40]
Exercise[41,42]
Nutriceuticals[43]
Fish oil[44]

References

1. **Puccio, M., and Nathanson, L.** (1997) The cancer cachexia syndrome. *Semin Oncol,* **24**, 277–87.
2. **Ma, G, and Alexander, H.R.** (1998) Prevalence and pathophysiology of cancer cachexia. In: Bruera E, Portenoy RK (eds) *Topics in Palliative Care,* Vol 2. New York: Oxford University Press, 91–129.
3. **Dunlop, R.** (1996) Clinical epidemiology of cancer cachexia. In: Bruera E, Higginson, I. (eds) *Cachexia–Anorexia in Cancer Patients.* Oxford: Oxford University Press, 76–82.
4. **Tisdale, M.G.** (1997) Cancer cachexia: metabolic alterations and clinical manifestations. *Nutrition,* **13**, 1–7.
5. **Dewys, W.D.** (1972) Anorexia as a general effect of cancer. *Cancer,* **45**, 2013–19.
6. **Vainio, A., and Auvinen, A.** (1996) Prevalence of symptoms among patients with advanced cancer: an international collaborative study. Symptom Prevalence Group. *J Pain Symptom Manage,* **12**, 3–10.
7. **Strasser, F., and Bruera, E.** (2002) Update on anorexia and cachexia. *Hematol Oncol Clin North Am,* **16**, 589–617.
8. **Bruera, E., and Sweeney, C.** (2000) Cachexia and asthenia in cancer patients. *Lancet Oncol,* **1**, 138–47.
9. **Klein, S., and Koretz, R.L.** (1994) Nutrition support in patients with cancer: what do the data really show? *Nutr Clin Pract,* **9**, 734–6.
10. **Kotler, D.P.** (2000) Cachexia. *Ann Intern Med,* **13**, 622–34.
11. **Gagnon, B., and Bruera, E.** (1998) A review of the drug treatment of cachexia associated with cancer. *Drugs,* **55**, 675–88.
12. **ASCO** (2001) Cancer-related weight loss.In: *Optimizing Cancer Care—The Importance of Symptom Management.* Dubuque, IA: Kendall/Hunt.
13. **Slaviero, K.A., Read, J.A., Clarke, S.J., and Rivory, L.P.** (2003) Baseline nutritional assessment in advanced cancer patients receiving palliative chemotherapy. *Nutr Cancer,* **46**, 148–57.
14. **Mahmoud, F.A., and Rivera, N.I.** (2002) The role of C-reactive protein as a prognostic indicator in advanced cancer. *Curr Oncol Rep,* **4**, 250–5.
15. **Bruera, E., Catz, Z., Hooper, R., Lentl, B., and MacDonald, R.N.** (1987) Chronic nausea and anorexia in patients with advanced cancer: a possible role for autonomic dysfunction. *J Pain Symptom Manage,* **2**, 19–21.
16. **Pereira, J., and Bruera, E.** (1996) Chronic nausea. In: Bruera E, Higginson I (eds) *Cachexia–Anorexia in Cancer Patients.* Oxford: Oxford University Press, 57–75.
17. **Higginson, I., and Winget, C.** (1996) Psychological impact of cancer cachexia on the patient and family. In: Bruera, E., Higginson, I. (eds) *Cachexia–Anorexia in Cancer Patients.* Oxford: Oxford University Press, 172–83.
18. **Klein, S., Simes, J., and Blackburn, G.** (1986) Total parenteral nutrition and cancer clinical trials. *Cancer,* **58**, 1378–86.
19. **McGeer, A.J., Detsky, A.S., and O'Rourke, K.O.** (1990) Parenteral nutrition in cancer patients undergoing chemotherapy: a metaanalysis. *Nutrition,* **6**, 233–40.
20. **Bruera, E., Macmillan, K., Hanson, J., Kuehn, N., and MacDonald, R.N.** (1990) A controlled trial of megestrol acetate on appetite, caloric intake, nutritional status, and other symptoms in patients with advanced cancer. *Cancer,* **66**, 1279–82.
21. **Loprinzi, C.L., Ellison, N.M., Schaid, D.J., *et al.*** (1990) Controlled trial of megestrol acetate for the treatment of cancer, anorexia and cachexia. *J Natl Cancer Inst,* **82**, 1127–32.
22. **Tchekmedyian, S., Hakman, M., Siau, J., *et al.*** (1992) Megestrol acetate in cancer anorexia and weight loss. *Cancer,* **69**, 1268–74.
23. **Heckmayr, M., and Gatzeneier, U.** (1992) Treatment of cancer weight loss in patients with advanced lung cancer. *Oncology,* **49**, 32–4.

24. **Feliu, J., Gonzalez-Baron, M., and Berrocal, A.** (1992) Usefulness of megestrol acetate in cancer cachexia and anorexia. *Am J Clin Oncol,* **15**, 436–40.
25. **Loprinzi, C.L., Schaid, D.J., Dose, A.N., *et al.*** (1993) Body composition changes in patients who gain weight while receiving megestrol acetate. *J Clin Oncol,* **11**, 152–4.
26. **Mantovani, G., Maccio, A., Lai, P., *et al.*** (1998) Cytokine activity in cancer-related anorexia–cachexia: role of megestrol acetate and medroxyprogesterone acetate. *Semin Oncol,* **25** (Suppl 6), 45–52.
27. **Ripamonti, C., Zecca, E., Brunelli, C., *et al.*** (1998) A randomized, controlled clinical trial to evaluate the effects of zinc sulfate on cancer patients with taste alterations caused by head and neck irradiation. *Cancer,* **82**,1938–45.
28. **Nelson, K.** (2000) The cancer anorexia–cachexia syndrome. *Semin Oncol,* **27**, 64–8.
29. **Moertel, C., Schutt, A.G., Reiteneier, R.J., and Hahn, R.G.** (1974) Corticosteroid therapy of pre-terminal gastrointestinal cancer. *Cancer,* **33**, 1607–9.
30. **Wilcox, J., Carr, J., Shaw, J., *et al.*** (1984) Prednisolone as an appetite stimulant in patients with cancer. *BMJ,* **200**, 27.
31. **Bruera, E., Roca, E., Cedaro, L., Carrarl, S., and Chaconk, R.** (1985) Action of oral methyl predisolone in terminal cancer patients: a prospective randomized double-blind study. *Cancer Treat Rep,* **69**, 751–4.
32. **Robustelli Della Cuna, G., Pellegrini, A., and Piazzi, M.** (1989) Effect of methylpredisolone sodium succinate on quality of life in pre-terminal cancer patients: a placebo controlled multicenter study. *Eur J Cancer Clin Oncol,* **29**, 1817–21.
33. **Popiela, T., Lucchi, R., and Giongo, F.** (1989) Methylprenisolone as palliative therapy for female terminal cancer patients. *Eur J Cancer Clin Oncol,* **25**, 1823–9.
34. **Thomas, D.A., and Kantarjian, H.M.** (2000) Current role of thalidomide in cancer treatment. *Curr Opin Oncol,* **12**(6), 564–573.
35. **Lissoni, P., Paolorossi, F., Tancini, G., *et al.*** (1996) Is there a role for melatonin in the treatment of neoplastic cachexia? *Eur J Cancer,* **32A**, 1340–3.
36. **Wigmore, S.J., Barber, M.D., Ross, J.A., *et al.*** (1995) Ibuprofen reduces energy expenditure and acute phase protein production compared with placebo in pancreatic cancer patients. *Br J Cancer,* **72**, 158–88.
37. **Strawford, A., Barbieri, T., Neese, R., *et al.*** Effects of nandrolone decanoate therapy in borderline hypogonadal men with HIV-associated weight loss. *J Acquir Immune Defic Syndr,* **20**,137–46.
38. **Bhasin, S., Storer, T.W., Javanbakht, M., *et al.*** (2000) Testosterone replacement and resistance exercise in HIV-infected men with weight loss and low testosterone levels. *JAMA* **283**, 763–70.
39. **Carbo, N., Lopez-Soriano, J., Tarrago, T., *et al.*** (1997) Comparative effects of beta2-adernergic agonists on muscle waste associated with tumour growth. *Cancer Lett,* **115**, 113–18.
40. **Heys, S.D., Walker, L.G., Smith, I., *et al.*** (1999) Enteral nutritional supplementation with key nutrients in patients with critical illness and cancer: a meta-analysis of randomized controlled clinical trials. *Ann Surg,* **229**, 467–77.
41. **Zinna, E.M., and Yarasheki, K.E.** (2003) Exercise treatment to counteract protein wasting of chronic diseases. *Curr Opin Clin Nutr Metab Care,* **6**, 87–93.
42. **Ardies, C.M.** (2002) Exercise, cachexia, and cancer therapy: a molecular rationale. *Nutr Cancer,* **42**, 143–57.
43. **McCarthy, D.O.** (2003) Rethinking nutritional support for persons with cancer cachexia. *Biol Res Nurs,* **5**, 3–17.
44. **Fearon, K.C.H., von Meyenfeldt, M.F., Moses, A.G.W., *et al.*, on behalf of the Cancer Cachexia Study Group** (2001) An energy and protein dense, high n-3 fatty acid oral supplement promotes weight gain in cancer cachexia. *Eur J Cancer,* **37** (Suppl 6), S27–8.

Chapter 8

Fatigue

Paul Walker and Eduardo Bruera

Attitude

To enable each student to:

- Recognize fatigue as a clinical problem which can sometimes be ameliorated.
- Appreciate the importance of a team approach to fatigue management, including a role for the patient and family members.

Skill

To enable each student to:

- Develop a differential diagnosis of chronic fatigue.
- Describe an approach to assess fatigue.
- Discuss strategies for energy conservation and life-style readaptation.
- Demonstrate the ability to meld non-pharmacological and pharmacological therapeutic approaches.

Knowledge

To enable each student to:

- Recognize the prevalence of fatigue.
- Recognize what is known about pathophysiology of cancer-associated fatigue.
- State current treatments of fatigue, and be aware of promising research leads.

Mrs I.M. is a 52-year-old woman with breast cancer. You are asked to see her in the outpatient clinic. She was diagnosed 5 years ago and at that time underwent a segmental resection followed by radiotherapy. She has since developed extensive bone metastases. During the interview Mrs I.M. states that she is easily tired and has no energy. She has been unable to do much to care for herself, and increasingly family members have been playing a more active role in her care. You learn that she spends most of her time in bed, only making short ventures from the bedroom to bathe and to spend brief periods of time interacting with her family. A symptom assessment tool is administered and from this you determine that her other symptoms are in good control. Specifically she has not expressed a depressed mood, anxiety, pain, nausea, or shortness of breath. She reports some difficulty getting restful sleep.

Question 1. What is the clinical problem?

Cancer-associated fatigue is the tentative diagnosis. Cancer-associated fatigue is defined as a subjective state of overwhelming sustained exhaustion and decreased capacity for physical and mental work, which is not relieved by rest.[1] Fatigue is notable for being the most frequently reported symptom in cancer patients.[2] Research studies report that over 70 per cent of cancer patients experience fatigue.[3,4] Fatigue has been reported to be a distressing symptom and to have a great impact on a patient's daily life.[5,6] There is a strong relationship between fatigue and poor performance status and overall quality of life.[7] This distressing symptom is also a significant component of the spectrum of HIV disease and is a common malady in the general population. A lifestyle survey reports that 20 per cent of men and 30 per cent of women 'always' feel tired.[8]

Question 2. How would you investigate the fatigue?

It is important to ask about fatigue or it may be missed by the clinician. The diagnosis is made by patient report. Asking 'Do you feel tired or fatigued?' gives permission for the patient to discuss this problem further.[9] Asking how it has affected her activities assesses the impact of fatigue on the patient's quality of life. Valid tools to assess fatigue are numerous and include the Visual Analog Scale, the Brief Fatigue Inventory, the Fact-F, and the Piper Fatigue Scale.

Treatment of cancer is often associated with the development of fatigue. Between 8 and 90 per cent of patients receiving chemotherapy develop fatigue, which often peaks within days of the treatment.[10–12] Studies of patients receiving radiation therapy found fatigue present in 60–93 per cent of subjects.[13–15] Radiation-associated fatigue usually accumulates over time and is at its most severe near the end of treatment. Fatigue is reported after surgery and bone marrow transplantation, and is expected with the use of biological response modifiers such as interleukins and interferon-α. Severe fatigue occurs more frequently with advanced cancer (78 per cent) and non-small-cell lung cancer (50 per cent) than with other cancers, such as prostate cancer and breast cancer.[3] Fatigue is known to increase with the progression of cancer. Although fatigue in cancer patients is exceedingly common, it is worthwhile to rule out other possible causes of fatigue. Conditions that cause chronic fatigue are numerous and include the following:

- sleep disorders
- psychiatric disorders, notably a masked depression or anxiety
- metabolic abnormalities
- endocrine problems
- anaemia
- drugs
- various infections
- neurological disorders
- cardiopulmonary disorders
- poor nutrition.

A comprehensive history and physical examination may give an indication of conditions that may be contributing to the patient's lassitude. Screening laboratory investigations such as complete blood cell count, electrolytes, serum calcium, creatinine, glucose, and transaminases are appropriate. If signs and symptoms of hypothyroidism are present, obtaining a thyroid-stimulating hormone level may be indicated.

After taking Mrs I.M.'s history, you find nothing further to implicate as the cause of her weakness. Specific questioning reveals no history or indication of psychiatric disorders. No drugs can be implicated and there are no symptoms indicative of infection. There is no past medical history of cardiopulmonary or neurological diseases. Physical examination gives no further leads. The cardiopulmonary examination is unremarkable. The patient is afebrile. Laboratory investigations show no evidence of hypercalcaemia, anaemia, electrolyte abnormalities, glucose elevation, hypothyroidism, liver failure, or renal failure. An admission chest radiograph shows no evidence of pulmonary infiltrates. She has not received surgery, radiotherapy, or chemotherapy within the last 4 years. You feel confident that the common causes of chronic fatigue can be excluded from your differential diagnosis. It appears likely that she suffers from fatigue due to cancer.

Question 3. Describe the pathophysiology of cancer-associated fatigue.

The profound fatigue and weakness so commonly seen in cancer remain for the most part a mystery. The specific mechanisms causing fatigue remain essentially unknown. Some cancer treatments, notably chemotherapy and radiation, can produce fatigue.[16] Current theory links cancer asthenia with a similar mechanism purported to play a role in producing the anorexia–cachexia syndrome and the profound fatigue and fever associated with some infectious diseases. An immune response to the tumour resulting in activation of macrophages and release of cytokines is central to the current model, as is the release of tumour by-products. Mediators released by the patient's immune cells, such as tumour necrosis factor, IL-1, IL-6, and interferon-γ are known to cause marked fatigue when administered to animals and humans.[16–18] A relationship between IL-1 levels and fatigue was noted in a study of men undergoing radiation therapy for localized prostate cancer.[19] In a similar fashion, a study involving lung cancer patients receiving chemotherapy observed a relationship between fatigue and IL-6 levels.[20] Tumour by-products, labelled by one author as 'asthenins', have also been purported as a cause of fatigue.[21]

Owing to the similarity of mechanisms thought to be involved, some authors view anorexia–cachexia and fatigue as points on a spectrum resulting from this process (see Chapter 7), and some authors have called it the cachexia–anorexia–asthenia complex.[22] However, it is not clear why some tumours cause asthenia independent of signs of cachexia. For example, fatigue without significant cachexia is common in advanced breast cancer while non-small-cell lung cancer patients suffer more from weight loss. How this cascade of chemical mediators produces weakness and fatigue is unknown. Various authors speculate that it may be due to functional or structural abnormalities produced in muscle tissue, the result of high levels of lactic acid, or secondary to malnutrition as a result of altered metabolism. The possible role of psychological disorders also remains unclear, but descriptive studies show that fatigue rarely occurs alone. It is usually associated with pain, insomnia, or sleep disturbance.[23] In addition, a multivariate analysis correlated fatigue with depression and pain.[24]

Question 4. How might you consider managing this problem?

Non-pharmalocogical therapies[25,26]

Exercise has been shown to have the strongest evidence of benefit.[6] A structured aerobic exercise programme has been shown in several trials to reduce fatigue and emotional distress and to improve quality of life in cancer patients who exercised during treatment. Exercise regimens usually included walking or cycling.[27–32] Patients with advanced disease may benefit from referral to physical therapy or rehabilitation medicine for determining a safe exercise prescription.

Other non-pharmacological treatments include sleep therapy, nutritional counselling, and 'restorative therapy'.[25] The last group may include walking or sitting in a natural environment, gardening, quiet or spiritual time, meditation, or volunteer activities unrelated to the illness. Open communication is important, as patients who are educated and knowledgeable about their medical treatment have shown more favourable outcomes.[33]

Pharmacological therapies

It is important to consider stopping or reducing drugs such as benzodiazepines, antihistamines, barbiturates, β-blockers, and opioids that act centrally and may cause fatigue.[26]

To date, drug treatment has been relatively unsuccessful in reversing cancer-associated fatigue. The use of corticosteroids or nutritional interventions for the treatment of fatigue has not been subjected to randomized controlled trials. In studies of cachexia, corticosteroids and progestational agents have been reported to improve levels of activity and well-being. These drugs are discussed in more detail in Chapter 7.

Erythropoietin has been shown to increase haemoglobin, quality of life, and, in a few studies, fatigue in patients receiving concomitant chemotherapy. Its efficacy in relieving fatigue in other settings remains to be established.[34–38] Erythropoietin at doses of 10 000 U subcutaneously three times a week or 40 000 U weekly was shown to raise haemoglobin levels and decrease transfusion requirements. A further study found that the increase in quality of life was highest when the haemoglobin level rose from 11 to 12 g/dl.[39] Treatment with erythropoietin is expensive, costing $250–1000 per week.[9]

Fatigue related to depression is best managed with an antidepressant. However, in a trial in which oral paroxetine 20 mg daily was administered in a double-blind placebo-controlled fashion for fatigue related to chemotherapy, significant reduction in symptoms of depression was seen but there was no significant improvement in fatigue.[40]

Future directions

There is much interest in the use of psychostimulants. Oral methylphenidate 5–20 mg/day improves fatigue in AIDS patients and has manageable side effects.[41] Preliminary studies have been encouraging but the results of controlled studies are not conclusive.[42,43] At present there is interest in the use of modafinil for the fatigue of multiple sclerosis.[44,45] Donepezil is a further agent requiring investigation.[46] Investigating and treating hypogonadism with agents such as testosterone is a new area of promise for managing cancer fatigue and requires further study. Two agents favoured by health food store consumers, ginseng[47] and levocarnitine, are also under investigation.[48]

You decide to give Mrs I.M. a trial of oral methylphenidate 10 mg each morning. Over the next 2 days, you notice that she is a little brighter and more inclined to take part in her daily care. However, she continues to complain of lack of energy and tiredness. A family member takes you aside and asks you what can be done, as nothing has helped so far.

Question 5. How would you reply to the family member? What would you propose for Mrs I.M.'s management at this point?

First, the methylphenidate should be titrated upwards, balancing dose with effect and adverse effects. In addition, counselling of the patient and family could help in dealing with this problem. It is important that they understand that this symptom is directly related to the cancer and that it is likely to persist or worsen. Some degree of acceptance of this condition can go a long way to developing an altered lifestyle as a successful adaptation in this problem. The multidisciplinary team plays an extremely important role in this process of adaptation. Energy conservation strategies need to be discussed and implemented. Providing devices such as a raised toilet seat, reaching aids, a walker, or a wheelchair can help to maintain endurance. Many patients find massage and relaxation techniques both enjoyable and beneficial in making the physical and mental adaptation to a lifestyle that becomes increasingly bedridden. Assisted exercise and strategies to avoid pressure ulcers may increase physical comfort and preserve function. It would be important for Mrs I.M. and her family to explore enjoyable activities that provide social interaction without causing excess fatigue. This not only prevents isolation, but can offer opportunities for life appreciation and meaning through vicarious experiences.

Over the course of 3 weeks, the methylphenidate dose was increased to a total of 60 mg daily; it was not associated with side effects but unfortunately was ineffective for her fatigue. Mrs I.M. is seen by members of the multidisciplinary team on your recommendation. At a team meeting, various nurses, a physiotherapist, and an occupational therapist compare notes and develop energy conservation strategies that can be offered to Mrs I.M. The social worker, pastoral care worker, and psychologist discuss approaches to counselling, aiding Mrs I.M. and her family in dealing with this situation. On implementing these strategies it is found that some are not workable, but overall there appears to be an improvement in enjoyment of life and ability to cope for both Mrs I.M. and her family.

References

1. **Cella, D., Peterman, A., Passik, S, *et al.*** (1998) Progress toward guidelines for the management of fatigue. *Oncology (Huntingt)*, **12**, 369–77.
2. **Glaus, A., Crow, R., and Hammond, S.** (1996) A qualitative study to explore the concept of fatigue/tiredness in cancer patients and healthy individuals. *Support Care Cancer*, **4**, 82–96.
3. **Stone, P., Richardson, A., Ream, E., *et al.*** (2000) Cancer-related fatigue: inevitable, unimportant and untreatable? Results of a multi-center patient survey. *Ann Oncol*, **11**, 971–5.
4. **Volgelzang, N.J., Breitbart, W., Cella, D., *et al.*** (1997) Patient, caregiver, and oncologist perceptions of cancer-related fatigue. Results of a tripart assessment survey. The Fatigue Coalition. *Semin Hematol*, **34** (Suppl 2), 4–12.

5. **Richardson, A.** (1995) Fatigue in cancer patients: a review of the literature. *Eur J Cancer Care,* **4**, 30–2.
6. **Manzullo, E.F., and Escalante, C.P.** (2002) Research into fatigue. *Hematol Oncol Clin North Am,* **16**, 619–628.
7. **Curt, G.A.** (2000) The impact of fatigue on patients with cancer. Overview of FATIGUE 1 and 2. *Oncologist,* **5** (Suppl 2), 9–12.
8. **Cox, B., Blaster, M., Buckle, A.,** ***et al.*** (1987) The health and lifestyle survey. In: Blacter M (ed) *Health Promotion Research Trust.* London: Tavistock/Routledge, London, 252–63.
9. **ASCO** (2001) Fatigue. In: *Optimizing Cancer Care—The Importance of Symptom Management.* Dubuque, IA: Kendall/Hunt.
10. **Blesch, K., Paice, J., Wickham, R.,** ***et al.*** (1991) Correlates of fatigue in people with breast or lung cancer. *Oncol Nurs Forum,* **18**, 81–7.
11. **Myerowitz, B., Watkins, I., and Sparks, F.** (1983) Quality of life for breast cancer patients receiving adjuvant chemotherapy. *Am J Nurs,* **183**, 232–5.
12. **Jamar, S.** (1989) Fatigue in women receiving chemotherapy for ovarian cancer. In: Funk S, Campagne M, *et al.* (eds) *Key Aspects of Comfort: Management of Pain Fatigue and Nausea.* New York: Springer-Verlag, 224–8.
13. **Irving, D., Vincent, I., Graydon, J.,** ***et al.*** (1994) The prevalence and correlates of fatigue in patients receiving treatment with chemotherapy and radiation therapy: a comparison with the fatigue experienced by health individuals. *Cancer Nurs,* **17**, 367–78.
14. **King, K.B., Nail, L.M., Kreamer, K.,** ***et al.*** (1985) Patients' descriptions of the experience of receiving radiation therapy. *Oncol Nurse Forum,* **12**, 55–61.
15. **Irvine, D., Vincent, L., Bubel, N.,** ***et al.*** (1991) A critical appraisal of the research literature investigating fatigue in the individual with cancer. *Cancer Nurs,* **14**, 188–98.
16. **Watanabe, S., and Bruera, E.** (1996) Anorexia and cachexia, asthenia, and lethargy. *Hematol Oncol Clin North Am,* **10**, 189–206.
17. **Beutler, B., and Cerami, A.** (1987) Cachetin: more than a tumor necrosis factor. *N Engl J Med,* **315**, 379–85.
18. **Morant, R.** (1991) Asthenia in cancer patients: a double-edged inflammatory response against the tumor? *J Palliat Care,* **7**, 22–4.
19. **Greenberg, D.B., Gray, J.L., Mannix, C.M.,** ***et al.*** (1993) Treatment-related fatigue and serum interleukin-1 levels in patients during external beam irradiation for prostate cancer. *J Pain Symptom Manage,* **8**, 196–200.
20. **Rigas, J.R., Hoopes, P.J., Meyer, L.A.,** ***et al.*** (1998) Fatigue linked to plasma cytokines in patients with lung cancer undergoing combined modality therapy. *Proc Am Soc Clin Oncol,* **17**, 68A.
21. **Theologides, A.** (1982) Asthenia in cancer. *Am, J Med,* **73**, 1–3.
22. **MacDonald, N., Alexander, H.R., and Bruera, E.** (1995) A National Cancer Institute of Canada workshop on symptom control and supportive care in patients with advanced cancer: methodological and administrative issues. Cachexia–anorexia–asthenia. *J Pain Symptom Manage,* **10**, 151–5.
23. **Jacobensen, P.B., Gover, T., Johnson, B.A.,** ***et al.*** (1999) Fatigue in women receiving adjuvant chemotherapy for breast cancer: characteristics, course, and correlates. *J Pain Symptom Manage,* **18**, 223–42.
24. **Bower, J., Ganz, P., and Desmond, K.** (2000) Fatigue in breast cancer survivors: occurrence, correlates, and impact on quality of life. *J Clin Oncol,* **18**, 743–53.
25. **Mock, V., Atkinson, A., Boasevick, A.,** ***et al.*** (2000) *NCCN Practice Guidelines for Cancer-Related Fatigue.* Rockledge, PA: National Comprehensive Cancer Network.
26. **Portenoy, R.K., and Itri, L.M.** (1999) Cancer-related fatigue. Guidelines for evaluation and management. *Oncologist,* **5**, 1–10.
27. **Mock, V., Cameron, L., Tompkins, C.,** ***et al.*** (1997) *Every Step Counts: A Walking Exercise Program for Persons Living with Cancer.* Baltimore, MD: Johns Hopkins University.
28. **MacVicar, M.G., Winningham, M.L., and Nickel, J.L.** (1986) Promoting the functional capacity of cancer patients. *Cancer Bull,* **338**, 235–9.

29. **Mock, V., Burke, M.B., Sheeham, PK., *et al.*** (1994) A nursing rehabilitation program for women with breast cancer receiving adjuvant chemotherapy. *Oncol Nurs Forum,* **21**, 899–907.
30. **Dimeo, F.C., Stieglitz, R., Novelli-Fischer, U., *et al.*** (1999) Effects of physical activity on the fatigue psychologic status of cancer patients during chemotherapy. *Cancer,* **85**, 2272–7.
31. **Schwartz, A.L.** (2000) Daily fatigue patterns and effects of exercise in women with breast cancer. *Cancer Pract,* **8**, 16–24.
32. **Dimeo, F., Rumberger, B., and Keul, J.** (1998) Aerobic exercise as therapy for cancer fatigue. *Med Sci Sports Exerc,* **30**, 475–8.
33. **Johnson, J.E., Nail, L.M., Lauver, D., *et al.*** (1988) Reducing the negative impact of radiation therapy on functional status. *Cancer,* **61**, 46–51.
34. **Demetri, G.D., Kris, M., Wade, J., *et al.*** (1998) Quality of life benefit in chemotherapy patients treated with epoetin alfa is independent of disease response or tumor type: results from a prospective community oncology study. *J Clin Oncol,* **16**, 3412–25.
35. **Gabrilove, J.L., Einhorn, L.H., Livingston, R.N., *et al.*** (1999) Once-weekly dosing of epoetin alfa is similar to three times-weekly dosing increasing hemoglobin and quality of life. *Proc Am Soc Clin Oncol,* **18**, 574A.
36. **Glaspy, J., Bukowski, R., Steinberg, D., *et al.*** (1997) Impact of therapy with epoetin alfa on clinical outcomes in patients with non-myeloid malignancies during cancer chemotherapy in community oncology practice. *J Clin Oncol,* **15**, 218–34.
37. **Littlewood, T.J., Bajetta, E., Nortier, J.W.R., Vercammen, E., and Rapoport, B.** (2001) Effects of epoetin alfa on hematologic parameters and quality of life in cancer patients receiving non-platinum chemotherapy: results of a randomized, double-blind, placebo-controlled trial. *J Clin Oncol,* **19**, 2865–74.
38. **Fallowfield, L., Gagnon, D., Zagri, M., *et al.*** (2002) Multivariate regression analyses of data from a randomised, double-blind, placebo-controlled study confirm quality of life benefit of epoetin alfa in patients receiving non-platinum chemotherapy. *Br J Cancer,* **87**, 1341–53.
39. **Cleeland, C.S., Demetri, G.D., Glaspy, J., *et al.*** (1999) Identifying hemoglobin level for optional quality of life: results of a incremental analysis. *Proc Am Soc Clin Oncol,* **18**, 574.
40. **Morrow, G.R., Hickok, J.T., Raubertas, R.F., *et al.*** (2002) Effect of an SSRI antidepressant on fatigue and depression in seven hundred thirty-eight cancer patients treated with chemotherapy: a URCC CCOP study. *Proc Am Soc Clin Oncol,* **20**, 384a (abstr 1531).
41. **Breitbart, W., Rosenfeld, B., Kaim, M., and Funesti-Esch, J.** (2001) A randomized, double-blind, placebo-controlled trial of psychostimulants for the treatment of fatigue in ambulatory patients with human immunodeficiency virus disease. *Arch Intern Med,* **151**, 411–20.
42. **Bruera, E., Driver, L., Barnes, E.A., *et al.*** (2003) Patient-controlled methylphenidate for the management of fatigue in patients with advanced cancer: a preliminary report. *J Clin Oncol,* **1**, 4439–43.
43. **Bruera, E., Driver, L., Vacero, V., *et al.*** (2005) Patient controlled methylphenydate for cancer related fatigue. A randomized controlled trial. *Proc Am Soc Clin Oncol,* **23,** 7405 (abstr 1531).
44. **Rammohan, K.W., Rosenberg, J.H., Lynn, D.J., *et al.*** (2002) Efficacy and safety of modafinil (Provigil) for the treatment of fatigue in multiple sclerosis: a two center phase 2 study. *J Neurol Neurosurg Psychiatry,* **72**, 179–83.
45. **Zifko, U.A., Rupp, M., Schwarz, S., Zipko, H.T., and Maida, E.M.** (2002) Modafinil in treatment of fatigue in multiple sclerosis. Results of an open-label study. *J Neurol,* **249**, 983–7.
46. **Bruera, E., Strasser, F., Shen, L., *et al.*** (2003) The effect of donepezil on sedation and other symptoms in patients receiving opioids for cancer pain: a pilot study. *J Pain Symptom Manage,* **26**, 1049–54.
47. **Bahrke, M.S., and Morgan, W.R.** (2000) Evaluation of the ergogenic properties of ginseng: an update. *Sports Med,* **29**, 113–33.
48. **Graziano, F., Bisonni, R., Catalano,V., *et al.*** (2002) Potential role of levocarnitine supplementation for the treatment of chemotherapy-induced fatigue in non-anaemic cancer patients. *Br J Cancer,* **86**, 1854–7.

Chapter 9

Anxiety and depression

Kurt Skakum and Harvey Max Chochinov

Attitude

To enable each student to:

- Appreciate the important influence of psychological factors on suffering.
- Be aware of the often unrecognized nature of anxiety and depression in the palliative care population.

Skill

To enable each student to:

- Be able to recognize factors that result in the development of anxiety and mood disorders.
- Demonstrate techniques that decrease the uncertainty patients have which often contributes to the development of anxiety and depression.
- Be able to recognize and diagnose mood and anxiety disorders in palliative care patients.
- Be able to appropriately utilize both pharmacological and non-pharmacological approaches to treat mood and anxiety disorders.

Knowledge

To enable each student to:

- Describe the incidence of common psychiatric disorders in persons with advanced cancer.
- Describe the mechanism of action of various antidepressant medications.
- Describe the role of psychotherapeutic interventions in the treatment of this population of patients.

Introduction

The diagnosis of a fatal illness is a devastating event. In addition to the medical and physical sequelae of such a diagnosis, there are various psychological and emotional consequences to be considered. This chapter will address the emotional aspects of care for patients with advanced illness.

Mood and anxiety disorders occur commonly in medically ill populations. Major depression is frequently underdiagnosed and, even when recognized, often undertreated.[1] Many health care professionals believe that depression is a natural reaction to a bad situation and therefore does not require focused clinical attention. This belief can cause further unnecessary suffering by the patient and their family.

Case 1

Mr. P. is a 63-year-old married man who worked in construction until his diagnosis of non-small-cell lung cancer 3 years ago. He was subsequently subject to the full panorama of cancer therapy; surgery, radiotherapy, and three chemotherapy regimens. Mr. P. is currently receiving single-agent vinorelbine. He was referred for psychiatric assessment because he did not appear to be coping well with his condition. Up until his diagnosis, he had been healthy and self-sufficient.

The oncologist involved in his treatment recognized a change in his usual ability to cope with his treatments and deteriorating health status. In the course of the oncologist's psychological assessment, Mr P. stated that he had been 'unhappy for a long time'. He related thoughts of hopelessness and worthlessness, and was preoccupied with thoughts of loss, including loss of his job, loss of money spent on an intensive search for a cure, loss of health, loss of independence, and loss of a future. In addition to the prominent negative thoughts, Mr. P. was also suffering from several physical symptoms. He had been experiencing a lack of sleep, characterized by difficulty falling asleep and trouble staying asleep throughout the night, decreased energy, decreased appetite, decreased concentration and forgetfulness, decreased libido, and worry about being a burden on his wife. He had not been contemplating ending his life, but did have frequent thoughts that he 'may be better off dead'.

His medications included lorazepam, zopiclone, acetaminophen with codeine, ranitidine, montelucast, dexamethasone, and vinorelbine. He stopped consuming alcohol and decreased his smoking when he was diagnosed with cancer. There was no history of street drug use; he did report recent erectile dysfunction.

He has been married twice, with his first marriage ending when he discovered that his wife had been unfaithful. He has three children with whom he does not have a close relationship. He describes his second marriage to a woman 15 years his junior as 'the best thing that ever happened to me', but is concerned, based on previous experience and his current condition, that she will not stay in the relationship.

Question 1. What psychiatric diagnosis would you consider in Mr P.'s case?

Mr P. exhibits many characteristics associated with a major depression. The diagnosis of major depression, according to the *Diagnostic and Statistical Manual of Mental Disorders, Fourth Edition*,[2] requires that a patient experience five or more symptoms during the same 2-week period, representing a change from a previous level of functioning. At least one of the symptoms must be either depressed mood or loss of interest or pleasure. For depressed mood to be considered a symptom of major depression, it must be experienced most of the day nearly every day for the duration of that 2-week period. Loss of interest or pleasure must also be present most of the day nearly every day. The other diagnostic symptoms of depression include significant change in appetite or body weight, insomnia or hypersomnia, psychomotor agitation or retardation, fatigue or loss of energy, feelings of worthlessness or inappropriate or excessive guilt, diminished ability to think or concentrate or indecisiveness, and recurrent thoughts of death (not simply a fear of dying) or recurrent suicidal ideation, with or without a specific plan or attempt. The symptoms must cause impairment in psychosocial functioning and are not due to the direct effects of a substance or medical condition.

Some of the symptoms of depression closely resemble symptoms that are commonly present in patients with an advanced illness. For example, loss of appetite, weight loss, sleep disturbance, difficulty in thinking or concentrating, and fatigue may be directly caused by lung cancer.

According to the diagnostic criteria, these symptoms should not be counted towards a diagnosis of major depression. How to approach these non-specific symptoms in suspected cases of depression in patients who are medically ill has been the subject of considerable debate. Some will ascribe these somatic symptoms to depression, regardless of there being a possible medical explanation. Endicott[3], on the other hand, believed that somatic symptoms of depression in medically ill patients could be substituted by other non-physical psychological symptoms. Asking patients if they are feeling depressed most of the time is a highly sensitive and efficient way of screening for depression in this patient population. This by no means replaces the need for careful diagnostic evaluation, but speaks to the importance of asking patients about their mood state as an initial step towards identifying major depression.[4]

Consider the case of fatigue in a patient receiving chemotherapy. Although fatigue is a symptom of depression, it could just as easily be a side effect of cancer treatment. The rationale behind the Endicott substitutions is that those somatic symptoms that can easily be explained by a medical illness should be replaced with non-somatic symptoms i.e. depressed appearance, social withdrawal, brooding, self-pity or pessimism, and lack of reactivity of mood.

Question 2. Is the presence of depression a normal and expected part of the experience of the palliative care patient?

Episodic appearance of depressed mood is thought of as understandable when present in a person with serious medical illness. Probably all patients with a fatal disorder will experience considerable sadness at various times. If lingering sadness is accompanied by other depressive symptoms, the diagnosis of major depression should be considered. The danger of not considering this diagnosis is unnecessary and prolonged suffering. Depression is commonly present in people with advanced illness of any aetiology.[5,6] Studies of the prevalence of major depression in medically ill populations of patients have reported a wide range (1–40 per cent). One 30-month study of elderly patients with medical illness found only two factors that predicted mortality: severity of medical illness and the presence of depression.[7]

Question 3. What are the medical causes of depression?

There are many medical illnesses that have been associated with the onset of depression (Table 9.1).[8] These illnesses must be properly diagnosed and treated in order to alleviate the symptoms of depression. Complete resolution of depressive symptoms may also require concurrent antidepressant therapy. Similarly, there are several classes of medication that have been found to trigger or worsen episodes of depression.[5,8] Agents sometimes encountered in palliative care practice are listed in Table 9.2.

If the initiation of treatment with a particular medication appears to coincide with the development of symptoms of depression, then consideration should be given to switching to an agent that does not cause depression. Sometimes, however, the medication is an absolute requirement. For example, patients with a brain tumour receiving radiotherapy require steroid medication to relieve swelling and increased intracranial pressure. These steroids can cause depression (and other psychiatric symptoms such as anxiety, mania, sleep disturbance, delirium, and psychosis). In these cases the medication should be kept to the minimum effective dosage, administered at a time of day that will minimize adverse effects, and concurrent treatment of the psychiatric symptoms should be initiated.

Table 9.1 Medical conditions associated with depression

Endocrine abnormalities	**Cancers**[a]
Hyperthyroidism	Oat cell carcinoma
Hypothyroidism	Pancreatic carcinoma
Adrenal dysfunction	Central nervous system tumours
Acromegaly	Lymphoma
Insulinoma	Leukaemia
Hypopituitarism	**Collagen–vascular disease**
Neurological abnormalities	Systemic lupus erythomatosus
Parkinson's disease	Giant cell arteritis
Alzheimer's disease	Rheumatoid arthritis
Huntington's disease	**Infectious disease**
Multiple sclerosis	Infectious mononucleosis
Cerebrovascular accidents	Hepatitis
Metabolic disorders	Tuberculosis
Electrolyte disturbances	AIDS
Uraemia	Influenza
Wilson's disease	Syphilis
Pernicious anaemia	Encephalitis

[a]The table lists those medical conditions, including cancers, where depression may be particularly prevalent.

Table 9.2 Medications associated with depression

β-Blockers	Clonidine	Thiazide diuretics
Digitalis	Oral contraceptives	Levodopa
Glucocorticoids	Anabolic steroids	Benzodiazepines
Cimetidine	Ranitidine	Cyclosporin
Antipsychotics	NSAIDs	Ethambutol
Sulfonamides	Baclofen	Metaclopramide
Cocaine	Amphetamines	Vincristine
Vinblastine	Asparagines	Intrathecal methotrexate

NSAIDs, non-steroidal anti-inflammatory drugs.

Question 4. Once the diagnosis of depression is made, what should the initial treatment be?

Mild to moderate depression can be treated with medications, psychotherapy, or a combination of both. Severe depression requires medication with or without psychotherapy. There are many classes of antidepressant medications and many types of psychotherapy. These approaches are not mutually exclusive, and often work best if applied together.

The Canadian Network for Mood and Anxiety Treatments (CANMAT) has developed guidelines for the diagnosis and pharmacological treatment of depression.[9] This publication classifies treatments as first, second, or third line, based on the available research regarding their effectiveness and tolerability.

CANMAT guidelines for the first-line treatment of mild to moderate depression includes those antidepressant medications that have been the subject of randomized placebo-controlled trials to establish efficacy and a generally tolerable side-effect and safety profile. These medications are:

- the serotonin specific reuptake inhibitors (SSRIs) including fluoxetine, fluvoxamine, paroxetine, citalopram and sertraline
- the norepinephrine and dopamine reuptake inhibitor (NDRI) bupropion
- the reversible monoamine oxidase inhibitor (RIMA) moclobemide
- serotonin-2 antagonist/reuptake inhibitor (SARI) nefazadone
- the serotonin and norepinephrine reuptake inhibitor (SNRI) venlafaxine.

Second-line antidepressants are those that have been the subject of either randomized placebo-controlled trials or 'non-randomized studies and substantial panel opinion' and/or a less tolerable side-effect profile. These medications include the heterocyclic and most of the tricyclic antidepressants. Specifically, the second-line choices include trazadone, amitriptyline, clomipramine, desipramine, doxepine, imipramine, maprotiline, and trimipramine. While not included in the CANMAT recommendations, psychostimulants have been used effectively in the treatment of chronically ill cancer patients who can medically tolerate the stimulant effects of such medications. Psychostimulants have been shown to be effective in improving appetite, feelings of weakness, concentration, and energy level, and appear to have a shorter latency of therapeutic onset.[5] This makes them an especially important consideration amongst patients with a very limited life expectancy.

Third-line antidepressants are those that have little research-based evidence to support their efficacy, but whose use is supported by significant clinical experience. Medications may also be considered as third-line agents because they have a less tolerable side-effect or safety profile. These medications include nortryptiline, protryptiline, amoxapine, and the monoamine oxidase (MAO) inhibitors phenelzine and tranylcypromine.

There are other considerations in selecting an antidepressant for a palliative care patient. Side-effect profile is an important factor. For example, one would not choose bupropion in a patient with a brain tumour and seizures, because of its tendency to lower the seizure threshold and therefore increase the risk of seizures. Considering the use of a psychostimulant may be appropriate in a palliative care patient population because of their rapid onset of action in alleviating symptoms of depression. Unlike typical antidepressants, psychosimulants can yield improvements within days of starting treatment or achieving adequate dosing levels. Side effects of psychostimulants can be used to the advantage of the patient. For example, chronically ill patients often have fatigue and decreased appetite. If one selects an antidepressant that is activating rather than sedating, or is appetite stimulating, then the patient will be much more tolerant of the antidepressant treatment while benefiting from these secondary effects.

Some clinicians will occasionally use psychostimulants in combination with SSRIs. This usually happens under the following circumstances:

- a more rapid response to treatment is being sought because of either profound suffering or overt suicidality
- electroconvulsive therapy is not considered viable within the particular clinical circumstance

- the depression is associated with a significant debilitating loss of energy (e.g. sedation secondary to opioids)
- the patient does not demonstrate evidence of delirium, which can progress to an agitated paranoid state with the addition of psychostimulants
- the patient's life expectancy is anticipated to exceed the therapeutic latency time of the SSRI (i.e. a minimum of 2–3 weeks).

A typical instance where such a combination might be used is a depressed patient with a brain tumour, demonstrating psychomotor slowing and attention and concentration difficulties. Stimulants have the potential of improving mood, mental speed, attention, and concentration.

One must ensure that the antidepressant medication is pharmacodynamically and pharmacokinetically compatible with the other medications that the patient is taking. Many antidepressants interfere with the metabolism of drugs through effects on the cytochrome *P*-450 system. Appropriate steps must be taken to prevent excessive risk of adverse events as a result of drug–drug interactions. Potential changes in the metabolism of both chemotherapeutic agents and antidepressants may occur because of effects on this enzyme system. These effects should be considered and monitored. A very recent small study ($n = 12$) showed that co-administration of paroxetine with tamoxifen lowered the measurable level of one of the active metabolites of tamoxifen.[10] Examples of antidepressants with fewer drug interactions include citalopram, sertraline, and venlafaxine.

Based on all the available information, you make several decisions about Mr. P.'s psychiatric treatment. First, you advise his oncologist that the steroids may be contributing to the mood difficulties. You recommend that the dexamethasone dose be adjusted to the minimum effective dose. Secondly, you make the decision that he may benefit from a trial of an antidepressant medication. You start him on sertraline, an SSRI medication (other reasonable choices include paroxetine, fluoxetine, fluvoxamine or citalopram), and make arrangements to see him again in 2 weeks.

In follow-up 2 weeks later, Mr. P. explains to you that he has tolerated the medication well, having experienced no noticeable side effects. However, he has not noticed any significant improvement in his mood or accompanying physical or cognitive symptoms of depression.

Question 5. What is your next step in the management of Mr. P.?

Typically, 2 weeks is not a sufficient time period to expect dramatic improvement in symptoms of depression. It may be beneficial to collect a collateral history from Mr. P.'s wife as she may have noticed some initial symptom relief that Mr. P., because of his negative outlook, may not have appreciated. Patients often notice some initial small improvements, such as improved sleep or energy. In the face of these improvements, it is reasonable to wait for a total of 3–4 weeks before considering any change to his treatment. However, if no such improvements take place within that time frame, it may then be beneficial to consider additional options. There are four possible available options.

Optimization

Optimization involves increasing the dose of the initial medication. Each of the SSRIs has a therapeutic dosage range. It is not known to which dose an individual patient will ultimately respond.

This option is most often utilized when a patient has had a partial response to the initial dose of medication.

Switching

Switching involves changing to a different antidepressant medication. There is evidence to show that switching to a different SSRI medication may be beneficial. Commonly, patients are switched to a different class of medication within the first-line treatment group (i.e. venlafaxaine, bupropion, nefazadone, or moclobemide).

Augmentation

Augmentation is defined as adding another medication, which is not an antidepressant, that will increase the effectiveness of the antidepressant agent. Common augmentation agents include lithium, methylphenidate, tri-iodothyronine, L-tryptophan, and pindolol.

Combination

Combination is defined as adding another medication which is known to have antidepressant effects in its own right. To utilize this approach, one must ensure that there are no known dangerous drug interactions.

> After 3 weeks of treatment with sertraline Mr. P. has only shown a partial response. He continues to tolerate the medication well. You decide to proceed by optimizing the dose of sertraline. Therefore you increase the dose from 50 to 100 mg daily. Mr. P. informs you that in addition to his symptoms of depression, he and his wife are now having more arguments. He believes that the arguments are a direct result of his insecurity in the relationship. He recognizes that this concern is excessive and unnecessary. He finds his sessions with you to be very beneficial because he is able to obtain a different perspective on his problems. Through empathic questioning over three more sessions, you are able to help Mr. P. understand that his insecurities stem from his own concerns about his situation and prognosis, not from any objective evidence that his wife has stopped caring about him. A meeting is arranged with Mr. P. and his wife. The goal of this meeting is for Mr. P. to express some of his concerns about the relationship in an environment with an impartial third party. Prior to this meeting Mr. P. informs you that his mood, worry, and concentration have all improved. Because of these changes he feels confident in talking with his wife about the relationship. During the session with his wife present you facilitate an open, caring, and productive discussion about the nature of depression and its effect on thinking and Mr. P.'s concerns about their relationship. Through this discussion Mr. P. is reassured that his wife remains committed to their relationship despite his failing health.

Question 6. What about psychotherapy?

As with antidepressant medications, there are a number of different forms of psychotherapy that may have a role in the treatment of patients in a palliative care setting. Initially, crisis management oriented interventions may be the most appropriate. Other types of psychotherapy that have been found helpful in palliative care populations include individual and group psychotherapies, existential psychotherapy, cognitive–behaviour therapy, interpersonal therapy, supportive psychotherapy, and, less commonly, psychodynamic psychotherapy.[11]

Psychotherapy with palliative care patients focuses on several main themes. One common theme is that of loss. The loss of health and a heightened sense of vulnerability and mortality can have devastating effects on the patient's sense of worth and identity. Frequently, the diagnosis of an advanced illness is accompanied by the need for treatment that may be difficult and can cause further losses. For example, the patient may not be able to continue working, supporting one's family, or participating in usual activities or routines. This can diminish the patient's sense of dignity or overall meaning in life. Psychotherapy that addresses these issues, and interventions that engender a sense of meaning and purpose, may help patients to come to terms with these losses and feel more in control of their life and the process of dying.

Palliative care patients are at varying stages of coming to terms with the inevitability of their own death. In psychological terms, this task can be understood as anticipatory grieving. Various stages of grief have been identified and described, with each stage addressing an element of the psychological challenges associated with accommodating to loss.[12] While not meant to be proscriptive, in that not all patients necessarily experience nor sequentially move through each stage, this does provide a helpful conceptual framework. The first stage is often described as a numbness or a feeling of unreality. This leads to a state of physical restlessness, which can appear as indecision or anxiety. The next phase of grief is one of disorganization and despair. If patients are not able to move through this phase, they may become depressed. The final phase of grief is that of recovery and reorganization. For dying patients, this may refer to those who are able to accommodate to and, in varying degrees, accept their circumstances. Patients may need help in navigating their way through any of these various psychological challenges, providing another role for psychotherapy.

Empowerment can safeguard patients against a sense of despair and lack of control. It can be instilled in patients by giving them information, knowledge, and control. Patients should be provided with information about their illness, the available treatment options, the risks and potential benefits of each of these options, and a realistic prognosis. Sensing that one lacks control over life is a particularly difficult facet of living with an advancing illness, and can engender further suffering. This can be addressed by allowing the competent patient to make decisions about which treatment options to pursue, based on the information that has been provided. This may also mean allowing the patient to decide when to forgo treatment and which palliative care options are still worth pursuing.

Case 2

Ms H. is a 49-year-old married woman with a recent diagnosis of metastatic breast cancer. She lives with her husband of 21 years and their three children, aged 18, 15 and 9. Until recently, she worked as an accountant for a large North American firm. She had stopped working shortly before the diagnosis was made because of diffuse pain that she attributed to arthritis. It was during the investigations for arthritis that the diagnosis of breast cancer was confirmed.

Prior to her cancer diagnosis, she had been in good health. Her only medical problem has been hypothyroidism, which has been followed and treated by her family physician. She has had no past surgeries. She does not smoke. Until recently she consumed only small amounts of alcohol on an infrequent basis. Since her diagnosis, she has increased her alcohol intake; now drinking three alcoholic beverages each evening. However, neither she nor her husband feels that this amount of alcohol has adversely affected her or their relationship. She does not use recreational drugs, herbal remedies, vitamin supplements, or over-the-counter medication. She has never had difficulties that would have suggested the need for psychiatric consultation.

The confirmation of her diagnosis has required her to attend the hospital and clinic on many occasions. As the investigations began to reveal the extent of her illness, she became increasingly anxious. The anxiety grew to the point of needing her husband or a friend to accompany her to each appointment.

She has found that her anxiety grows as she gets closer to the hospital. At times the anxiety has been so severe that she has had 'anxiety attacks'. She describes these episodes as extremely distressing, both mentally and physically. When they occur, she experiences a sudden onset of fear that she is dying and feeling that she is losing control, and at times she worries that she is having a heart attack. These fears are associated with physical symptoms including chest pain, shortness of breath, heart palpitations, dizziness, sweating, and nausea. The symptoms are most frequently triggered by the sight of the hospital, but occasionally they occur 'out of the blue'. The entire episode lasts only 20 min but leaves her feeling emotionally and physically exhausted and embarrassed by her lack of self-control.

Question 1. What is the most likely diagnosis of these "episodes"?

At this early point in the history, although the episodes appear to be consistent with panic attacks, it is not possible to make a definitive diagnosis. Panic attacks are defined[2] as a discrete period of intense fear or discomfort, during which at least four of the following symptoms develop abruptly and reach a peak within 10 min:

- palpitations or accelerated heart rate
- sweating
- trembling or shaking
- shortness of breath
- feeling of choking
- chest pain or discomfort
- feeling dizzy, light-headed, unsteady, or faint
- derealization or depersonalization
- fear of losing control or going crazy
- fear of dying, parasthesias
- chills or hot flushes.

However, the presence of panic attacks is not sufficient to make a diagnosis of panic disorder. Panic attacks can occur in the context of several other psychiatric disorders. For example, it is quite common for patients with major depression to experience panic attacks. These episodes also occur with other anxiety disorders, such as social phobia, generalized anxiety disorder, obsessive–compulsive disorder, and post-traumatic stress disorder.

Further history indicates that Ms H. has not experienced symptoms of major depression. She reveals that even between episodes of panic, she worries about having another attack or that she may be 'losing her mind'. In fact, the fear of having another attack has caused her to return home halfway to an appointment at the hospital on at least two occasions. She does not spend a significant amount of time worrying about trivial matters, is not easily startled, and does not worry about participating in activities in public. She has never had difficulty in giving important presentations to large groups of people. Other than a fairly regimented daily schedule, she does not have behavioural rituals that must be performed to relieve anxiety.

Based on this further information the most likely diagnosis is that of panic disorder. Given her avoidance of the hospital, she may be developing agoraphobia (an abnormal fear of being helpless in an embarrassing or inescapable situation that is particularly characterized by the avoidance of open or public places) along with panic disorder.

Before the diagnosis of panic disorder can be confirmed, certain medical illnesses need to be eliminated as causes of the panic attacks. Examples of illnesses that can cause panic attacks include:[8]

- endocrine conditions such as hyperthyroidism, hypothyroidism, hyperparathyroidism, or adrenal dysfunction
- vestibular dysfunction
- seizure disorders
- central nervous system stimulant intoxication
- central nervous system depressant withdrawal
- cardiac conditions such as arrhythmias.

Question 2. What is the prevalence of anxiety disorders in the palliative care population?

Symptoms of anxiety and depression often co-occur in patients with advanced illness. These problems are frequently the catalyst for referral to psychiatry. Compared with depression, severe anxiety is less likely to be dismissed as a normal reaction to having an advanced illness. One study of the prevalence of psychiatric disorders in cancer patients found that 21 per cent had symptoms of anxiety.[13] Other studies have found significant increases in anxiety disorders in populations of cancer patients compared with the general population.

Question 3. Once the medical conditions have been eliminated as potential causes, how is panic disorder treated?

Untreated panic disorder may interfere with the patient's ability to obtain adequate treatment and can lead to increased morbidity. The ultimate goal of Ms H.'s treatment is to quell her anxiety, improve her quality of life, and enable her to attend her appointments. This means initiating measures to decrease both the frequency and intensity of the panic attacks.

The treatment of panic disorder comprises several approaches, beginning with providing reassurance. Patients can benefit greatly by being reassured that what they are experiencing is a panic attack and not a life-threatening event such as a myocardial infarction.

For those patients whose anxiety is not relieved by reassurance, further treatment is necessary. Both pharmacological and psychotherapeutic treatments can be effective in the treatment of anxiety disorders.

SSRIs have been shown to be effective in decreasing the frequency and intensity of panic attacks. However, these medications require a period of weeks to have their optimal effect. In addition to the delay in onset of effectiveness, SSRI medications can have troubling side effects in patients with anxiety, which could enhance the problem. Some of these side effects include headache, nausea, somnolence, dizziness, diarrhoea, tremor, and anticholinergic effects such as dry mouth, constipation, urinary retention, and blurred vision. Starting with small doses of medication and increasing the dose slowly in small increments can minimize the severity of the side effects. Symptoms of anxiety disorders tend to respond more slowly than mood symptoms to SSRI medication. Therefore it is important to utilize longer trials of these medications before deeming them unsuccessful. A typical trial of SSRI in the treatment of panic disorder could last as long as 8–12 weeks.

Tricyclic antidepressants have also demonstrated efficacy in the treatment of panic disorder. This class of medication tends to be less well tolerated with more drug interactions than SSRIs and therefore is not used as frequently.

Benzodiazepines can also be used to treat panic disorder. These medications have been used with both regular daily dosing and as-needed dosing schedules. Shorter-acting benzodiazepines, such as lorazepam, can be used to terminate a panic attack after it has begun. Longer-acting benzodiazepines may be more beneficial in the prevention of panic attacks when taken regularly throughout the day.

Benzodiazepine medications can induce both tolerance and dependence. However, this is less of a concern when prescribing this class of medication to palliative care patients. When prescribing this class of medications, the relative benefits of a sense of well-being and mastery and control over symptoms on the one hand, and the risk of dependence, side effects, and cognitive clouding on the other, should be considered. It is important to remember that patients who have been on benzodiazepine medications for a long time can suffer withdrawal symptoms if the medication is abruptly discontinued. If benzodiazepine medications need to be discontinued, the process should involve a gradual tapering over a period of weeks. Little benefit may be gained by attempting to discontinue the medication in a palliative care patient who has been on benzodiazepines for many years.

With certain patients in whom panic attacks are frequent and severe, it may be beneficial to start both an SSRI and a benzodiazepine. The benzodiazepine may help to decrease the frequency and severity of panic attacks while waiting for the SSRI to become effective, which may take 2–3 weeks. Buspirone, a non-benzodiazepine anxiolytic, can sometimes be helpful for the treatment of anxiety. It is usually most beneficial in patients who have not previously been given benzodiazepines.

Several psychotherapeutic approaches can be beneficial to patients with panic disorder. The psychotherapeutic understanding of panic is the catastrophic misinterpretation of bodily symptoms. With this understanding, cognitive techniques can be employed to decrease distorted interpretations of these bodily symptoms. It is also possible to employ behavioural techniques such as relaxation exercises, biofeedback, meditation, and exposure therapy to decrease the occurrence of panic attacks.

> Ms H. is started on a low dose of paroxetine (10 mg). This dose is titrated up in 10-mg increments after the first and third weeks of treatment. She experiences mild nausea for 4 days after each dose increase. Because she was informed of the likelihood of this occurring, she is able to cope with the side effects until they resolve. With medication and psychotherapy sessions addressing the cognitive distortions that occur in panic attacks, Ms H. notices weekly improvement in both the frequency and intensity of panic attacks. Over the course of 4 weeks she is able to report that she is no longer experiencing panic attacks.

Case 3

Mr V. has endured 4 years of therapy for prostate cancer. He has been married for 31 years and has three children. He describes his marriage as having had its rough times, usually because of his drive to succeed in his work. However, he feels that he and his wife are close and very committed to each other. His oldest son is married and has two sons. Mr V. adores his young grandchildren and spends every Saturday with them. Mr V.'s career has been spent in the insurance industry, and he ultimately rose to the position of vice-president of a company. He had to stop work 3 months ago after the bone pain he had been experiencing for 8 months could no longer be adequately controlled with medications that would not impair his concentration or ability to be productive.

Mr V. was originally diagnosed following a routine physical examination at age 57. His treatment was intensive, including surgery, radiation, and chemotherapy. This was a difficult time in his life, but he managed to face it as another challenge. Following the initial treatment, Mr V. thought that he might be cured. Unfortunately, investigations a year later revealed wide spread metastases. He has had several rounds of different therapies over the past 3 years, none of which has been successful in containing his prostatic cancer.

Owing to the extent and severity of his symptoms, Mr V. was admitted to hospital. Subsequent investigations indicated that further aggressive treatment would carry substantial risk and would be unlikely to provide any benefit. After long discussions with Mr V. and his family, the decision was made to admit him to the palliative care unit where you work as a house officer.

On your fifth day of working with Mr V. he reveals to you that he has had some very disturbing thoughts. Since admission to the unit he has been preoccupied with thoughts of death and dying, and thoughts that there is little point or purpose in his going on living. This disturbs him because he does not want his grandchildren, who have been visiting him regularly, to be burdened with images of him as a weak person. He confides in you that he has even had thoughts that 'perhaps it would be better if I ended my life right now, instead of waiting for it to happen'.

Question 1. Given his current situation, should his attitude be considered normal?

Patients at the end of life commonly experience thoughts of death and even occasional thoughts that dying might ultimately offer relief. This is not uncommon and does not necessarily reflect the presence of a comorbid psychiatric illness. On the other hand, fixedly held suicidal ideation and perseveration about thoughts of death are most often associated with a mental disorder such as major depression.[5] In this case, Mr. V. does not meet the diagnostic criteria for depression. He denies feeling depressed most of the time (a reasonable screening approach to help identify depression in patients who are terminally ill)[4] and does not have prominent neurovegetative symptoms of depression. He also does not endorse a pervasive sense of hopelessness, helplessness, or worthlessness, symptoms that should raise clinical suspicion regarding major depression in this patient population.

Many patients will openly discuss their fears if approached by an empathic and caring health care professional. These discussions frequently disclose that the patients are less afraid of death, and more concerned about the process of their dying. In anticipating death and given the opportunity to discuss these issues, patients may raise many questions such as: 'How will death come?' 'What will I experience?' 'How well will I handle it?' 'Am I ready for it?' 'Will I suffer?' Without answers to these questions, both uncertainty and distress can heighten and become intolerable.

Some dying patients may also sense that life itself has lost all meaning and purpose. Without meaning and purpose, or feeling that there is simply no reason to face another day, patients are more apt to report a sense of hopelessness. Hopelessness has been shown to correlate highly with suicidal ideation and thoughts of hastened death.[14] In fact, hopelessness, loss of dignity, and despair may be a painful triad that determines whether terminally ill patients do or do not wish to carry on living in the face of a foreshortened life expectancy.

Question 2. What therapeutic options or approaches should be considered at this time?

The first step in dealing with Mr. V.'s situation is to respond to his many questions with open and honest discussions about the process of dying that include as much detail as he is able to process at any one time. Patients often need to have many conversations about these issues. There are several reasons for this. The medical condition may limit abilities to attend to conversations for extended periods of time. Pain, fluctuating levels of consciousness, drowsiness, side effects of analgesics, and other medications can all prevent optimal levels of concentration or contribute to memory impairment. These discussions can be expected to cause a marked emotional response. To defend against feeling overwhelmed, patients will often psychologically distance themselves from the full impact of this information. In some instances, the process of dissociation will leave the patient listening but not really hearing or understanding the information. As discussions are repeated, and the information carefully reviewed in tolerable increments, emotional distancing will lessen, and patients will be better able to listen, understand, and integrate what they are being told.

To preserve Mr. V.'s dignity, therapeutic approaches must include a genuine exploration of how meaning and purpose can be reintroduced into his life.[15] A commitment to this process, along with an acknowledgement of who Mr. V. is as a person, may heighten his sense of being valued as an individual. This process can help patients reconnect with a part of themselves that feels untouched by their illness and defines their core sense of self. Mr. V.'s role as grandfather, for example, defines part of his core identity. Reinforcing the ongoing importance of this role, even with the involvement of his family if necessary, can provide a tangible reason to continue living. Even in the face of death, Mr. V. has something to contribute and pass along to those he cares about most, including being able to provide a role model of how one copes with vulnerability, deteriorating health, and, inevitably, facing death.

Look to the future

There are exciting advances coming to the treatment of palliative care patients who are suffering from anxiety and depression. Psychopharmacology is a rapidly changing field. New antidepressant medications are becoming available and are being studied at an impressive rate. Recent advances include antidepressant medications such as mirtazepine and the atypical neuroleptic medications (the potential appetite-stimulating aspects of mirtazapine and olanzapine are of interest; clinical trial data are awaited). The atypical neuroleptics have shown promise in patients with psychosis, delirium, and mood disorders. Medications of this class tend to have fewer extrapyramidal and dystonic side effects. These types of drug have yet to be thoroughly studied in the context of end-of-life care.

There is a growing literature regarding the use of meaning-enhancing psychotherapies in palliative care. Psychotherapeutic approaches that help patients regain a sense of meaning or purpose could bolster their chances of being able to die with dignity. Ongoing attempts to understand the inner life of dying patients and their families will pave the way to future therapeutic options, which will better serve the needs of those who are dying, those who love them, and those charged with the responsibility of providing them with quality end-of-life care.

References

1. **Katon, W.** (1987) The epidemiology of depression in medical care. *Int J Psychiatry Med,* **17**, 93–112.
2. **American Psychiatric Association** (1994) *Diagnostic and Statistical Manual of Mental Disorders* (4th edn). Arlington, VA: APPI.
3. **Endicott, J.** (1984) Measurement of depression in patients with cancer. *Cancer,* **53**, 2243–8.
4. **Chochinov, H.M., Wilson, K., Enns, M., and Lander, S.** (1997) Are you depressed? Screening for depression in the terminally ill. *Am J Psychiatry,* **154**, 674–6.
5. **Wilson, K., Chochinov, H.M., de Faye, B., and Breitbart, W.** (2000) Diagnosis and management of depression in palliative care. In: Chochinov HM, Breitbart W (eds) *Handbook of Psychiatry in Palliative Medicine.* Oxford: Oxford University Press, 25–50.
6. **Chochinov, H.M., Wilson, K.G., Enns, M., and Lander, S.** (1994) The prevalence of depression in the terminally ill: effects of diagnostic criteria and symptom threshold judgements. *Am J Psychiatry,* **151**, 537–40.
7. **Ganzini, L., Smith, D.M., Fenn, D.S., and Lee, M.A.** (1997) Depression and mortality in medically ill older adults. *J Am Geriatr Soc,* **45**, 307–12.
8. **Stoudemire, A., and Daniel, J.S.** (1995) Psychological factors affecting medical condition (psychosomatic disorders) In: Kaplan HI, Sadock BJ (eds) *Comprehensive Textbook of Psychiatry* (6th edn). Philadelphia, PA: Williams and Wilkins, 1595–7.
9. **Canadian Network for Mood and Anxiety Treatments** (1999) *Guidelines for the Diagnosis and Pharmacological Treatment of Depression* (revised). Toronto: CANMAT.
10. **Stearns, V., Johnson, M.D., and Rae, J.M.** (2003) Active tamoxifen metabolite plasma concentrations after co-administration of tamaxifen and the selective serotonin reuptake inhibitor paroxetine. *J Natl Cancer Inst,* **95**, 1758–64.
11. **Rodin, G., and Gillies, L.** (2000) Individual psychotherapy for the patient with advanced disease. In: Chochinov HM, Breitbart W (eds) *Handbook of Psychiatry in Palliative Medicine.* Oxford: Oxford University Press, 189–96.
12. **Ross, E.K.** (1970) *On Death and Dying.* London: Tavistock.
13. **Derogatis, L.R., Morrow, G.R., Fetting, J.,** ***et al.*** (1983) The prevalence of psychiatric disorders among cancer patients. *JAMA* **249**, 751–7.
14. **Chochinov, H.M., Wilson, K.G., Enns, M., and Lander, S.** (1998) Depression, hopelessness, and suicidal ideation in the terminally ill. *Psychosomatics,* **39**, 366–70.
15. **Chochinov, H.M.** (2002) Dignity conserving care: a new model for palliative care. *JAMA,* **287**, 2253–60.

Chapter 10

Grief

S. Lawrence Librach and Michéle Chaban

Attitude

To enable each student to:

- Identify the personal impact of loss for the palliative care patient and his or her family.
- Describe the physician's responsibility for ensuring adequate assessment and management of the grief process.
- Identify that the care provided by a physician or other health care provider may be influenced by his or her experiences of loss.

Skill

To enable each student to:

- Assess an individual experiencing loss in order to understand the current status of the grief response.
- Counsel individuals experiencing normal grief behaviours.
- Provide access to informational, emotional, practical, and social support to an individual.

Knowledge

To enable the student to:

- Define grief, mourning, and bereavement.
- Describe and differentiate between normal and complicated grief processes.
- Discuss how children are affected by death and how they grieve.
- Describe how professional caregivers may be affected by a patient's death.

Introduction

> There are tears in all things including joy and sorrow, birth and death.
>
> Steve Jenkinson

All of us will experience losses during our lifetimes and thus experience subsequent grief. The features, depth, and length of the grieving process are uniquely personal and relate to a number of factors. For the terminally ill patient and family, the illness and dying experience are replete with losses and grief. Grief does not wait for the death of the patient, but develops as patient and family confront a variety of successive losses in physical, psychological, and social spheres. This grief can have a profound and lasting impact on family members if it is not resolved in an effective and healthy manner. All physicians and other professional caregivers need to understand the basics of grief, an approach to managing grief as a normative process, and an understanding of complicated grief.

Elizabeth is a 44-year-old school teacher who has breast cancer with metastases to the brain, bone, and liver. She previously received palliative chemotherapy with limited response. She spends most of her time in bed at home and requires assistance with her daily care. She and her family are aware that her disease is very advanced.

Elizabeth is married. Her husband, Mel, has taken time off work to be with her. They have two daughters, Jennifer who is 8 and Alexandra who is 19. Alexandra attends university in another city and Jennifer is in elementary school.

As her physician, you make a home visit. During that visit, Elizabeth states that she is worried about how her family will cope following her death. She fears that her husband will be very lonely. In private conversation, Mel tells you that he is frequently tearful when he thinks about losing his wife. Although it has been difficult, they have together initiated funeral arrangements. Alexandra expresses that she feels sad when she looks at family photographs.

Question 1. How are grief, bereavement, and mourning defined?

Grief is the reaction to any loss. It is not only an emotional and psychological response but also has physical and social issues as part of the response. Any loss during life can induce grief, which really is a normative process. **Bereavement** is the state of having suffered a loss. **Mourning** describes the intrapsychic and cultural processes that occur when one suffers a loss.

Question 2. What indications are there that Elizabeth and her family are experiencing anticipatory grief?

The grief process

There is no firm agreement on a unified theory of the process of grief. It is difficult to standardize an emotional constellation when grief, as a response to loss and death and death's circumstances, is as individualized as we are. Several authors who have studied grief and bereavement[1–6] have developed the concepts of phases of grief and mourning. One suggests that grief and grief work should be viewed as a practical process that takes place over time and has certain tasks that need accomplishing.[6] These tasks include:

- recognizing the reality of the loss
- experiencing the emotional pain of the loss
- assuming a new reality
- investing emotional energy in other relationships.

Although these tasks apply to those who are grieving for someone who is deceased, these processes may also relate to the person who is dying as well as to his or her family members who are actively experiencing successive losses and anticipating the final loss—the death of the patient. This so-called anticipatory grief period demands as much attention as the bereavement period to prevent or reduce a harmful grief reaction. It is no longer sufficient simply to provide supportive grief counselling to families after death has taken place.

> Elizabeth and her family are expressing feelings of sadness and are occasionally tearful when they contemplate her anticipated death; these responses suggest the presence of anticipatory grief.
>
> Over the next week, Elizabeth's condition deteriorates further. She becomes unresponsive and dies several days later at home. Her funeral is held 3 days after her death. One week following the funeral, her husband comes to see you at your office. He complains of heartburn. You inquire as to how he is coping with his wife's death. He tells you that he is also experiencing decreased concentration and mild insomnia. He finds himself thinking frequently about his wife and often becomes tearful at those times. He has been invited by friends to come to dinner but he has no desire to do so. He wonders if how he is feeling is normal and asks if and when these symptoms will go away.

Question 3. What would you tell Elizabeth's husband about his manifestations of his grief?

Manifestations of grief[7] may involve psychological, physical, and social components.

Psychological manifestations

Avoidance phase

- The avoidance phase may be characterized by shock, denial, and disbelief. These will be experienced by patients as they first hear the diagnosis and later as they cope with 'bad news' about disease progression and changes in roles, independence, and emotions. Family members undergo similar but individualized experiences.
- This numbing experience may initially be intellectualized, but that defence mechanism usually fails quickly as the next phase of reality develops.
- Decision-making during this phase is often difficult.
- There is some experiential evidence that if the dying process is managed well, this avoidance phase is limited and shortened.

Confrontation phase

- During this phase, those who grieve confront the reality of the loss.
- This is accompanied by extremes of emotion: sadness, anxiety, fear, anger and guilt.
- Anger may be with oneself over a perceived lack of a certain appropriate response, over a perceived ability to have averted the illness, or over relationship issues that have not been resolved.
- Anger displaced to others, including professional caregivers, is also very common.
- Spiritual angst may manifest as anger with God.
- Restlessness, irritability, and panic may occur.
- There is often a feeling of loss of control, and decision-making during this phase may be difficult, requiring more time.

Re-establishment phase

- Grief over a particular issue begins to decline although the loss is never forgotten.
- The dying process for the patient may constantly remind him or her about these losses.
- Both patient and family reinvest emotional energy into hope, role maintenance, and, with some further adjustment and adaptation, social and emotional activities.
- Grief lessens in the bereavement period, allowing family members to reinvest physical, psychological, and emotional energy in other and new relationships as they learn to live without the deceased.

Physical and physiological manifestations

- Anorexia
- Gastrointestinal disturbances such as dysphagia and diarrhoea
- Insomnia
- Fatigue and generalized weakness
- Anxiety-related symptoms such as palpitations and shortness of breath
- Sighing and crying
- Sexual dysfunction including loss of libido and erectile dysfunction
- Headaches

Some of these symptoms may be the result of disease states and may be more likely to develop in vulnerable populations such as those with pre-existing conditions or those who are elderly. Treatment of these physical symptoms may require some investigation if they are persistent.

Social manifestations

- Restlessness and inability to sit still
- Lack of ability to initiate and maintain organized patterns of activity, leading to decreased productivity, decreasing social interactions, difficulty fulfilling social roles, etc.
- Social withdrawal and isolation

> Elizabeth's husband should be reassured that his symptoms and feelings are normal and not unexpected following his wife's death. You tell him that they will probably dissipate over time, although you are not able to give him a specific time frame. You provide him with an antacid and ask him to check back with you if the heartburn persists.

Question 4. What factors may you be thinking about at this time that may influence Mel's grieving process and resolution?

Factors influencing grief and its resolution

Characteristics of the individual

- The nature of the relationship with the deceased
- Unresolved issues with the deceased

- Coping strategies
- Personality and current or past major psychiatric illness
- Past experiences with illness and death
- Age and development
- Physical illnesses that may impede grieving or add risk
- Culture and religiosity
- Social isolation
- History of harm or abuse
- History of post-traumatic stress disorder and/or compassion fatigue

Characteristics of the deceased

- Personality
- The nature of the relationship
- Age at death
- History of harm or abuse
- History of post-traumatic stress disorder

Characteristics of the death

The acute death that is unexpected does not allow family members the opportunities to express grief openly pre-mortem or the time to develop coping mechanisms to deal with grief. This may make grief more prolonged and difficult for the bereaved.

The family system

The family can be defined as those closest to the patient in knowledge, care, and affection. This may include the biological family, the family of acquisition (related by marriage/contract), the family of choice, and friends (including pets). The patient defines who will be involved in his or her care and/or present at the bedside. Each family is a system with a variety of rules, roles, and behaviours that govern family members and their interaction with themselves and others. Some families work well and cope well with stress and grief, while others are very dysfunctional. The hallmark of the healthy family is the ability to cope with crises. Dying, death, and grief all present challenges to a family. A number of issues impact on the development and resolution of grief in a family.[8]

- Emotional support is the most influential type of support provided by families. The family's listening ear and empathy reinforce the sense of belonging. A lack of this support will complicate grief.
- For adults, a strong marriage or partnership arrangement with open direct communication, flexible boundaries, and strong loyalties over time is beneficial.
- Negative, critical, or hostile family relationships have a stronger impact on health than positive supportive ones.
- Family psychoeducation appears to be the most effective and efficient type of family intervention. Bringing a family together to educate them about grief and facilitating healthy approaches to resolving issues works better than individual counselling alone.

- Families with serious problems such as addiction and drug abuse, family violence, other history of harm (e.g. Holocaust or genocide experiences), a history of significant mental illness, or other significant dysfunction will need expert counsellors.

System induced trauma/harm

Dying persons and their families are sometimes battered by the health system. Bad news poorly delivered, false hope, withdrawal or abandonment by professional caregivers, lack of support for emotional and psychological needs, unresolved unnecessary physical suffering such as pain, and lack of honesty and clarity are all issues that may harm patients and families and increase grief. By taking a comprehensive, holistic, and communicative approach that diminishes the possibility of harm, grief can be dealt with effectively.

> Elizabeth's husband asks if he could see you regularly for a while for support. He feels that it would be helpful for him to come in and speak with you. You agree to this arrangement.

Question 5. What approach would you take to assist Mel with his grieving process?

Normal or uncomplicated grief

Deal with issues of loss and grief throughout the illness and provide good end-of-life care

Good end-of-life care with attention to all the components of physical, psychological, social, and spiritual issues will help most patients and families to cope with their grief. Early intervention to provide psychoeducational support to patient and family is important. The goal of this intervention is to teach the family to discover their own values and beliefs about dying and death, to teach family members new values and beliefs, and to teach the dying person how to mentor their family with regard to how he or she is to be remembered and about the emotional, spiritual, or financial legacy being left to the family.

Family sessions are also important to assess family functioning, to identify possible factors that may have a significant impact on grief, and also to mobilize resources to deal with issues of loss and grief. If the patient and family are from a culture that is not familiar, develop cultural competence in issues of grief and death rites for that culture and pass on information and educate other caregivers. Early intervention with a family often smoothes the course of family grief during the bereavement period.

Enhance coping skills

Learning how to grieve is a skill set that is developed over a lifetime.[9] Taking an approach to grief that is person-centred in the context of the family avoids the isolation and marginalization that often comes with grieving. Exploring how each person views death, how each person chooses to grieve, and how that impacts on the family as a whole is an essential part of assessing how a family grieves. Some families have healthy grieving strategies; some families need help to develop healthier strategies. Stressing the uniqueness of grief for each family member and the normative nature of grief is also helpful, since family members sometimes think they are 'going crazy'.

When grief work is done effectively before the dying person dies, there is time to develop new ways of being and new roles, functions, and strategies within a family. As death approaches, more energy should be devoted to preparing the family for what they will experience after the death of their loved one.

Do some initial bereavement counselling at the time of the patient's death

Just before and immediately after the patient's death, whether it has occurred at home or in an institution, briefly counsel families about important issues such as initial reactions of shock, what to expect at funerals, interventions with children, the need for tears and emotions, the time frame of grief, and the availability for some follow-up.

Avoid prescribing medications to alter grief especially in the early phases of acute grief

Family members will often request a sedative or tranquillizer to help someone avoid the emotional extremes of fresh grief. This should be avoided, as these medications may actually cloud the person's natural expressions of grief and his or her ability to cope with the emotional extremes. Later on in grief, antidepressants should be avoided unless there is firm evidence of clinical depression. Brief courses of mild tranquillizers later on in grief may help if there are problems of insomnia.

Allow sufficient time to grieve

The general public usually has a very contracted time frame for grief. Employers often assume that grieving employees can be ready to work and as productive as usual after having had a few days off. In most individuals, working through the tasks of grief takes about a year. For some, especially those who have been well prepared for the experience of grief, this period can be much shorter. Fresh grief with prolonged denial, frequent emotional extremes, and other behaviours should not be seen beyond 6–9 months. Naturally, grieving will be heightened and present at times of birthdays, anniversaries, high holidays and/or holy days on the calendar, as well as anniversary dates for the family, especially in the first 1 or 2 years after the death. Inform and prepare the family for this. Suggest ways in which anniversaries may be occasions for celebratory commemorations.

Provide grief counselling as necessary

- Reach out and follow up with family members after a month. This can be done by telephone call or by a sympathy card. The message should be one of reassurance about the normal ebb and flow of grief over time, hope, empathy for the grief, giving permission to grieve, and commitment for further help if necessary.
- If family members return for further follow-up, provide enough time to listen to them. Remember that grief is individual to each person.
- Maintain a family systems perspective in all the interventions.
- Identify the tasks of grief.
- The most important grief counselling skill is the skill of listening and normalizing the grief experience. Allow the bereaved to review their perceptions of what happened. Encourage verbalization of feelings. Identify the normal components of grief. Avoid being judgemental or falsely reassuring. Maintain hope. Allow the repetition of their stories and perceptions. Stress the individuality of the grief experience.

- Tolerate reactions such as anger, tears, and guilt. Listen and react with empathy.
- Identify unresolved issues and those issues that have been resolved.
- Identify whether elements of post-traumatic stress disorder, depression, compassion fatigue or suicidal ideation are present.
- Encourage the bereaved to deal with spiritual issues by consulting experienced clergy or by reading self-help books[10] that may help them deal with these issues.
- Refer early if grief is becoming complicated or if there is significant family dysfunction.
- Let people grieve in the environments that they live in. As a clinician, try to work where people live rather than bringing people to where you work. Teach their community and peers about their suffering. Help to create a supportive community for them where they work or go to school. Use school or occupational health counselling resources as necessary.

Ask for help

Be aware of counselling resources in your area. Ask for psychiatric consultation if there is major depression, suicidal risk, severe family dysfunction, a history of family abuse, violence, or addiction.

> You see Elizabeth's husband every 2–3 weeks for a period of three months since his wife's death. He then indicates that he is feeling better and wishes to stop seeing you a regular basis. Ten months pass before he again presents to your office. This time he tells you that he has not been doing well. He states that he feels depressed, that he has no enjoyment from life, that he cries at the drop of a hat, and that he cannot 'stop thinking about her' (his wife). You are quite concerned by his presentation.

Question 6. What is complicated grief? When would you consider making a diagnosis of complicated grief?

In most family members, grief involves a normal, if somewhat volatile, process that resolves over time. The time frame for most persons for active grief is about a year. However, there are some people whose grief becomes complicated and in whom resolution of grief becomes difficult. The reasons for complicated grief may relate to the impact of the factors discussed earlier, to the avoidance of the pain of grief, to excessive guilt, to denial of the loss and trauma, and to being socially isolated. Grief may be absent, delayed, greatly inhibited, chronic, or conflict ridden.

Question 7. How would you proceed to manage this situation?

Some diagnostic criteria have been proposed for diagnosing unresolved grief.[11]

- Clinical depression
- History of prolonged or delayed grief
- Excessive symptoms of guilt and self-reproach.
- Somatic symptoms similar to those of the deceased
- Extreme anniversary reactions

- Unwillingness to part with the deceased's belongings
- A feeling that the death was very recent even if it was remote
- Minor events trigger major grief expression
- Extreme social withdrawal that persists
- Self-destructive impulses
- Elements of a post-traumatic stress disorder

Unresolved grief may be associated with suicide, psychiatric illnesses and perhaps even increased mortality. If grief is going poorly, expert counselling help should be obtained.

> You assess Mel for other symptoms and signs of clinical depression including suicidal ideation. You are prepared to treat him with an antidepressant. In addition to follow-up with yourself, you refer him to a social worker who specializes in bereavement counselling.

Question 8. How do children understand death and express their grief?

Children have the same tasks as adults in the grieving process but their developmental stage, relationship with the deceased, and the circumstances of the death affect their ability to conceptualize, understand, and express grief. Children do express their feelings of grief differently from adults. Children often do not display their feelings as openly as adults. They can often immerse themselves in their usual activities while harbouring strong feelings of anger and continuing fears of abandonment and death. Although a child's grief may appear more intermittent and brief than an adult's grief, it usually lasts longer and requires constant support and monitoring by knowledgeable family and community supports. As children grow and develop, they often revisit their grief at significant life events. Also, such children often have difficulty in articulating their feelings and may express their grief through behaviours such as aggressive and destructive actions, difficulty in bonding with new caregivers, school phobias and other school problems, or overly attention-seeking actions.[12] Children may also become devoted to becoming 'the good child', convinced that a family member's death was caused by his or her not being 'good enough' in the first place. All these extremes need to be monitored. School systems, family systems, and health care systems can work collaboratively to create a caring environment in which the child can grieve and thrive.

Children's understanding of death depends on their developmental stage.[13]

- Children aged 0–3 years do not have clear concepts of death. The emotional expression and dependable presence of loved ones are more important than the words used. Since these children may equate death with sleep, explanations that compare death to sleep should be avoided. Otherwise abnormal fear of sleep or night-time may occur. Children in this age group may sense the grief in others, and protecting them from the pain of grief may lead to physical and emotional changes such as weight loss, anorexia, sleep disturbance, listlessness, and other changes in activity.
- Children aged 3–6 years often consider death as a reversible event. They frequently have images from television cartoons that death is temporary. They also may express 'magical thinking', believing that they caused the death in some way or that they can reverse the death. They may regress and show disturbances in eating, sleeping, and toileting.

- Children aged 6–9 years may be more aware of the finality of death but do not believe that it is universal. In their grief they can become aggressive or overly clingy.
- By age of 9 or 10 years, most children understand that death is final and universal.

Alexandra, Elizabeth's 19-year-old daughter, called you 6 weeks after her mother's death. She was worried about her younger sister, Jennifer. She tells you that Jennifer is afraid to be away from home for extended periods of time and her grades have been falling at school.

Question 9. How would you handle this situation?

The tasks of grieving in children are similar to those in adults. The first task for them is to understand and make some sense of the loss.[14] The approach to this depends on their age and verbal skills. Preparation for an impending death is an important way of beginning this process. Waiting until the death occurs may lead to more extreme bereavement reactions. The second task relates to expression of emotions in regards to the loss. Facilitating and validating these responses is important. Allowing children to see others grieve makes them feel normal in their own grief. The third task is to commemorate the loss in some way. This may be through participation in funerals or even through some other commemorative activity such as drawing pictures, writing a diary, or planting a tree. Finally, the fourth task is to learn to go on with life despite the loss.

Children should be told about death in language that is appropriate for their development. There are quite a number of age-specific resource books and visual media available to assist in the discussion of dying and death. The parents should be coached to do this education, as it is important for children not to feel isolated from their family and for them to see parental and family grief. They should be reassured that they did not cause the illness or death, that they could not have prevented it, and that they cannot bring back the deceased.[15]

Children's attendance at funerals is also important. They can participate and observe the family and community grief responses. They need to be prepared in advance for what they are to see and can be encouraged to participate in the service if they are old enough and if that participation fits with family values and culture. At all times during the funeral children should be supervised by someone they trust who can explain the rituals and deal with their questions.

Indicators of atypical grief in children may include:

- continued denial of the death
- prolonged anger
- school problems that are not resolving
- behavioural problems that did not exist before
- persistent physical symptoms such as sleep disturbances, eating disorders, etc.
- social withdrawal
- disabling or persistent regression.

Children displaying any of the above should be referred to experienced counsellors for management, since unresolved grief may lead to serious emotional and psychological problems and even suicide.

The clinician's grief

You had spent much time with Elizabeth and her family prior to her death and with her husband after her death. She had been a patient of yours for over 10 years and you had come to know her and her family well. You felt it a great honour to care for her during her cancer illness but at the same time you identify that it was stressful and that you were going to miss visiting her.

Working with those who have serious illnesses and who are dying can be stressful and full of grief for the professional caregiver. There are certain personal and professional values, beliefs, and practices that accompany our specific approaches to delivering health care interventions. Underlying these approaches are very real personal experiences that have determined them. In the presence of death, we all feel helpless at first. Then, with experience and time, we begin to develop a sense of what to do. Vachon[16] and others have also pointed out the effect of grief leading to staff stress in health care professionals caring for the dying. Figley's[17] concept of 'compassion fatigue' captures the essence of caregiver burden as it presents in both psychological intensity and the exhaustion felt by those committed to caring for the dying. This may be complicated by other stress factors such as insufficient personal or vacation time, a sense of failure, unrealistic role expectations, anger towards the system, and personal issues. Unresolved grief in caregivers may lead to burnout.

Caregivers must, like the patients and families they serve, learn to grieve effectively. The naturally occurring social supports of family, colleagues, and friends are the best remedy for recovery from this trauma. Effective grieving in caregivers may involve:

- discussion with colleagues and friends
- seeking out humour in everyday life
- time for oneself for pleasurable activities
- religion
- sufficient personal and vacation time
- attending funerals and memorial services for patients who have touched you in a particular way
- being part of institutional memorial services.

Summary

The untreated or undertreated process of dying can negatively impact on grief and bereavement. This may have a negative impact on the social role and function of the bereaved survivors, resulting in increased dependency and reduced social and occupational abilities. Early intervention strategies of working with dying, death, and grief in a family helps enhance the family's sense of competency, self-worth, self-esteem and autonomy, while avoiding feelings of helplessness and hopelessness which tend to enhance or compound grief.

References

1. **Lindemann, E.** (1944) Symptomatology and management of acute grief. *Am J Psychiatry*, **101**, 141–8.
2. **Bowlby, J.** (1961) Processes of mourning. *Int J Psychoanal*, **42**, 317–40.

3. **Bowlby, J.** (1973–1982) *Attachment and Loss.* Vols 1, 2, 3. New York: Basic Books.
4. **Parkes, C.M.** (1975) *Bereavement: Studies of Grief in Adult Life.* New York: International Universities Press.
5. **Rando, T.A.** (1984) *Grief, Dying and Death: Clinical Interventions for Caregivers.* Champaign IL: Research Press.
6. **Worden, J.W.** (1982) *Grief Counselling and Grief Theory: A Handbook for the Mental Health Professional.* New York: Springer.
7. **Rando, T.A.** (1984) *Grief, Dying and Death: Clinical Interventions for Caregivers.* Champaign IL: Research Press, 28–41.
8. **Campbell, T.L, and McDaniel, S.H.** (2001) Family systems in family medicine. *Clin Fam Pract,* **3**, (1), 13–54.
9. **Jenkinson, S.** (2000) Lecture on Griefwork with Men. Humber College, Toronto, Canada.
10. **Kushner, H.S.** *When Bad Things Happen to Good People.* New York: Schocken Books.
11. **Rando, T.A.** (1984) *Grief, Dying and Death: Clinical Interventions for Caregivers.* Champaign IL: Research Press, 63–64.
12. **Zeitlin, S.V.** (2001) Grief and bereavement. *Prim Care* **28**, 415–25.
13. **Stuber, M.L.** (2001) What do we tell the children: understanding childhood grief. *West J Med,* **174**, 187–91.
14. **Fox, S.S.** (1988) Helping children deal with death teaches valuable skills. *Psychiatric Times,* August 10–11.
15. **Wolraich, M.L., Aceves, J., Feldman, H.M., *et al.*** (2000) American Academy of Pediatrics Committee on Psychosocial Aspects of Child and Family Health. The pediatrician and childhood bereavement. *Pediatrics,* **105**, 445–7.
16. **Vachon, M.L.S.** (1978) Motivation and stress experienced by staff working with the terminally ill. *Death Educ,* **2**, 113–22.
17. **Figley, C.R.** (1995) *Compassion Fatigue: Coping with Secondary Traumatic Stress Disorders in Those Who Treat the Traumatized.* New York: Brunner–Mazel.

Chapter 11

Sleep

Srini Chary

> Sleep that knits up the raveled sleeve of care, the death of each day's life, sore labour's balm, balm of hurt minds, great nature's second course, chief nourisher in life's feast.
>
> (William Shakespeare, *Macbeth* Act II, Scene 2)

Attitude

To enable each student to:

- Understand the relation between pain, other symptoms, psychosocial problems, existential distress, and disturbed sleep.
- Recognize that it is critical for symptom control to ensure that patients have a regular period of good rest.

Skill

To enable each student to:

- Understand the physiology of sleep and demonstrate skills in integrating the use of drugs and non-drug techniques to assist with evening sleep or to correct the day–night reversal pattern.

Knowledge

To enable each student to:

- Describe the pathophysiological reasons for sleep disorders and, based on this background, learn a classification of specific sleep disturbance syndromes.
- Recognize that sleep disorders characterized by reversal of the day–night sleep pattern are very common in patients with advanced cancer and other serious illnesses.
- Describe the role of hypnotics and other medications in alleviating sleep problems and describe how to select the proper medication to assist sleep.

Introduction

Patients with a wide variety of chronic illnesses frequently complain of insomnia and daytime drowsiness. These problems, coupled with pain, depression, and other symptoms, increase the quotient of human misery. Reduced sleep also has profound biological effects including insulin resistance and increased cardiovascular disease.[1]

Strangely, while each of us can personally testify to the effects of a poor night's sleep on performance and mood, little research and resultant evidence-based advice is available on the management of sleep disorders in the chronically ill. This chapter will illustrate the importance of sleep and incorporate some of what is known in guidelines for patient management; the importance of non-pharmacological measures will be stressed, together with the importance of quantifying sleep disorders and integrating them into the identification and treatment of other problems, notably depression.

> Mr S.T. is a 59-year-old government employee who has lost 5 kg over the past 3 months. In addition to poor appetite and fatigue, he presents with a nagging back pain. A smoker for many years, he states that the back pain is mild during the day, but seems to accentuate at night. Previously without sleep problems, he now has difficulty falling asleep, and recently has started waking during the night with ruminations about his health. Both he and his fellow employees note that the calibre of his work has dropped. Mr S.T., a formerly placid individual, is now often irritable and subject to bursts of anger.

Question 1. Mr S.T. presents with symptoms of a serious illness. While organizing a diagnostic work-up, what advice will you offer him?

While undertaking a diagnostic work-up, you will take steps to address Mr S.T.'s immediate sources of distress, which include pain, insomnia, anxiety, and possible depression. Mr S.T. commences on regular acetaminophen (paracetamol), with an opportunity to receive acetaminophen with codeine if pain is not relieved and is interfering with sleep or work. You discuss the importance of sleep with Mr S.T. and relate both his level of anxiety and his increasingly poor performance at work to sleep loss. He is missing the restorative power of sleep.

We spend 75 per cent of our sleep time in a state of 'non-rapid-eye-movement sleep' (NREM), a phase of global inhibition of central nervous system (CNS) activities. The second intermingled phase of sleep, 'rapid-eye-movement sleep' (REM) is not a time of CNS quiescence; rather dreaming and fluctuating autonomic nervous system activity is noted during this phase. Normally, a 'good sleep', with a consequent feeling of vigour to approach the tasks of the day, requires maintenance of a coordinated pattern of NREM–REM sleep. In Mr S.T.'s situation, both the total period of sleep and probably the sleep architecture have been disturbed, leading to a vicious circle of increased anxiety, irritability, and poor work performance. Common causes of sleep disturbance in patients with chronic illness are given in Table 11.1.

Interference with sleep is commonly noted in cancer patients, particularly those experiencing pain.[2] The pain threshold is reduced, while insomnia may interfere with opioid action. Patients who sleep poorly commonly experience more pain during the day. Less sleep–more pain–less sleep is another of the vicious circles which often bedevil our patients. Another vicious circle

Table 11.1 Common causes of sleep disturbance in patients with chronic illness.

Precipitating factor	Possible cause
Insomnia	
Anxiety	Primary disorder; related to illness; direct effects of tumour on CNS?
Depression	Related to illness; direct effects of tumour on CNS?
Pain	Related to direct tumour effects; diagnostic or treatment interventions
Cognitive impairment disorders	As disease advances, hallucinations and delirium commonly occur, particularly in the older populations (see Chapter 24); dementia may complicate patient management
Other disturbing symptoms	Nausea and vomiting; respiratory distress; changes in urination or bowel function
Medications	Corticosteroids; bronchodilators; activating antidepressants; analgesics; adverse reactions; sedative-hypnotics (or withdrawal); stimulants
Other	Poor sleep hygiene; conditioned insomnia; sleep–wake schedule problems
Excessive sleep during the day	
Insufficient sleep	
Movement disorder	Restless legs syndrome (RLS) Periodic limb movements in sleep (PLMS)
Respiratory disorder	Obstructive sleep apnoea
Other	Sleep–wake schedule disorders; medications (e.g. opiates) Direct effects of CNS tumour

Adapted with permission from Sateia MJ, Santulli RB (2003) Sleep in palliative care. In: Doyle D, Hanks GWC, MacDonald N (eds) *Oxford Textbook of Palliative Medicine* (3rd edn). Oxford: Oxford University Press, Chapter 8.16.

links sleeplessness and fatigue. They are clearly linked in disorders such as fibromyalgia, while poor sleep and fatigue are also twinned in cancer patients. Most patients with serious chronic illness and many geriatric patients sleep poorly. Sleep hygiene problems exist across the spectrum, and specific features stand out in certain disorders (cancer, congestive heart failure, chronic respiratory disease). For example, dyspnoea, which is sometimes related to position and probably arouses anxiety, may require careful blending of therapies to relieve the primary symptom and resultant insomnia, i.e. more emphasis on non-pharmacological agents and judicious timing of bronchodilator therapy. It is important to ask about prior sleep disturbance, often as noted by a sleeping partner. For example, a specific syndrome, sleep apnoea, is common and may be accentuated as illness progresses.

Anxiety and depression, prevalent across the spectrum of chronic illness, interfere with sleep. As with pain, patients may enter a vicious circle: less sleep–more risk of depression. It is possible that the wide variety of chemical changes associated with the presence of tumours and other illnesses, such as generation of cytokines both by the tumour and as part of the host response, specifically influence the sleep–wake cycle. Chronic inflammation and its products (e.g. certain cytokines and C-reactive protein)[1,3] are associated with a poor prognosis in virtually all chronic illnesses. These in turn produce sleep alterations which in true vicious circle mode may influence the course of a disorder.

Question 2. How will you obtain a sleep history from Mr S.T.?

There are important specific components of a sleep history. First, ask about sleep; many physicians do not.[4] As emphasized elsewhere, using a symptom scale including inquiries on sleep, daytime drowsiness, and the level of possible contributory symptoms will sharpen both the patient's and doctor's concern about adequate sleep. If the patient has a sleep problem, the following questions are relevant.

- How many hours of sleep does he normally obtain?
- When does he usually go to bed?
- Has he had prior difficulty with sleep?
- Is there any past psychiatric history?
- Is there a history of possible drug or alcohol abuse?
- Sleep pattern: Does he fall asleep readily? Awaken during the night? Get up when aroused?
- Prior patterns: sleep disturbance in the past is usually exacerbated in the chronically ill.
- Environment: comfortable bed, noise, light, odours.

Alcohol may assist with falling asleep, but rapid rebound often occurs. What measures has Mr S.T. adopted to help himself sleep?

> You quickly determine that Mr S.T. has never encountered difficulty in sleeping prior to his illness, and has no significant past history of contributory ill health. He does not drink alcohol, smoke, or take tea, coffee, or soft drinks. He goes to bed at his usual time (11 p.m.), setting an alarm for his usual time of waking (6 a.m.). If he cannot sleep, he lies in bed willing himself to fall asleep. He is frequently roused during the night by back discomfort. Once awake, he is beset by ruminations on his growing life concerns

Question 3. How would you advise Mr S.T. concerning his problem with sleep?

In addition to ensuring that he begins a pain management routine, you suggest a variety of specific measures.

Non-drug sleep hygiene

> You advise Mr S.T., a sedentary man, to keep active during the day, cutting back on naps, and increasing his level of mild exercise. You encourage him to walk more during the day; however, you caution him to cancel this advice if walking increases his pain. You suggest that willing himself to sleep is probably counterproductive. Rather, you suggest that he arise from bed when he cannot sleep and use distraction therapy, including relaxing, (sometimes dull) reading, and listening to soft music. Mr S.T. turns out to be a 'clock watcher'. You suggest that he remove this metronome of failure from visual contact and accentuate positive stimuli to sleep, including comfortable room temperature and ventilation, the presence of a soft breeze (through open windows or a gentle fan), and a comfortable mattress. You recommend that he delay attempts to sleep for an hour beyond his usual bedtime, allowing himself an extra hour of sleep in the morning.

You could recommend the use of relaxation tapes (often available through local palliative care programmes). Professional counselling in behaviour therapy or self-hypnosis could also help. Non-pharmacological measures for combating insomnia are given in Table 11.2.

If simple measures are unsuccessful and if your clinic resources will allow, consultation with a sleep expert (a clinical psychologist or an internist with special expertise) is in order. The specialist

Table 11.2 Non-pharmacological advice for combating insomnia

- Maintain as regular a sleep–wake schedule as possible, particularly with respect to the hour of morning awakening
- Avoid unnecessary time in bed during the day; for bedridden patients, provide as much mental (conversations, reading) and physical stimulation during daytime hours as conditions permit
- Nap only as necessary, and avoid napping in the late afternoon and evening whenever possible
- Keep as active a daytime schedule as possible; this should include social contacts and, when able, light exercise
- Try to maintain a light–dark cycle similar to the outdoor environment; during the daytime, let as much outdoor light as you can into your room and if possible go outside (including on the balcony); at night, try to maintain a dark environment by closing the curtains or blinds
- Minimize night-time sleep interruptions due to medication, noise, or other environmental conditions
- Avoid lying in bed for prolonged periods at night in an alert and frustrated or tense state; read or prepare a light snack or engage in other relaxing activities (out of bed when appropriate) until drowsiness ensues
- Remove unpleasant conditioned stimuli, such as clocks, from sight and sound
- Try listening to relaxing music
- Try to tune out problems and concerns of the day before trying to sleep. Reflecting on pleasant events in your family or the world at large may help. You may want to consult professional help to guide you in meditation, yoga, or self-hypnosis techniques
- Avoid stimulating medication and other substances (e.g. caffeine in coffee and tea, nicotine), particularly in the hours before bedtime.
- If you enjoy a hot beverage after 4:00 pm, try decaffeinated coffee or tea or a herbal tea
- Avoid drinking liquids before bed as you may be disturbed in the middle of night.
- Maintain adequate pain relief through the night. If specific symptoms interfere with sleep, discuss with your nurse and doctor.
- Use sleep medication as indicated after proper evaluation of the sleep problem and avoid over-usage

Adapted with permission from Sateia MJ, Santulli RB (2003) Sleep in palliative care. In: Doyle D, Hanks GWC, MacDonald N (eds) *Oxford Textbook of Palliative Medicine* (3rd edn). Oxford: Oxford University Press, Chapter 8.16.

can guide the patient and family in the use of tailored behavioural therapy (e.g. relaxation hypnosis) and possibly identify and remedy unresolved anxiety–depression.

Pharmacological help

If Mr S.T. were a patient in whom you did not suspect serious underlying illness, and who was not about to undergo a sequence of unpleasant tests, you would stress proper sleep hygiene and eschew the use of hypnotics or antidepressants unless a specific diagnosis of endogenous anxiety or depression were present. However, this is not the situation with Mr S.T. Therefore you suggest that he start on low doses of zopiclone, a hypnotic with an intermediate length of action. You suggest a dose of 7.5 mg at night. Zaleplon may be better in some individuals as this short-acting agent may cause less daytime somnolence.[5] Variation in response occurs; alternatives can be used if the patient's response to the primary choice is unsatisfactory.

You decide to forego benzodiazepines, as the non-benzodiazepine hypnotics zopiclone, zolpidem, and zaleplon are believed to cause less disturbance of normal sleep architecture, dependency, and rebound insomnia, and there is less risk of drug interactions[6] (the last belief may change as further experience with these relatively new agents informs clinical practice[7]).

Question 4. Mr S.T.'s ESAS scores for depression are low, and you do not think he is clinically depressed. If he were depressed, would this alter your approach?

A choice of a sedative antidepressant such as trazodone, or a newer agent mirtazapine, would be reasonable in place of zopiclone[8,9]. The combined effects of these two drug classes are not yet clear. One may need to be cautious about using mirtazapine with chemotherapy patients, as it may have a bone marrow suppressive effect.[10]

> You arrange a series of tests as quickly as possible. Chest radiography reveals the presence of a left hilar mass and a widened mediastinum. Bone radiographs are normal, but a bone scan reveals multiple areas of increased uptake throughout the pelvis and the thoracolumbar spine. After a biopsy, a diagnosis of small-cell carcinoma of the lung is established.
>
> Mr S.T. is placed on a course of chemotherapy, with good effect. The chest radiograph returns to normal, while a repeat bone scan shows diminution in uptake associated with complete relief of the patient's pain. Mr S.T. gains weight, returns to full employment, and, while he recognizes that he has an ultimately fatal disorder, is encouraged by the reversal of his immediate problems. The zopiclone dose is tapered over 2 weeks, and then stopped.
>
> Six months later Mr S.T. returns to your office. Once again, his complaints relate primarily to sleep. On this occasion, he describes a chaotic pattern of sleep disturbance. He falls asleep without undue difficulty, but his sleep is disturbed by unusual thoughts and dreams which cause him to awaken. He does not return to sleep easily. Upon awakening, he notes that he has a frontal headache which improves during the course of the morning. On his own, he once again commenced zopiclone, this time with poor results.

Question 5. What advice do you offer Mr S.T.?

In view of the underlying diagnosis, Mr S.T. again presents with ominous symptoms. You must rule out a metabolic or organic cause related to recurrence of small-cell lung carcinoma.

A CT scan of the brain is rapidly arranged which confirms the presence of multiple brain metastases. Mr S.T. commences on dexamethasone, together with radiation therapy. Headaches rapidly improve, and the nightmares disappear. However, once again, Mr S.T. notes that he cannot readily fall asleep.

Question 6. What is happening? How will you counsel Mr S.T.?

The dose and timing of the dexamethasone, a drug with a long half-life, may contribute to the problem. The patient is well launched on a course of radiation therapy and is free of symptoms, apart from sleep disturbance. An attempt to taper the dexamethasone as rapidly as safely tolerated is reasonable, and you advise Mr S.T. that he should only take dexamethasone (previously ordered in four daily doses) once daily in the morning. You tell him that dexamethasone has a long period of action which will protect him throughout the day, but that increases in levels in the drug associated with doses late in the day may have disturbed his sleep.

Mr S.T. returns to a reasonable state of health which continues for a further 3 months. He presents once again with a history of return of back pain, now severe, dry cough, and weight loss of 5 kg associated with poor appetite and a general sense of ill health and fatigue. Investigations confirm the presence of widespread bone metastases, liver metastases, and lymphangitic carcinomatosis within the lung. A trial of palliative chemotherapy is associated with adverse effects, but no relief of symptoms. Pain relief is obtained with palliative radiotherapy, the use of sustained release morphine, reaching a dose of 90 mg every 12 h, and ibuprofen 400 mg three times daily. His cough improves with nebulization with normal saline 15 ml every 2 h when he is awake. Mr S.T. continues to lose weight, has little energy, and exhibits a pattern of increased drowsiness during the day and poor sleep at night. He will doze off for 1–3 h, awaken for a similar period of time, and then doze off again.

Question 7. You have controlled pain and cough. How can you further help Mr S.T. to obtain a good night's rest?

The necessary doses of opioids which Mr S.T. is taking may adversely affect his sleep patterns. Opioids are not classic hypnotics as, while they may cause drowsiness, they are not usually associated with restoring the normal sleep architecture. Initially, they tend to suppress REM activity and have a variable effect on NREM sleep patterns.[3] Moreover, the daytime drowsiness and napping secondary to opioid therapy will disturb the day–night pattern of rest. Although there is no research on rotating opioids to assist sleep, the benefits of alternating opioids when faced with undue adverse effects in other situations suggest that the trial of a sister opioid may be worth considering.

The use of CNS stimulants may be somewhat controversial in Mr S.T.'s case, as he has a history of anxiety. In other patients, CNS stimulants such as methylphenidate (starting with 5 mg in the morning and 5 mg at noon) can improve sleep, as daytime alertness is improved. The half-life of methylphenidate is short; therefore the stimulatory effects of a mid-day dose will be fully dissipated by the early evening. Methylphenidate may be safely used in patients who do not have a past history of paranoia or aggressive behaviour, who are not delirious (and are not likely to become so), and who present no significant risk associated with cardiac adrenergic stimulation[11].

In the case of Mr S.T., you decide not to recommend methylphenidate. You change morphine to hydromorphone. You suggest that Mr S.T. may once again start zopiclone and, again, studiously apply principles of good sleep hygiene.

Future directions

First and foremost, sleep problems must be a priority for research. The evidence base informing practice is modest. A recent Cochrane Review entitled 'Benzodiazepines and related drugs for insomnia in palliative care' concluded that 'despite a comprehensive search, no evidence from randomized controlled trials was evident'[12] They are concerned that any conclusions can be drawn; for the present we depend upon small studies, and extrapolation from research involving non-palliative care patients.

As stressed in this chapter and elsewhere in the text, depression commonly accompanies insomnia. Will sedative antidepressants such as mirtazapine used alone or in combination with zopiclone advance the field? Clinical trials are required.

Methylphenidate to improve daytime sleepiness is underused, in part because of its somewhat controversial use in children with attention-deficit disorder and its amphetamine pedigree. Modafinil is a newer agent which can combat daytime somnolence. Trials comparing it with methylphenidate are awaited.

Melatonin is a staple of health food stores and is widely used without medical supervision. Does it help? Data obtained in geriatric populations is equivocal; studies in chronically ill populations are yet to be carried out. Two caveats are obvious.

- Over-the-counter melatonin is an unregulated substance; content may vary from brand to brand.
- Melatonin is a hormone with multiple actions. Are these actions helpful in chronic illness states?

The above melange of promise and uncertainty illustrates the neglected state of sleep research, in sharp contrast with the importance of sleep. Hindu writings view sleep as an active process and spent in three states: wakefulness, dreaming sleep, and dreamless sleep. Hindu writings also recognize the clinical importance of sleep: 'who is moderate in sleep and wakefulness becomes ... the destroyer of pain' (*Bhagavad Gita*). To date the wisdom of ancient Hindu culture reflected in this quote is not sufficiently observed in modern medical practice.

References

1. **Anonymous** (2003) *National Sleep Disorders Research Plan*. Bethesda, MD: US Department of Health and Human Services, National Institutes of Health.
2. **Davidson, J.R., MacLean, A.W., Brundage, M.D., and Schulze, K.** (2002) Sleep disturbance in cancer patients. *Soc Sci Med*, **54**, 1309–21.
3. **Sateia, M.J., and Santulli, R.B.** (2003) Sleep in palliative care. In: Doyle D, Hanks GWC, MacDonald N (eds) *Oxford Textbook of Palliative Medicine* (3rd edn). Oxford: Oxford University Press, Chapter 8.16.
4. **Everitt, D.E., Avorn, J., and Baker, M.W.** (1990) Clinical decision-making in the evaluation and treatment of insomnia. *Am J Med*, **89**, 838.
5. **Patat, A., Paty, I., and Hindmarch, I.** (2001) Pharmacodynamic profile of zaleplon, a new non-benzodiazepine hypnotic agent. *Hum Psychopharmacol*, **16**, 369–92.

6. **Wagner, J., and Wagner, M.L.** (2000) Non-benzodiazepines for the treatment of insomnia. *Sleep Med Rev*, **4**, 551–81.
7. **Hesse, L.M., von Moltke, L.L., and Greenblatt, D.J.** (2003) Clinically important drug interactions with zopiclone, zolpidem and zaleplon. *CNS Drugs*, **17**, 513–32.
8. **Theobald, D.E., Kirsh, K.L., Holtsclaw, E. *et al.*** (2003) An open-label, crossover trial of mirtazapine (15 and 30 mg) in cancer patients with pain and other distressing symptoms. *J Pain Symptom Manage*, **25**, 7–8.
9. **Antilla, S.A., and Leinonen, E.V.** (2001) A review of the pharmacological and clinical profile of mirtazapine. *CNS Drug Rev*, **7**, 249–64.
10. **Kast, R.** (2001) Mirtazapine may be useful in treating nausea and insomnia of cancer chemotherapy. *Support Care Cancer*, **9**, 469–70.
11. **Bruera, E., and Watanabe, S.** (2002) Psychostimulants as adjuvant analgesics. *J Pain Symptom Manage*, **9**, 412–15.
12. **Hirst, A., and Sloan, R.** (2002) Benzodiazepines and related drugs for insomnia in palliative care. *Cochrane Database Syst Rev*, **4**, CD003346.

Chapter 12

Dyspnoea

Deborah Dudgeon

Attitude

To enable each student to:

- Demonstrate an appreciation of the suffering associated with dyspnoea and its devastating impact on the quality of life of the person and family

Skill

To enable each student to:

- Identify the physical findings associated with the clinical syndromes of superior vena cava syndrome, pleural effusion, collapse of lung, and pulmonary embolus.
- Demonstrate the appropriate techniques for positioning patients to minimize shortness of breath.
- Be able to use the various drugs that are helpful in combating the sensation of dyspnoea. Specifically, students will learn that dyspnoea should be treated with opioids in similar fashion to the way opioids are used in pain control.

Knowledge

To enable each student to:

- Describe the pathophysiology of dyspnoea.
- Describe the appropriate investigations and treatment of a person with suspected chronic obstructive pulmonary disease (COPD), superior vena cava syndrome, pleural effusion, loss of lung volume, radiation pneumonitis, and lymphangitic carcinomatosis.
- Describe the treatment of dyspnoea when it is not possible to treat the underlying disease.
- Describe the appropriate use of oxygen.
- Describe the management of 'death rattle'.

Mr G.R. is a 68 year-old-man whom you first started seeing 2 years ago. At that time he gave you a history of a recurrent cough productive of whitish sputum and slowly progressive shortness of breath. He was able to walk up the flight of stairs in his home but had to stop at least once to catch

Continued

his breath. He had smoked one to two packs of cigarettes per day for the previous 40 years. At the time you had taken a chest radiograph and pulmonary function tests and made a diagnosis of severe COPD. Despite extensive counselling he had not stopped smoking and had declined nicotine replacement therapy. In testing he had had a good response to a bronchodilator and so you had started him on an anticholinergic and a β-agonist on an as-needed basis. You gave him influenza and pneumococcal vaccinations and enrolled him on a rehabilitation programme.

Question 1. What is dyspnoea and how common is it?

Dyspnoea is an uncomfortable awareness of breathing. Dyspnoea, like pain, is multidimensional in nature, having not only physical elements but also affective components, which are shaped by previous experience. Stimulation of a number of receptors, responding to biochemical, mechanical, vascular, and psychogenic changes, can alter ventilation and result in the sensation of breathlessness.[1] Exertional dyspnoea is caused by increased ventilatory demand, impaired mechanical responses, or a combination of the two.[2] The only reliable measure of dyspnoea is the patient's self-report as no test correlates well with the feeling of breathlessness. It is a very common symptom in people with advanced disease. The prevalence of dyspnoea varies with the underlying disease: COPD, 95 per cent; congestive heart failure, 61 per cent; stroke, 37 per cent;[3] amyotrophic lateral sclerosis, 47–50 per cent; dementia, 70 per cent;[4] cancer, 46–70 per cent.[5,6]

Question 2. What are the risk factors for the development of COPD?

Cigarette smoking is the most important risk factor for the development of COPD. It is estimated that 15 per cent of one pack per day smokers and 25 per cent of two pack per day smokers will develop COPD. Other risk factors include second hand smoke, air pollution, occupational exposure, and α_1-antitrypsin deficiency.[7] Smoking cessation is the single most important therapeutic intervention. Studies show that forced expiratory volume in 1 second (FEV_1) may decrease by >75 ml/year in smokers; the age-related decline in non-smokers is only 30 ml/year.[7]

Question 3. What abnormalities might you see on a chest radiograph of someone with COPD?

The chest radiograph of someone with COPD will often have flattened diaphragms and an increased anteroposterior diameter.

Question 4. What pulmonary function tests would you do to determine if someone had COPD?

COPD is a disease state characterized by cough, dyspnoea, sputum production, and air-flow obstruction, and is most frequently caused by chronic bronchitis and emphysema.[8]

Pulmonary function tests are important for diagnosis, for assessment of severity and prognosis, and to follow the progression of the condition. Air-flow obstruction is best assessed by FEV_1 and lung volume with forced vital capacity (FVC). The diagnosis is established when FEV_1/FVC is ≤70 per cent of predicted value. Staging of COPD is based on FEV_1. A person is considered to have a moderate degree of COPD if FEV_1 is ≥50 per cent, severe if it is 35–49 per cent and very severe if it is ≤34 per cent.[8]

Question 5. How is 'a good response to a bronchodilator' defined?

A post-bronchodilator increase in FEV_1 of >15 per cent is considered a significant response to a bronchodilator.[7]

Question 6. What are the management goals in COPD?

Management goals in COPD are:

- to lessen airflow obstruction and improve symptoms
- to decrease airway inflammation
- to avoid secondary complications
- to maintain functional capacity
- to improve quality of life.

Question 7. Why would you have started Mr R on an anticholinergic drug and a β-agonist drug?

Anticholinergic drugs cause bronchodilatation by blocking cholinergic-mediated increases in bronchomotor tone and the vagally mediated bronchoconstriction induced by non-specific airway irritants. β_2-Agonists induce bronchodilation by stimulating β_2-adrenergic receptors in the airways. Anticholinergics have a slower onset of action and a longer half-life than β-agonists. They are also thought to have greater bronchodilator effects and fewer side effects than β_2-agonists and therefore are recommended for initial routine therapy, with β_2 agonists used on an 'as needed' basis.[7,9]

Question 8. Why give Mr R. vaccinations or enrol him in a rehabilitation programme?

As every respiratory infection can lead to airway inflammation and further deterioration in lung function, routine vaccinations are recommended in many countries. The influenza virus may cause COPD exacerbations and, as the vaccination is 70 per cent effective in reducing the morbidity of influenza, it is recommended that COPD patients receive yearly prophylaxis against the disease. *Streptococcus pneumoniae* is the most common community-acquired pneumonia and therefore pneumococcal vaccination every 10 years is recommended.[9]

Patients with advanced COPD usually severely limit their activity because of breathlessness with mild to moderate exercise. This lack of exercise leads to deconditioning and a further worsening of their breathlessness. Pulmonary rehabilitation programmes are designed to maintain an individual's maximum level of independence and functioning. Patients are taught the proper technique for using an inhaler, nutritional guidelines, exercise programmes for aerobic training, breathing and relaxation exercises, and energy conservation techniques. These programmes have demonstrated improvements in exercise endurance with decreased sensations of breathlessness.[7,10]

Many patients obtain relief of dyspnoea by leaning forward while sitting and supporting their upper arms on a table. This technique is effective in patients with emphysema as it improves the length–tension state of the diaphragm which increases efficiency. Pursed-lip breathing is also helpful as it slows the respiratory rate and increases intra-airway pressures, thus decreasing small-airway collapse during periods of increased dyspnoea.

> During the past year Mr R. has required admission to hospital three times for treatment of pneumonia. Following his last admission he was discharged with continuous oxygen at 3 l/min via nasal prongs. He is now finding it difficult to walk slowly without experiencing some breathlessness and finds that he is spending most of his time in his house. His most recent FEV_1 was 900 ml. He had been sleeping with two pillows at night and had lost 10 pounds in weight over the last year. Despite all these problems he had only managed to quit smoking completely 2 months previously.

Question 9. What are the indications for oxygen therapy in COPD patients?

Oxygen therapy in COPD patients with daytime hypoxaemia is the only treatment that has been shown to prolong life.[9] Current indications for long term oxygen therapy are:

- continuous oxygen
  - $PaO_2 \leq 55$ mmHg or oxygen saturation ≤88 per cent at rest
  - PaO_2 56–59 mmHg or oxygen saturation 89 per cent if any of the following are present:[9]
    - polycythaemia (haematocrit >56 per cent)
    - cor pulmonale
    - pulmonary hypertension
- non-continuous oxygen
  - $PaO_2 \leq 55$ mmHg or oxygen saturation ≤88 per cent during exertion
  - $PaO_2 \leq 55$ mmHg or oxygen saturation ≤ 88 per cent during sleep.

Question 10. Given Mr R.'s FEV_1, what is his prognosis?

The 1-year mortality is 30 per cent in COPD patients with $FEV_1 \leq 1$ litre. This information is not widely known. COPD patients with this finding have a prognosis certainly worse than the prognosis of many cancers.

Question 11. What are the possible consequences of malnutrition in a COPD patient? Are there any interventions that might help?

Malnutrition in COPD patients is associated with respiratory muscle wasting and weakness. There is evidence in COPD patients that re-feeding, exercise reconditioning, and anabolic steroids improve exercise tolerance.[10–12] Unfortunately, specific programmes designed to build up respiratory muscle strength are uncommon. At this time it is reasonable to try anti-cachexia measures as outlined in Chapter 7.

Mr R. presents to your office in significant distress. He relates that his shortness of breath has worsened over the past few weeks. He now has to sit up in a chair to sleep and is unable to lie flat for even a short period of time. His wife needs to help him with his bath and combing his hair, as even that amount of exertion causes him to become short of breath. He says he noticed some puffiness around his eyes about a week ago. He has lost another 10 pounds in weight in the past month. He denies any fever or night sweats, and his cough is productive of white sputum with occasional blood streaks.

On examination he does appear much thinner. He is using his accessory muscles for inspiration and has some nasal flaring. He has slight periorbital oedema and increased venous markings on his chest. When you raise his arm the veins do not flatten until his arm is above his head. The jugular venous pressure (JVP) is 8 cm above the sternal notch. After lying flat he becomes flushed and sits bolt upright to catch his breath. He has no lymphadenopathy. His liver is enlarged with a span of 14 cm. There is no detectable splenomegaly.

The laboratory findings show that his liver function is abnormal. His chest radiograph shows bilateral hilar adenopathy, which is worse on the right and extends to the azygous vein region.

Question 12. What is the clinical syndrome?

Mr R. has a superior vena cava syndrome. The physical findings are periorbital oedema, increased venous markings on the chest, delayed venous return, increased JVP, and inability to lie flat without becoming very short of breath and flushed.

Question 13. What are the most likely diagnoses? Do you need further diagnostic tests? What are they?

The most frequent neoplasms associated with the syndrome are lung, lymphomas, and tumours metastatic to the mediastinum.

If an underlying malignancy is present, a plain chest radiograph will often show the abnormality. Except in extreme circumstances, it is important to obtain a histological diagnosis before the initiation of any cancer treatment. In a case such as the scenario presented by Mr R., you will want to establish a definitive diagnosis very quickly. An open biopsy will give you the required information.

You arrange for a thoracic surgeon to perform a mediastinoscopy with biopsy. The pathologist is alerted that you need a diagnosis on the same day and that lymphoma is a possibility. However, the pathological diagnosis is small-cell carcinoma of the lung.

Question 14. What type of treatment would you initiate?

Mr R. is already receiving oxygen and with it he is not hypoxaemic. Once the diagnosis is made, dexamethasone can be used to decrease the swelling around the tumour and improve venous return. Dexamethasone is not recommended prior to diagnosis as lymphomas are usually very steroid sensitive, and shrinkage of the lymphoma would make it more difficult to diagnose or characterize histologically. Diuretics are also not indicated as they decrease venous return, further reducing preload with the potential to precipitate shock. Diuretics may also increase the risk of thrombosis. Small-cell lung cancer is very sensitive to chemotherapy. The disease responds as quickly to chemotherapy as to radiotherapy; the former is the preferred treatment owing to the systemic nature of small-cell carcinoma.

Mr R. received a course of dexamethasone, cisplatin, and VP-16. Within 24 h of his first treatment his wife noted that his face was less swollen. During his stay in hospital a CT of the chest and abdomen was performed. A mass in the area of the azygous vein, bilateral hilar adenopathy, and several liver metastases were identified. When he was discharged a week later, he could lie flat without any shortness of breath. His chest radiograph showed a 50 per cent reduction in the size of the tumour.

He received three further cycles of chemotherapy with an apparent complete response. He was back to his baseline breathlessness and had gained 10 pounds. He remained this way for about 4 months, but then returned to your office with worsening shortness of breath and a new onset of haemoptysis.

On examination, he is distressed, is using his accessory muscles, and has a respiratory rate of 28 bpm. His trachea is deviated to the right. His entire right thorax is dull to percussion, with absent tactile and vocal fremitus, and no audible air entry.

Question 15. What is the clinical syndrome?

Mr R. has signs of loss of lung volume on the right side. This can be caused by external compression of the mainstem bronchus or by an endobronchial lesion causing obstruction and collapse of the lung.

Question 16. What are the diagnostic tests?

A mass large enough to cause collapse of a lung will usually be evident on a plain chest radiograph, but a CT scan is more definitive. A bronchoscopy is necessary to demonstrate an endobronchial lesion.

Question 17. What are your treatment options?

External beam irradiation, laser therapy, electrocautery, cryotherapy, endobronchial irradiation, photodynamic therapy, and tracheobronchial stents are used to relieve endobronchial obstructions in appropriate cases.

A chest radiograph is obtained. It shows total collapse of the right lung with a marked increase in the hilar adenopathy, greatest on the right side.

Although further chemotherapy is an option for treatment of Mr R.'s tumour, he has adamantly stated that he wants no more of 'that poison' (despite his having few side effects and the tumour responding very well to his previous course of treatment). Therefore it is decided that he will receive external beam irradiation in an attempt to shrink the tumour and open the right mainstem bronchus.

The tumour proves to be very radiosensitive and within a week his breathing has again returned to baseline. On examination there is good air entry on the right side of his chest.

Unfortunately, he returns in 4 weeks with marked breathlessness. Before examining him, you wonder whether radiation pneumonitis could be causing his breathlessness, but the physical examination supports another diagnosis.

On examination he is very distressed, is using his accessory muscles, and has a respiratory rate of 36 breaths per minute (bpm). His trachea is deviated to the left (not to the right as previously). His entire right thorax is dull to percussion. There is decreased tactile and vocal fremitus on the right side. You note that his liver is now extending down to his umbilicus and is very hard and irregular.

Question 18. What is radiation pneumonitis?

Radiation pneumonitis is an acute inflammatory response to radiation treatments that include the lung in the field of radiation treatment. The clinical syndrome usually occurs 1–3 months after completion of radiation. The rate of symptomatic pneumonitis ranges from 1 to 34 per cent, with radiological changes from 13 to 100 per cent depending on the dose and fractionation schedule.[13]

Question 19. What signs and physical findings might be present?

Symptoms can include low-grade fever, congestion, cough, dyspnoea, and pleuritic chest pain. Physical signs in the chest are usually absent, but could include consolidation, pleural friction rub, or evidence of pleural effusion.[14]

Question 20. How would you treat it?

Corticosteroids are the mainstay of treatment for radiation pneumonitis. In more severe cases, oxygen and even ventilatory support (in a person with an otherwise good prognosis) may be required.[1]

Question 21. What is the clinical syndrome?

Mr R.'s clinical findings are consistent with a pleural effusion.

Question 22. What are the diagnostic tests?

A chest radiograph would confirm your clinical impression.

Question 23. What treatment would you initiate?

A thoracentesis is indicated for diagnostic and therapeutic reasons. [NB. Rapid removal of fluid (>1.5 litres) can induce pulmonary edema; one may need to stop earlier if increasing dyspnoea is noted.] The most probable cause of the pleural effusion is progression of intrathoracic malignancy, but pleural fluid cytology, measurement of lactic dehydrogenase levels, protein, pH, cell count and culture, and sensitivity would help to confirm this. Removal of the pleural fluid should help to relieve Mr R.'s shortness of breath. Occasionally, dyspnoea will not be relieved by removal of the fluid as the lung has collapsed or is too fibrosed to re-expand. If there is significant improvement in Mr R.'s shortness of breath, you would insert a chest tube for further drainage and pleurodesis. Pleurodesis involves injecting a chemical, such as doxycycline or talc, into the pleural space, when it has been completely drained, to create inflammation and stick the pleural surfaces together so that fluid cannot re-accumulate. As pleurodesis is often painful, intrapleural lidocaine is administered before instillation of the sclerosing agent to reduce local pain. Patients should also be premedicated and have adequate analgesic available after the procedure.[1]

A chest radiograph demonstrated a large right-sided pleural effusion that was pushing the mediastinum to the left and causing the trachea to deviate to the left. There was also evidence of a diffuse infiltrative process in the left lung, consistent with lymphangitic spread of the tumour.

A chest tube was inserted and over 3 days a total of 2.5 litres of fluid was drained. Unfortunately, Mr R. remained quite short of breath, pausing to catch a breath after speaking only a sentence. A repeat radiograph demonstrated a re-expansion of his right lung and no significant pleural fluid, but the diffuse infiltrative process was present in both lungs. Pleurodesis with doxycycline was performed to prevent the re-accumulation of fluid in the right pleural space.

Question 24. What is lymphangitic carcinomatosis of the lung?

Lymphangitic carcinomatosis of the lung is a term used to describe infiltration of the lymph system of the lung by tumour.

Question 25. What are the treatment options?

The most effective approach is oncological treatment directed against the underlying tumour; however, as in this case, that is often not possible. Although there are no randomized trials, anecdotal evidence suggests that there is benefit from corticosteroids and diuretics.

Question 26. What options for management are there when you are unable to treat the underlying disease?

A Cochrane Review of the literature confirmed that oral or parenteral opioids are effective in relieving the sensation of shortness of breath.[15] In an emergency opioids are given by an intravenous or subcutaneous route. This is because the onset of action is 10 min for intravenous administration and 30 min for subcutaneous administration. Opioids can be given orally if rapid control of breathlessness is not required. The authors of the Cochrane Review found no evidence to support the use of nebulized opioids; nebulized morphine was no more effective than nebulized saline for the relief of breathlessness.[15] The proposed mechanisms for the effects of opioids on dyspnoea include an alteration in the perception of breathlessness, a decrease in the ventilatory drive and the response to stimuli such as hypoxia and hypercapnia, and a decrease in oxygen consumption at any given level of exercise.

Some health professionals fear that the respiratory-depressant effects of opioids will induce respiratory failure and hasten death. The Cochrane Review identified 11 studies that contained information on blood gases or oxygen saturation after intervention with opioids.[15] Only one study reported a significant increase in $Paco_2$ but it did not rise above 40 mmHg.[16] Whether clinically significant hypoventilation and a consequent increase in $Paco_2$ develop following opioid therapy depends on the history of previous exposure to opioids, the rate of increase of the opioid dose, and possibly the route of administration as well.[17] The goal is clearly to decrease the distressing sensation of breathlessness. In a situation such as this, as with a person in pain, it is appropriate to use opioids to relieve suffering.

You prescribe morphine 5 mg orally every 4 h and 2.5 mg orally every 2 h as needed for breathlessness. You also order a trial of prednisone 50 mg orally daily and furosemide (frusemide) 40 mg orally daily for 3 days and change Mr R.'s bronchodilators so that they are now given by nebulizer every 4 h.

Four hours after you have left the ward, you receive a call from the nurse that Mr R. is in extreme distress. You have previously discussed the extent of his disease and the fact that there is no further disease-oriented treatment. Mr R. has clearly stated that he does not want to be resuscitated or to have any life-prolonging measures; he just wants to be kept comfortable.

When you enter the room he gasps, 'I can't breathe! I feel like I'm choking! Do something!' He is sitting bolt upright and leaning forward. His wife has been called to the hospital. The nurse has placed an over-bed table in a position that allows him to rest on it.

On examination he is very distressed. His respiratory rate is 48 bpm. He has evidence of central cyanosis and has marked indrawing of his intercostal muscles with paradoxical movement of the diaphragm. His lungs have diffuse crackles scattered throughout. His JVP is elevated to his jaw when he is sitting upright. He has a loud P2 heart sound.

Mr R. is very distressed and requires reassurance that he will not choke to death. It is important that someone stays with him while drugs are prepared and tests arranged. While the nurse is preparing the morphine you have ordered, you measure some arterial blood gases. He is already receiving oxygen via nasal prongs at 5 l/min.

Question 27. How would you treat his dyspnoea?

Mr R. is hypoxic and requires an increase in his oxygen to raise his oxygen saturation to >90 per cent. Patients can also obtain some relief with a cool fan blowing on their face. It is thought that this effect is mediated through stimulation of the receptors of the trigeminal nerve.[18]

Question 28. Are there other medications in addition to opioids that have shown benefit for treatment of breathlessness?

Although not commonly used, the current evidence supports the administration of phenothiazines, such as promethazine or chlorpromazine, alone or in combination with morphine for the treatment of dyspnoea.[1] A double-blind placebo-controlled randomized trial demonstrated that a combination of morphine and promethazine significantly improved exercise tolerance without worsening dyspnoea compared with placebo, morphine alone, or a combination of morphine and prochlorperazine.[19] Clinical trials to determine the effectiveness of anxiolytics have had conflicting results and there is little support for their use in the treatment of chronic breathlessness.[1] Anecdotally, they are useful for people who have acute severe breathlessness.

Mr R. shows signs of right heart failure, probably secondary to a large pulmonary embolism. You prescribe intravenous furosemide, salbutamol, and ipratropium bromide by nebulizer and give him morphine 5 mg intravenous push (IVP). After 10 min he is still very breathless and so you repeat the morphine 5 mg IVP. After a further 10 minutes his breathing is more settled, but he says

Continued

he is still not comfortable and so you repeat the morphine 5 mg IVP. Following this last dose, his respiratory rate is 24 bpm and he says that he is more comfortable. You increase his routine morphine dose to 20 mg orally every 4 h with 10 mg orally every 2 h as needed. Over the next 24 h he needs about four extra doses of morphine and says he is still not comfortable with his breathing. You change the morphine to 10 mg subcutaneously and add the phenothiazine, methotrimeprazine (laevomepromazine) 2.5 mg subcutaneously every 6 h. This combination settles him and he says that he is very comfortable.

Unfortunately, over the next few days his condition deteriorates further. He is no longer responding. He is very congested and quite restless. His family is very distressed as it sounds as if he is 'drowning in his own fluid!'

Question 29. Is there anything you can prescribe?

The 'death rattle' is very distressing for the family or others at the bedside. At times simple repositioning of the patient can help to relieve the secretions. Suctioning of secretions is generally not recommended, as it can be very uncomfortable for the patient and can cause significant agitation and distress. Medications such as hyoscine hydrobromide, atropine sulphate, glycopyrrolate, and hyoscine butylbromide are usually effective and prevent the need for suctioning.[20]

You prescribe hyoscine hydrobromide 0.3–0.6 mg subcutaneously every 3 h as needed. He receives one dose and his respiration becomes less noisy and laboured. He dies peacefully 12 h later with his family at his bedside.

Conclusion

The aetiology and treatment of the symptom dyspnoea have received relatively little attention in research and the literature. More studies need to be conducted to determine the aetiology of breathlessness and the receptors responsible for the sensation in different disease states. It may then be possible to give more targeted therapies that are directed at interrupting those specific receptors.

References

1. **Dudgeon, D.** (2002) Managing dyspnea and cough. *Hematol Oncol Clin North Am,* **16**, 557–77.
2. **O'Donnell, D.E.** (1999) Exertional breathlessness in chronic respiratory disease. In: Mahler D (ed) *Dyspnea.* New York: Marcel Dekker, 97–147.
3. **Zeppetella, G.** (1998) The palliation of dyspnea in terminal disease. *Am J Hosp Palliat Care,* **15**, 322–30.
4. **Voltz, R., and Borasio, G.D.** (1997) Palliative therapy in the terminal stage of neurological disease. *J Neurol,* **244** (Suppl 4), S2–10.
5. **Dudgeon, D.J., Kristjanson, L., Sloan, J.A., Lertzman, M., and Clement, K.** (2001) Dyspnea in cancer patients: prevalence and associated factors. *J Pain Symptom Manage,* **21**, 95–102.
6. **Reuben, D.B., and Mor, V.** (1986) Dyspnea in terminally ill cancer patients. *Chest,* **89**, 234–6.
7. **Cordova, F.C., and Criner, G.J.** (1997) Management of advanced chronic obstructive pulmonary disease. *Compr Ther,* **23**, 413–24.

8. **Celli, B.R.** (1998) Standards for the optimal management of COPD. A summary. *Chest,* **113** (Suppl), 283S–7S.
9. **Donado, J.R., and Hill, N.S.** (1998) Outpatient management. *Respir Care Clin North Am,* **4**, 391–423.
10. **O'Donnell, D.E., McGuire, M., Samis, L., and Webb, K.A.** (1995) The impact of exercise reconditioning on breathlessness in severe chronic airflow limitation. *Am J Respir Crit Care Med,* **152**, 2005–13.
11. **Whittaker, J.S., Ryan, C.F., Buckley, P.A., and Road, J.D.** (1990) The effects of refeeding on peripheral and respiratory muscle function in malnourished chronic obstructive pulmonary disease patients. *Am Rev Respir Dis,* **142**, 283–8.
12. **Schols, A.M., Soeters, P.B., Mostert, R., Pluymers, R.J., and Wouters, E.F.** (1995) Physiologic effects of nutritional support and anabolic steroids in patients with chronic obstructive pulmonary disease. A placebo-controlled randomized trial. *Am J Respir Crit Care Med,* **152**, 1268–74.
13. **Movsas, B., Raffin, T.A., Epstein, A.H., and Link, C.J.J.** (1997) Pulmonary radiation injury. *Chest,* **111**, 1061–76.
14. **McDonald, S., Rubin, P., Phillips, T.L., and Marks, L.B.** (1995) Injury to the lung from cancer therapy: clinical syndromes, measurable endpoints, and potential scoring systems. *Int J Radiat Oncol Biol Phys,* **31**, 1187–1203.
15. **Jennings, A.L., Davies, A., Higgins, J.P.T., and Broadley, K.** (2001) Opioids for the palliation of breathlessness in terminal illness. *Cochrane Review* **4,** Oxford: Update Software.
16. **Woodcock, A.A., Johnson, M.A., and Geddes, D.M.** (1982) Breathlessness, alcohol and opiates. *N Engl J Med,* **306**, 1363–4.
17. **Dudgeon, D.J., and Rosenthal, S.** (1996) Management of dyspnea and cough in patients with cancer. *Hematol Oncol Clin North Am,* **10**, 157–71.
18. **Schwartzstein, R.M., Lahive, K., Pope, A., Weinberger, S.E., and Weiss, J.W.** (1987) Cold facial stimulation reduces breathlessness induced in normal subjects. *Am Rev Respir Dis,* **136**, 58–61.
19. **Light, R.W., Stansbury, D.W., and Webster, J.S.** (1996) Effect of 30 mg of morphine alone or with promethazine or prochlorperazine on the exercise capacity of patients with COPD. *Chest,* **109**, 975–81.
20. **Dudgeon, D.** (2001) Dyspnea, death rattle, and cough. In: Ferrell BR, Coyle N (eds) *Textbook of Palliative Nursing.* New York: Oxford University Press, 164–74.

Chapter 13

Cough

Natalie Whiting

Attitude

To enable each student to:

- Characterize the impact of cough on patients and their caregivers.
- Construct an individualized approach to the assessment and treatment of cough based on stage of underlying illness, potential risks and benefits of treatment, and patient's and family's goals of care.

Skill

To enable each student to:

- Use non-pharmacological interventions to alleviate cough.
- Apply, when possible, an evidence-based approach with medications useful to relieve cough.
- Recognize situations in which cough suppression is inadvisable.

Knowledge

To enable each student to:

- Describe the pathophysiology of cough.
- Classify the causes of cough in patients with advanced cancer.
- Identify the reversible causes of cough and their treatment.

Mr A. is a 72-year-old, retired cabinet-maker, who was diagnosed with squamous cell carcinoma of the lung 18 months ago. At the time of diagnosis he was found to have a 10 cm tumour in the lower lobe of the left lung. The mediastinal lymph nodes were negative for malignancy. Because of pre-existing poor cardiac and lung function, he was not a candidate for surgical resection of the tumour. Instead, he received local radiotherapy treatment, at a dose of 5500 cGy in 20 fractions, which resulted in partial regression of his lung primary. Since his treatment, he has had mild dyspnoea on exertion and a 10-kg weight loss, but otherwise has been stable.

Mr A. lives in an apartment with elevator access. He has been married to L., his second wife, for 6 years, and she is very supportive. Together they have four grown children from previous marriages. A nurse from a community agency visits Mr A. at home twice a week.

Over the past month he has developed a dry nagging cough that keeps him up at night and causes soreness of his abdominal wall muscles. He finds it difficult to catch his breath during a coughing spell, and is frightened that he will choke. His wife finds it difficult to calm him during these episodes.

Question 1. What is the pathophysiology of cough?

Coughing is a reflex action that serves both a protective and cleansing function for the respiratory tract. It prevents the entry of potentially harmful material into the airways and lungs, and clears away excess mucous and foreign particles.[1]

Cough usually results from stimulation of receptors in the larynx, pharynx, and proximal tracheobronchial tree; irritation of small airways and alveoli does not induce cough. However, stimulation of receptors in the pleura, pericardium, diaphragm, sinuses, and tympanic membranes may also lead to cough. Information from these areas is carried to the 'cough centre' in the brainstem (medulla). When the cough centre is activated, an efferent loop integrates respiratory muscle, bronchial tree, and laryngeal activity, causing forceful expiration of air against and through the glottis. Cough may also be produced voluntarily, bypassing the brainstem cough centre.

Inadequate respiratory muscle strength, inability to appose the vocal cords (because of vocal cord paralysis), or the presence of thick dehydrated respiratory secretions can compromise a person's ability to cough effectively. Conversely, overly vigourous coughing can have distressing consequences including rib fractures, pneumothorax, incontinence, and patient/family fatigue.

Question 2. How significant a symptom is cough in patients with lung cancer?

Cough is one of the most common and severe symptoms in lung cancer, and is often not as well controlled as other symptoms. In a study of patients with non-small-cell lung cancer, cough affected more than 60 per cent of patients at initial presentation. Before the time of death, 80 per cent of patients in this group had suffered from cough.[2] Chronic cough can interfere with sleep, cause pain, precipitate vomiting, interfere with speech, and lead to pathological fracture. Episodes of uncontrolled coughing are frightening and can generate a fear of choking. Although cough is less prevalent in cancers that are not of lung origin, chronic cough still affects about a third of patients with advanced cancer of any type.[3] The incidence in patients with endstage non-respiratory disease approaches that of lung cancer.

Question 3. How do you classify the many causes of cough in cancer patients?

Cancer may cause cough directly by direct tumour invasion of the bronchial mucosa. It may also cause cough indirectly by predisposing patients to other conditions such as infection, radiation pneumonitis, pulmonary embolus, or aspiration. Medical conditions unrelated to cancer may also cause cough in cancer patients. When possible and appropriate, treatment for cough should address the underlying cause (Table 13.1).

Table 13.1 Causes of cough in advanced cancer[1,3,5]

Directly caused by cancer	Indirectly caused by cancer	Unrelated to cancer
Airway, parenchymal or pleural tumour	Pulmonary emboli	Respiratory infection
Lymphangitic carcinomatosis	Pulmonary aspiration	COPD
Superior vena cava syndrome	Adverse effects of chemotherapy/radiotherapy	Asthma
Mediastinal tumour	Weakness and dehydration (can lead to retention of thickened mucous)	Gastro-oesophageal reflux
Pleural or pericardial effusion		CHF
		Medications
		Post-nasal drip

Question 4. What information will you want to obtain from this patient on history?

What is the nature of the cough?

- productive or non-productive
- what material is expectorated (bloody, purulent).

Are there any symptoms to suggest a reversible cause?

- fever and purulent sputum might suggest infection
- cough triggered by eating or drinking might suggest gastric reflux and aspiration
- shortness of breath, orthopnoea, or pedal oedema might suggest congestive heart failure (CHF).

Is the patient taking any medication that could induce cough?

- ACE inhibitors.

Does the patient have any underlying conditions (unrelated to the cancer) that might cause cough?

- CHF
- chronic obstructive pulmonary disease (COPD)
- asthma
- gastro oesophageal reflux
- smoking history.

Can the patient identify any triggers for the cough?

- environmental irritants
- use of supplemental oxygen.

What treatments have been tried and how effective were they?

Mr A. tells you he has not had any fever or chills recently. His cough is generally dry and does not produce any mucous. However, for the past week he has been coughing up some bright red blood four or five times a day, a tablespoon at the most.

He has a 40 pack-year history of smoking with subsequent COPD, and a dilated cardiomyopathy secondary to prior alcohol use. He stopped drinking all alcohol and lost interest in smoking a few months before his cancer diagnosis.

He has been taking two inhalers, a β-agonist and an anticholinergic agent, regularly for several years. For 2 weeks, he has also been using a sweet-tasting over-the-counter cough syrup containing dextromethorphan, at a dose of 30 mg by mouth every 4 h, with minimal improvement. At present he has home oxygen therapy, and uses 3 l/min unhumidified oxygen by nasal prongs on an as-needed basis.

You ask him a few additional questions and determine that he has not had any orthopnoea or recent swelling of his feet or legs. He is not on any non-steroidal anti-inflammatory drugs or anticoagulants that might increase his risk of bleeding. Although his nostrils are dry, he has not had any nosebleeds since starting on the oxygen.

Question 5. What specific findings will you look for on physical examination?

Given Mr A.'s history of heart and lung disease, you will want to look for signs of an acute exacerbation of either COPD or CHF. You will also want to rule out other common and potentially treatable causes of cough such as infection and aspiration.

Head and neck:

- lymphadenopathy, tracheal deviation, elevated jugular venous pressure (JVP), post-nasal drip, hoarseness of voice
- aspiration upon swallowing water.

Respiratory:

- use of accessory muscles of respiration, pursed lip breathing
- wheezes, crackles, decreased air entry, or bronchial breath sounds
- dullness on percussion of the lungs.

Cardiac:

- extra heart sounds (S3, S4), muffling of heart sounds, peripheral oedema.

On physical examination, there is no evidence of infection, acute COPD exacerbation, aspiration, or CHF.

Question 6. What investigations will you consider ordering?

You order a chest radiograph and compare it with the previous one. You measure Mr A.'s oxygen saturation on room air. His respirologist suggests a bronchoscopy to confirm the source of the haemoptysis and Mr A. agrees.

On room air at rest, his oxygen saturation is 96 per cent. Chest radiography shows an enlarged heart, a stable mass, and radiation fibrosis in the left lower lobe. There is an enlarging mass in the left hilum that suggests progression of his lung cancer. There is no evidence of pneumonia or pulmonary oedema. A bronchoscopy is performed which reveals a small amount of blood in the upper airway, including the trachea, and on the vocal cords. The site of haemoptysis is localized to a segment of the left upper lobe where there is a mass causing intraluminal narrowing of the bronchus.

Question 7. Is there a treatment you can offer to address the underlying cause of his cough and haemoptysis?

Thoracic reirradiation can be an effective treatment for palliation of cough and haemoptysis in patients with recurrent or progressive lung cancer. Several retrospective reviews demonstrate relief of cough following re-treatment in approximately 60 per cent of patients and relief of haemoptysis in 80–90 per cent.[6] There can be a risk of radiation pneumonitis if the cumulative radiation dose to the lung tissue is too high. Factors that determine whether re-treatment is possible include previous radiation dosage, overlap of treatment fields, and time elapsed since last treatment. Consultation with a radiation oncologist is essential and will help to quantify the potential risks and benefits.

In consultation with the radiation oncologist, you determine that a second course of palliative radiotherapy might improve Mr A.'s cough and decrease the risk of further haemoptysis. Mr A. tells you that he is still enjoying the quality of his day-to-day life, despite some limitation in activity. He is frightened by the coughing spasms and blood and would like them to be treated if possible. He did not have any significant side effects, except fatigue, after his last course of radiation and is willing to have another course. He tells you that he is 'not ready to give up fighting yet'. You suggest a consultation with a medical oncologist to explore coordinating chemotherapy with radiotherapy, and Mr A. agrees to consider this.

Question 8. What symptomatic measures can you suggest to help control his cough?

Non-pharmacological interventions

Environmental modifications:

- humidify living environment and supplemental oxygen
- avoid airway irritants such as perfumes and cigarette smoke
- consider positional factors—elevate head of bed for reflux or heart failure.

Other interventions

- chest physiotherapy and suctioning may help to clear mucus
- keep the mouth moist with adequate fluid intake and use of lozenges
- placement of an oesophageal stent may help to avoid aspiration if a tracheobronchial fistula exists
- injection of a paralysed vocal cord may strengthen the valsalva part of the cough reflex and thereby enhance the ability of the cough to clear secretions.

Pharmacological agents

In the same way that medications are used for pain control, medications used to treat cough should be dosed in a proactive rather than a reactive way. When possible, a regular dose of an antitussive should be used to prevent cough, with a smaller dose available for breakthrough as needed.

Demulcents

Demulcents are sugar solutions and are found in most-over-the counter cough syrups. They are often the base for cough syrups containing opioids or dextromethorphan. However, they may act to inhibit cough even in the absence of other pharmacologically active ingredients. Their mechanism of action is not fully known.

Demulcents may inhibit cough by:[7]

- increasing saliva production and swallowing
- providing a protective barrier over sensory receptors in the pharynx
- stimulating local nerve endings and inhibiting the cough reflex via a gating mechanism.

Opioids

All opioids have antitussive activity. Although codeine is commonly used to treat cough, it is not superior to other opioids and has no added benefit when a high dose of another opioid is already being used for analgesia.[1]

Opioids may inhibit cough by:[7]

- suppressing the cough centre in the medulla
- inhibiting opioid receptors in the lung periphery
- decreasing mucus production and stimulating ciliary mucous clearance.

Opioids used to treat cough produce the same side effects (nausea, drowsiness, constipation) as opioids used for other indications. These side effects should be anticipated and prevented whenever possible.

Dextromethorphan

Over 200 non-opioid antitussive medications have been identified, but only dextromethorphan has been shown to be as effective as codeine.[8] Dextromethorphan is active at central nervous system receptors that are separate from opioid receptors. A usual starting dose of dextromethorphan is 15–30 mg by mouth every 4 h. Side effects are uncommon at this dose.

Benzonatate

Benzonatate, an oral local anaesthetic, inhibits cough by anaesthetizing the vagal stretch receptors in the bronchi, alveoli, and pleura. It may also act centrally in the medullary cough centre.[5] The majority of evidence for its use is in non-cancer patients. There are three cancer case reports in which 100–200 mg by mouth three times a day was found to be effective for opioid-resistant cough within 24 h of initiation.[9] Benzonatate is not available in some countries, including Canada.

> Mr A. received a course of palliative radiotherapy, 2000 cGy in five fractions, to the hilum of his left lung with no side effects. His haemoptysis resolved within 48 h.
>
> Because he has tried dextromethorphan at a therapeutic dose with no effect, you decide to recommend an opioid preparation to treat his cough while the radiation therapy takes effect. He dislikes the taste of the cough syrup and so you initiate codeine tablets at a dose of 15 mg by mouth every 4 h with a breakthrough dose of 7.5 mg by mouth every 2 h as needed. You counsel him regarding potential opioid side effects and provide him with a prescription for a stool softener and stimulant laxative to prevent constipation. He takes the codeine regularly for 10 days, during which time his cough is well controlled.
>
> You see him in follow-up 3 weeks after the radiation therapy. By this time, he has been able to reduce the codeine to a single dose at bedtime with only occasional recurrence of his cough. He is sleeping better and the soreness in his abdominal muscles has resolved. He becomes anxious while recalling his earlier coughing spells. You ask him what was most frightening for him and he says: 'I worry that if it happens again I could choke to death. Just thinking about it makes me feel panicked all over again.'

Question 10. How will you counsel Mr A. regarding his fear of choking to death?

> After giving Mr A. an opportunity to summarize the events of the past month, you reflect on some of the emotions he has described. You begin by legitimizing and normalizing Mr A.'s fears of choking. In your position as a palliative care provider, you have encountered many other people with

respiratory illnesses who have experienced the same fears. You review with Mr A. and his wife what they should do if he has further coughing spells at home. This might include taking a breakthrough dose or calling the community nurse. You reassure Mr A. that there are a variety of medications available to treat cough and breathlessness which you can use in the future if necessary. You reinforce that, in your experience, these treatments are adequate to relieve symptoms, even in the last weeks or days of life. You make plans to follow up with Mr A., and give him a way of contacting the clinic if symptoms arise sooner. You arrange for him to meet the palliative care team's physiotherapist, who teaches him relaxation breathing techniques to use at home when he feels anxious.

Further clinical considerations

Before initiating an aggressive anti-tussive program, consider whether cough suppression is in the patient's best interest or if it might prevent clearance of infectious material or mucous which should be expelled.

Cough caused by bronchospasm may respond to inhaled bronchodilators such as anticholinergics or β-adrenergic agonists. These should generally be considered in any patient with a cough and a prior smoking history.

If an inflammatory cause or lymphangitic carcinomatosis is present, corticosteroids such as prednisone or dexamethasone may be beneficial.

For productive coughs, adequate hydration and chest physiotherapy may help to clear secretions. Over-the-counter syrups containing expectorants and mucolytics are often employed to 'thin' secretions, but there is little evidence of their efficacy.

At the end of life, when swallowing is compromised, cough may occur secondary to pooling of upper respiratory tract secretions and saliva. At this stage, use of anticholinergic agents may help to decrease mucus production and reduce the cough stimulus.

Future research directions

There is a theoretical possibility that opioid and non-opioid antitussives may act synergistically to inhibit cough.[1] However, the question has not been thoroughly addressed. Co-administration of dextromethorphan and opioids is a reasonable part of an overall antitussive regimen.

The use of nebulized local anaesthetics, such as lidocaine and bupivucaine, to suppress chronic cough has been described in case series. The effectiveness of these agents in cough secondary to malignant causes has not yet been studied.[10,11]

The antitussive properties of compounds with activity at different opioid receptor subtypes are currently being investigated in animal models.

References

1. **Hagen, N.A.** (1991) Management of cough in cancer patients. *J Pain Symp Manage*, **6**, 257–62.
2. **Muers, M.F., and Round, C.D.** (1993) Palliation of symptoms in non-small cell lung cancer: a study by the Yorkshire Regional Cancer Organization thoracic group. *Thorax*, **48**, 339–43.
3. **Donnelly, S., and Walsh, D.** (1995) The symptoms of advanced cancer. *Semin Oncol*, **22**, 67–72.
4. **Dudgeon, D.J.** (2002) Managing dyspnea and cough. *Hematol Oncol Clin North Am*, **16**, 557–77.
5. **Homsi, H., Walsh, D., and Nelson, K.** (2001) Important drugs for cough in advanced cancer. *Support Care Cancer*, **9**, 565–74.

6. **Gressen, E.L., Werner-Wasik, M., Cohn, J. *et al.*** (2000) Thoracic reirradiation for symptomatic relief after prior radiotherapeutic management for lung cancer. *Am J Clin Oncol*, **23**, 160–3.
7. **Fuller, R.W., and Jackson, D.M.** (1990) Physiology and treatment of cough. *Thorax*, **45**, 425–30.
8. **Eddy, N.B., Friebel, H., Hahn, K.J. *et al.*** (1969) Codeine and its alternatives for pain and cough relief. Potential alternatives for cough relief. *Bull WHO*, **40**, 639–719.
9. **Doona, M., and Walsh, D.** (1997) Benzonatate for opioid-resistant cough in advanced cancer. *Palliat Med*, **12**, 55–8.
10. **Howard, P.C., Cayton, R.M., Brennan, S.R. *et al.*** (1977) Lignocaine aerosol and persistent cough. *Br J Dis Chest*, **71**, 19–24.
11. **Sander, R.V., and Kirkpatrick, M.B.** (1984) Prolonged suppression of cough after inhalation of lidocaine in a patient with sarcoid. *JAMA*, **252**, 2456–7.

Chapter 14

AIDS

Daphne Lobb, Jacqueline Fraser, Millie Cumming, and Sharon Duncan

Attitude

To enable each student to:

- Be aware of the fluctuations in the course of AIDS, and in the uncertainty of prognosis.
- Recognize that medications are a major burden in AIDS, and that there is a need for frequent reassessment of medications with regard to the benefits versus burden of continuing medications.
- Understand that very active acute treatment can go hand in hand with palliative measures throughout the course of AIDS.
- Appreciate the complex nature of disease processes that may coexist in the course of AIDS.

Skill

To enable each student to:

- Describe the classes of medication that not only prevent or treat the active underlying condition but also increase comfort [e.g. prevention and treatment of *Pneumocystis carinii* pneumonia (PCP) results in less distressing dyspnoea].
- Describe the differential diagnosis for common syndromes in endstage AIDS (e.g. dyspnoea, altered mental state, diarrhoea).
- Articulate to patients and families the balancing of aggressive treatment while maintaining an overall focus on end-of-life care.

Knowledge

To enable each student to:

- Relate the pathophysiology of AIDS to its course and therapy.
- Describe the rationale behind the continuation or discontinuation of antiretroviral medications (ARVs) in endstage AIDS.
- Describe the classes of medication for prophylaxis and treatment of HIV-related illnesses.
- Be familiar with investigation and diagnosis of common HIV-related opportunistic infections and malignancies [e.g. PCP, cytomegalovirus (CMV), lymphoma].

Mr D.C. is a 41-year-old man who has been HIV positive for 15 years. He developed PCP 2 years ago at which time he was diagnosed with AIDS. He went on to develop Kaposi's sarcoma (KS) 1 year ago. He is presently receiving chemotherapy for this. He has received ARVs intermittently for the past 4 years. He has become resistant to many of them and most recently is struggling with side effects from the current regimen. His CD4 count is 40 cells/mm^3 (the normal CD4 count is 600–1000 cells/mm^3) and his viral load is >100 000 RNA copies/ml. (A higher viral load is associated with more active virus in blood and a poorer prognosis. The goal of ARVs is to achieve an undetectable viral load.) D.C.'s partner is also HIV positive but has not developed AIDS. His partner is exhausted because D.C. has only recently recovered from a bout of bacterial pneumonia.

D.C.'s family physician suggests that he go into the hospital's palliative care unit for a week of respite. This would give his partner a well-needed break, and while he is in hospital the physicians could reassess chronic neuropathic leg pain that has been increasing for the past few weeks. Currently he is receiving the following medications: didanosine (DDI) EC 400 mg orally daily; saquinavir HGC 1000 mg orally twice daily; Combivir® (lamuvudine and zidovudine) one tablet twice daily; co-trimoxazole DS one tablet daily; azithromycin 1200 mg orally weekly; gabapentin 300g orally three times daily; trazadone 200 mg orally at bedtime.

Note: The patient has not been taking his ARVs regularly and has skipped some doses.

Question 1. You are the admitting physician on the unit. What would you want to review with the patient on admission?

The patient should be aware of his progressive disease, understand the palliative care approach and benefits, and agree to the philosophy of care of the palliative care unit. In many units there is a policy that a do not resuscitate (DNR) order is in place prior to admission. Defining when a patient has entered the last days of life is more difficult owing to the effectiveness of newer antiretroviral therapies, the increasing life expectancy, and the resultant view of HIV illness as a chronic disease. Combining active aggressive therapy and a comfort-focused palliative approach represents a shift in care which is often unclear for both patients and their medical caregivers. However, there is a point when CD4 counts remain low, viral loads are rising, ARVs are failing, choices for new medications are running out, and symptom management becomes the paramount goal. These patients have often lived with the disease for many years and have had numerous episodes of serious illness (e.g. opportunistic infections, lymphomas, and KS) secondary to it. Patients are often unable to continue the complicated regimes of dozens of pills per day and stop their ARVs, with resulting worsening of their disease.

D.C. has had HIV for 15 years, has exhausted most of his ARV options, and is considering stopping them because of side effects. He knows he is much sicker than even 6 months ago. He is not completely comfortable with a DNR order, as he has relied on aggressive treatment in the past. However, he agrees to a DNR order for this admission and does not want to discuss the topic any further at this point.

You review the goals of respite. It includes a review of his symptoms, a rest for his partner and other caregivers for 1 week, and an opportunity for him to get to know the staff in case of future symptom management admissions. You introduce the team and indicate to the patient that they are here to be of support to his partner and family as well.

Table 14.1 Prophylaxis for opportunistic infection

Pathogen	Indication	Regimen
Pneumocystis carinii	CD4 cell count <200/ml or <14%, oropharyngeal candidiasis, or an AIDS-defining illness	Trimethoprim 160 mg/sulfamethoxazole 800 mg daily (if allergic, dapsone and pyramethamine)
Toxoplasma gondii	IgG antibody to toxoplasma and CD4 cell count <100/ml	Trimethoprim 160 mg/sulfamethoxazole 800 mg daily
Mycobacterium tuberculosis	5 TU Mantoux skin test >5mm or contact with active tuberculosis	Isoniazide 300 mg orally daily + pyridoxine 25 mg orally daily × 9 mos
Mycobacterium avium complex	CD4 cell count <50/ml	Azithromycin 1200 mg orally weekly

Question 2. When reviewing his medications you notice that he is on a number of antibiotics. Are these medications helpful and do they need to continue?

A number of opportunistic infections are common in HIV infection and their incidence correlates with the level of immunosuppression. Prophylactic treatment can prevent certain opportunistic infections and this prevention can greatly improve the quality of life (Table 14.1).

It is helpful to be familiar with late complications of HIV infection when working in palliative care (Table 14.2). As noted above, some of these late complications can be prevented with medications. For others, treatment is largely symptomatic and will be discussed in the remainder of this chapter.

Question 3. What questions would you ask with regard to his neuropathic leg pain?

A pain history should be taken with specific attention to quality of pain, change in pain, level of pain, and medication history, with particular focus on adjuvant analgesic medications and ARVs (see Chapter 3).

Question 4. What are potential causes of AIDS related neuropathic pain?

One of the most common causes of neuropathic pain in HIV is direct infection of the nerve with HIV or CMV. Another common cause is medication (especially ARVs and chemotherapeutic agents). Other causes are superimposed medical or metabolic processes (i.e. alcoholism, diabetes), or malignancies such as Kaposi's sarcoma, lymphoma, and squamous cell carcinoma.

You diagnose pain from HIV-related peripheral neuropathy. You decide to titrate D.C.'s gabapentin further as he is tolerating it very well and is only on a dose of 300 mg orally three times daily. You increase the dose over the first 4 days of admission to 500 mg orally three times daily and he feels significant improvement in pain. However, the day before the planned discharge, the patient develops severe diarrhoea.

Table 14.2 Late complications of HIV infection

CD4 <500/mm^3	B-cell lymphoma Cervical intra-epithelial neoplasia Idiopathic thrombocytopenic purpura Kaposi's sarcoma Oral hairy leucoplakia Pneumococcal pneumonia Pulmonary tuberculosis Thrush Herpes zoster
CD4 <200/mm^3	*Candida* oesophagitis Chronic cryptosporidiosis Cryptococcosis Disseminated/chronic herpes simplex HIV-associated dementia Miliary tuberculosis *Pneumocystis carinii* pneumonia Toxoplasmosis Wasting
CD4 <50/mm^3	Disseminated Mycobacterium avium Cytomegalovirus retinitis

Question 5. How would you investigate the diarrhoea?

Diarrhoea is common in HIV disease and has multiple causes. Since this symptom has a devastating effect on quality of life and can cause dehydration, lethargy, and further weight loss, vigorous intervention is necessary. Investigating the cause may lead to specific and effective treatment. Basic investigations include the following.

- Stool cultures including stool smear for cryptospiridial infection and a screen for *Clostridium difficile* toxin. It is important to exclude *C. difficile* as D.C. was recently treated with a course of antibiotics for a community-acquired bacterial pneumonia. Treatable pathogens include *Salmonella*, *Shigella*, *Campylobacter*, *Giardia*, and *C. difficile*. One of the most common pathogens with advanced HIV disease is *Cryptospiridium*, a protozoal infection that causes watery diarrhoea, malabsorption, weight loss, and malnutrition. Treatment is usually supportive (oral or intravenous hydration, antidiarrhoeal medication) as no antimicrobials have been proven effective (although some may be tried).
- Review of medications (is D.C. on any drugs that could contribute?).
- Any of his ARVs as well as his antibiotics for prophylaxis could be causing his diarrhoea. These would need to be reviewed with the patient, and changing or stopping them should be considered if no other cause is found.

Question 6. How would you manage the diarrhoea?

Once a definitive cause is found, specific treatment can be initiated. Adequate hydration is essential. Other interventions may include reducing peristalsis, increasing bulk, and reducing intestinal secretions. Loperamide 2 mg orally three times daily and after each loose bowel movement (not to exceed 16 mg/day) or diphenoxylate HCl 2.5–5.0 mg orally every 4–6 h (maximum 20 mg/day) may be effective by reducing peristalsis. Codeine 30–60 mg every 4 h as needed is often effective. Codeine may be prescribed in combination with loperamide or diphenoxylate. Psyllium, fibre, bran, and pectin can increase bulk and octreotide 100–200 mg s.c. three times daily can decrease secretions (a short course of 4–7 days is usually sufficient until the cause is identified and definitive treatment initiated). Lactose intolerance is common, and a lactose-free diet and lactase enzyme 1–4 tablets 15–30 min before meals can be effective. Absorption of slow release medications such as opioid analgesics is affected by reduced bowel transit time and thus immediate release medications should be considered in the presence of diarrhoea.

D.C.'s respite admission was extended for an additional 4 days in order to treat his diarrhoea before he returned home. Before leaving hospital, D.C. started to talk about restarting ARVs.

Question 7. If D.C. restarts ARVs, will he still be considered palliative and be considered for readmission?

Reinstitution of AIDS treatment should not affect a patient's access to palliative care. Successful ARV treatment can often extend life for many years and considerably improve a patient's quality of life. However, the time often comes when patients have exhausted use of ARVs. Their virus becomes resistant to most drugs and even the most complex combination of ARVs is no longer effective. At this point the decision to stop ARVs, although difficult emotionally, may be medically indicated. Some patients who have been on ARVs for some time and are still quite ill may choose to discontinue them because of side effects; when their viral loads rise and CD4 counts fall, they have to make difficult decisions about restarting them. In some cases even restarting ARVs is unsuccessful, but for many life can be prolonged. These patients still require symptom management. It is important to remember that ARVs need to be taken regularly in order to work effectively. If taken improperly (i.e. skipped doses) the virus can develop resistance rapidly. Because ARVs can only be taken orally, patients must be well enough to swallow and tolerate many pills daily.

D.C. is discharged from hospital after 11 days. His diarrhoea has stopped and he has decided to remain off ARVs for now. His partner has used the time to rest and is feeling stronger than when D.C. was admitted, but he still feels very stressed with the worry of continued decline of D.C.'s health. A second respite booking is considered for the future.

Six weeks later, D.C. is feeling unwell again. Over the last few days he has had low-grade fever, poor appetite, and poor energy. Overnight he develops a mild cough, and as the day progresses he becomes progressively more dyspnoeic until his partner becomes alarmed and brings him to emergency.

Question 8. If you were the first physician assessing D.C., what quick differential diagnosis might you consider for acute cough and dyspnoea in advanced AIDS?

- PCP is high on the list, particularly with D.C.'s history. PCP can masquerade as a variety of entities, and presentation may be subtle.

- Acute bacterial pneumonia is also possible; the most common pathogens are *Streptococcus pneumoniae*, *Haemophilus influenzae*, and *Staphylococcus aureus*.
- Other opportunistic pulmonary infections (cytomegalovirus, *Mycobacterium avium* complex, fungal or parasitic infections).
- Pulmonary KS is a possibility, particularly with D.C.'s history. Chest radiography may not be definitive, but CT may be helpful.
- You should consider other diagnoses that are relevant for both AIDS and non-AIDS patients such as pleural effusion, congestive heart failure, septicaemia, pulmonary embolus, reactive airways disease, or malignancy.

Question 9. Apart from the likely underlying cause of his current symptoms, what other factors might contribute to his dyspnoea?

- Fever and hypoxaemia can increase his ventilatory rate.
- Malnutrition causes weakening of his respiratory muscles and therefore can decrease his respiratory capacity.
- Anaemia is a common accompaniment of his medication regimen and of his chronic illness, resulting in less haemoglobin to transport his oxygen.
- Anxiety can markedly escalate the subjective feeling of dyspnoea.

Question 10. Given that he has recently had a DNR in place, how aggressive should you be in doing investigations? What investigations would you order?

Even in endstage AIDS, there are a number of treatable causes of acute illness; further, treatment of these underlying complications can result in improvement in symptoms (in this case dyspnoea). Therefore, if D.C. is in agreement with investigations, you would start with a total blood count and serum lactate dehydrogenase (LDH), which can be elevated in PCP, sputum stain and culture for bacteria, acid-fast bacilli, and fungi, blood cultures, chest radiography, and possibly specialized radiology procedures such as CT scan. If you have a strong index of suspicion that he has PCP, or is deteriorating despite the initiation of therapy, bronchoscopy is the safest and most reliable method of making a specific diagnosis. If possible, it is helpful to seek a consultation with an infectious disease specialist or a respirologist who is knowledgeable about AIDS.

Question 11. When investigations are completed and definitive therapy is underway, you are asked to decide whether D.C. should go to a medical ward or to a palliative care bed. What will your response be?

In the end, the decision may be determined by where a bed is available and the care philosophy associated with that place of care. The investigations and treatments are still well within the realm of palliative care because the goal of the therapy is to improve the patient's well-being. Some palliative care units will be very comfortable taking care of D.C. during this admission, whereas in some hospitals he could be cared for only on a medical ward.

D.C. was found to have a classic diffuse interstitial infiltrate on chest radiography, his serum LDH was elevated, and *P. carinii* was found in bronchoscopic washings. His oxygen saturation was <90% on room air. Consequently he was diagnosed as having severe PCP and he was placed on appropriate antimicrobials and also started on prednisone. However, he continued to deteriorate and was deemed to be in incipient respiratory failure. You raise the question with D.C.'s partner and family as to whether he is a candidate for intubation and ventilation. His partner and family have differing views about this; D.C. is somnolent and very dyspnoeic, and so he is unable to take part in the decision-making. Previously, D.C. had signed an Advanced Directive stating his desire for no cardiopulmonary resuscitation.

Question 12. Is D.C. a candidate for intubation and ventilation?

Once again, there is not a clear-cut answer. The chance of D.C. successfully weaning from the ventilator and leaving hospital is approximately 50% if intubation occurs within 3–5 days of the start of anti-PCP therapy. The scenario that D.C. finds himself in emphasizes the wisdom of embarking on these discussions ahead of time. There may be better guidance in decision-making if he has signed a detailed advanced directive rather than a less specific directive. A detailed advanced directive might give guidance as to whether a patient wishes comfort measures only, full medical care but no ICU/CCU admission, or full medical care including admission to ICU/CCU with or without intubation and ventilation. Without a definitive advanced medical directive, the clinician should have an open discussion with D.C.'s partner and family regarding the medical and ethical issues at play.

Fortunately, D.C. had previously indicated on his advanced directive that he still wished to consider intubation and ventilation; this was done, and 48 h later he was able to be weaned off the ventilator. He required several weeks of hospital care. He was aware that he did not recover nearly as well or as quickly from this episode of PCP compared with his first episode, and before discharge he revised his advanced directive to indicate that full medical therapy must exclude ICU/CCU and intubation and ventilation in the future.

Approximately 8 weeks later, D.C.'s partner calls the palliative care ward and asks to speak to a doctor about an urgent problem. He is very upset but is able to describe clearly that D.C. has 'not been himself' for the past few days. He says that D.C. has been vague mentally with some alteration in behaviour for the past few months, and there have been very distressing further changes within the past week. About a week ago D.C. became more confused and forgetful. The confusion has increased further over the last few days; now D.C. does not recognize friends and cannot feed and care for himself. He has not taken his medications for the last 2 days. D.C.'s partner further describes that, today, D.C. is drowsy and his speech is unintelligible. D.C.'s partner is distressed by these changes, and is frantic to know what could be causing them and whether it means that D.C. is dying.

The palliative care physician who takes this call reassures D.C.'s partner over the telephone that there is a bed available and that D.C. can be admitted to the palliative care unit today. Arrangements are made to bring D.C. to the hospital by ambulance, and once he arrives on the ward you assess him and speak to his partner who is quite distraught.

Your initial assessment of D.C. reveals that he is not oriented to person, time, or place. He is afebrile with a respiratory rate of 14 bpm and heart rate of 96 breaths/min. His physical examination reveals some findings seen previously, i.e. cachexia and KS lesions. His chest is clear and there are no significant abdominal findings. Neurological examination reveals decreased sensation to pain and light

Continued

touch in both legs (most marked in the feet) and generalized weakness, with no other focal findings. You step out of the room to speak to D.C.'s partner and write some orders based on your preliminary findings. D.C.'s partner is very emotional and you escort him to a private area where you can support him and talk about D.C.'s signs and symptoms. He pleads with you to tell him: 'Is this it? Is he dying? What's wrong with him? What are you going to do?'

Question 13. How will you describe your differential diagnosis and approach in terms of investigations at this time? What are your thoughts regarding the likely prognosis that would correlate with the possible diagnoses?

You will consider whether the neurological findings are attributable to delirium, dementia, or both. The cognitive and behavioural change exhibited by D.C. over the last few weeks is consistent with AIDS-related dementia. However, the recent rapid progression leads you to suspect that delirium is now superimposed on the pre-existing dementia. You describe to D.C.'s partner that there are numerous possibilities and that the prognosis varies considerably, depending on the specific diagnosis. You explain that you want to proceed with investigations that may assist in identifying the diagnosis.

D.C.'s partner wants to know everything about the possibilities and the types of tests you are considering.

The differential diagnosis is large at this point, as D.C. is susceptible to numerous infectious, metabolic, neoplastic, and other conditions associated with endstage AIDS that affect the central nervous system (CNS). The most common are as follows.

- Infection: meningitis, encephalitis, toxoplasmosis, other sepsis.
- Metabolic: renal failure, electrolyte abnormalities, hypoxaemia, medication administration errors, dehydration.
- Primary CNS pathology: cerebrovascular accident , progressive multifocal leucoencephalopathy (PML), lymphoma.

Investigations you may consider are blood cultures, complete blood count, electrolytes, chest radiography, CT scan of the head, lumbar puncture, and brain biopsy if appropriate (not in this case). In addition to these investigations, consideration of an infectious disease consultation may also be appropriate to ensure optimal assessment and opinion regarding diagnosis and treatment options.

Question 14. A medical student doing an elective in palliative care with you expresses some surprise at the aggressive approach to diagnosis and determining potential treatment options for this palliative patient. How do you address her questions about what seems to be aggressive medical care in a palliative setting?

The medical student's question again raises the issue of palliative care and AIDS, and the coexistence of supportive symptom management and aggressive investigation and treatment of potentially reversible medical problems. Upon reviewing with you the differential diagnosis for

D.C. at this time, the medical student understands that it is worthwhile considering tests such as lumbar puncture and CT scan of the head that may reveal reversible infection or treatable pathology (e.g. CNS lymphoma).

Results of the investigations reveal unremarkable blood tests, blood cultures, chest radiographs, and lumbar puncture. CT of the head reveals multifocal enhancing lesions consistent with CNS lymphoma and surrounding oedema without evidence of raised intracranial pressure or herniation. Lumbar puncture subsequently reveals cytology consistent with lymphoma. Although a brain biopsy was suggested by a neurologist to definitively confirm the diagnosis, D.C.'s partner and family feel that such a test would be too invasive at this time. You are able to reassure them that treatment of lymphoma can be pursued based on the investigations to date and that a brain biopsy is not required.

Question 15. What treatment options would you discuss with D.C. and his family?

Initiation of corticosteroid therapy to reduce cerebral oedema should be discussed and considered without delay. Corticosteroids can be cytotoxic in lymphoma, although their antineoplastic effect is short in duration. Referral to radiation oncology should be arranged to consider a course of radiation therapy. Ongoing supportive care in hospital should be anticipated as these treatments are commenced and as the efficacy of treatment is assessed. Given the poor prognosis associated with CNS lymphoma and the difficulty in home management prior to this admission, the option of hospice care should be discussed, either for care at discharge or for direct admission to hospice from home at a later date.

The radiation oncologist sees D.C. and discusses the prognosis and proposed radiation treatment with his partner and family. He explains that CNS lymphoma in the setting of AIDS is associated with a life expectancy of 2–4 months. It is carefully explained that the treatments such as corticosteroids and radiation are palliative in nature with the goal of reducing symptoms attributable to the CNS lymphoma. Within 24 h of initiation of dexamethasone, D.C.'s level of consciousness and cognitive function begin to improve. He remains an inpatient in the palliative care unit throughout a week-long course of radiation therapy, which is well tolerated, and ultimately is discharged home approximately 3 weeks after he was originally admitted. Dexamethasone 12 mg daily will be tapered over the next 3 weeks (the patient may be able to stop dexamethasone completely or may require a small ongoing dose if symptoms persist with tapering). D.C. and his partner agree that he should go on the waiting list for hospice care in the future, and are reassured to know that if managing at home were to become more difficult, the hospice was indeed another option for ongoing care.

Two months later, D.C.'s family physician requests an admission to the palliative care unit for symptom management. She reports that D.C. has continued to decline physically and cognitively. His pain is worse; he is not eating well, and he has lost 8 kg from his usual weight of 63 kg. His balance is poor and he has had some falls at home. His partner is exhausted, and the home care nurse is concerned about the patient's daily care needs as well as the risk of falling. D.C.'s mother, who has moved in to help with care, thinks that he needs to be admitted to hospital for nutritional support. On admission, D.C. appears vague and anxious. He is markedly cachectic and mildly dehydrated. He requires a one-person assist to transfer from his wheelchair to bed. He attempts to walk a few steps, but tends to fall to his left. He is noted to have oropharyngeal candidiasis and some KS lesions on his palate. When asked, D.C. affirms that his throat hurts, making it hard to swallow. He says that he is not hungry. D.C. is accompanied by his mother and his partner who state that he has been refusing food, and is taking only small amounts of liquids with his medications.

Question 16. How will you approach the management of D.C. at this time?

Pain needs to be managed, and a medication review with optimization of medications should be a priority. D.C.'s reluctance to eat may be due in part to mouth pain, and his oral thrush should be treated aggressively with the goals of improving comfort and oral intake. D.C. has been taking oral ketoconazole for 2 weeks. The oral route may no longer be reliable for absorption of his medications because of heavy overgrowth of *Candida*, and alternative routes may be more feasible. Amphotericin B given intravenously in a dose range of 0.3–0.5 mg/kg/day for 3–7 days, followed by an oral agent such as itraconazole 200 mg daily in refractory cases, is effective, but amphotericin B is often poorly tolerated. A recent alternative is caspofungin 50 mg i.v. daily for 10–14 days.

Although D.C. has AIDS-related dementia and CNS lymphoma, there may also be some superimposed delirium due to dehydration, infection, or other causes. Bloodwork should include complete blood count and differential white cell count, electrolytes, urea and creatinine, blood sugar, and blood cultures.

D.C.'s weight loss of >10% is significant and in advanced AIDS indicates wasting syndrome, with a high risk for further complications or death. Comfort and safety are paramount at this late stage of D.C.'s illness.

D.C. is mildly anaemic, but does not require transfusion. His sodium is low, his urea is elevated, and his blood sugar is within the normal range. Blood cultures are negative. He is rehydrated with normal saline, and his refractory candidiasis is treated with intravenous amphotericin B. Fortunately, he tolerates this well. He receives regular mouth care. The oropharyngeal candidiasis improves and he is able to swallow with less discomfort, but he remains uninterested in food. His mother is distressed about this and is concerned that D.C. is 'starving to death'. She asks for artificial feeding, but D.C.'s partner states that D.C. had previously told him that he did not want a 'feeding tube'.

Question 17. Is enteral or parenteral feeding indicated?

A discussion of the risks and benefits of enteral-parenteral feeding is given in Chapter 7. A nasogastric tube is contraindicated in the setting of persistent, although improved, oesophageal candidiasis in this patient. He has previously expressed a wish not to have a feeding tube placed. Parenteral nutrition would require central intravenous access, which carries significant risk of pneumothorax, line infection, thrombosis, etc. There is no clear evidence that parenteral nutrition improves survival time. Parenteral feeding is not indicated in a person who is in the final stages of disease. An appetite stimulant could be proposed, but should have been discussed earlier in the course of his illness as it may have been effective to encourage oral intake at that point. Megestrol acetate or a corticosteroid, such as prednisone or dexamethasone, may be beneficial in some patients to promote appetite and well-being. Earlier interventions with anabolic or amino acid supplements may have been helpful, but not at this point.

A family meeting is arranged to discuss the question of nutrition and artificial feeding. D.C. attends with his mother and partner. A palliative care physician, D.C.'s family physician, the unit social worker, and his nurse are also present. At the meeting, D.C. re-affirms that he does not want artificial feeding, but his mother says that he does not understand the consequences. However, his wish is supported by his family physician, who has documented a similar statement by D.C. in her practice notes, and by D.C.'s partner, who had made a promise to D.C. not to allow such interventions. There is a question as to D.C.'s current competence and decision-making ability; the discussion focuses on advanced directives, which are on record, naming D.C.'s partner as his substitute decision-maker. It is recognized that his mother is concerned about the weight loss and poor nutrition, and the team members counsel her as to the likely futility of artificial feeding at this stage and the inherent risks. She acknowledges that D.C. is swallowing better, but has a poor appetite. The care team agrees to start oral megestrol 160 mg twice daily, as long as D.C. can swallow. Mrs. C is willing to come in at mealtimes, and will make his favourite soup and puddings in small quantities. His nurse will also encourage small high-nutrient snacks. D.C. is tired, and his nurse takes him back to bed. The meeting goes on to discuss D.C.'s poor prognosis and imminent death. He and his partner have already made funeral arrangements. D.C. had hoped to die at home, but both his mother and his partner are feeling stressed and would prefer that he remain on the palliative care unit. They state that he appears quite content and may not be very aware of his surroundings. He has his own quilt and some familiar photographs in his room. The social worker discusses hospice and telephephones to find that there is still a considerable waiting list. They understand that he may not outlive the waiting list. It is agreed that he will remain on the palliative care unit in the meantime. At the end of the meeting, his mother and partner, although sad and overtly emotional, say that they feel relieved to have made some decisions.

Commentary

Palliative management of people with AIDS clearly has much in common with that of cancer and other endstage illnesses, but there are some special considerations. A mere 20 years ago, the first AIDS patients were being identified and treated for rapidly progressing disease. Hospice palliative care was an emerging humanistic response to the biomedical model of cure-oriented pathology-based medical management. The art of medicine was overshadowed by its science. To some extent, palliative AIDS care has shaped palliative care in general over the last two decades. The relative youth of AIDS patients, the 'peaks and valleys' course of the disease, and the responsibility to investigate more actively to identify reversible opportunistic infections have influenced the approach to all palliative patients, including those with metastatic cancer. People with cancer and AIDS are living longer in the palliative phase owing to pharmacological and other scientific advances. Active treatment is best administered in partnership with considerate caring. In the next two decades, there will be further advances in medical and pharmacological management to cure or control pathogens. There are also new challenges: the prevalent risks for HIV/AIDS are intravenous drug use and unprotected intercourse in a population that has few resources, multiple pathologies, is socially marginalized, and feels alienated within the existing hospital system. Palliative care has much to offer to people with AIDS … and people with AIDS can teach us much about palliative care.

Acknowledgements

The authors wish to thank Dr Lindsay Lawson, Dr Sylvia Guillemi, and Dr Fraser Norrie of St Paul's Hospital, Vancouver, BC, Canada, for their wise input into this chapter.

Bibliography

Anonymous (1995) *Comprehensive Guide for the Care of Persons with HIV Disease.* Toronto: Mount Sinai Hospital/Casey Hospice.

Anonymous (1998) AIDS care. In: *Medical Care of the Dying* (3rd edn). Victoria, BC: Victoria Hospice Society, 415–35. www.victoriahospice.com

Anonymous (1999) *Therapeutic Guidelines for the Treatment of HIV/AIDS and Related Conditions.* Vancouver, BC: British Columbia Centre for Excellence in HIV/AIDS, St Paul's Hospital. www.providencehealthcentre.org

Anonymous (2001) *HIV Care: A Primer and Resource Guide for Family Physicians.* Missisauga, Ontario: College of Family Physicians of Canada. www.cfpc.ca/English/cfpc/programs/patient%20care/hiv%20primer/

Bartlett, J.G. (1994) *The Johns Hopkins Hospital Guide to Medical Care of Patients with HIV Infection.* Baltimore, MD: Williams and Wilkins.

Coyne, P., Lyne, M., and Watson, A. (2002) Symptom management in people with AIDS. *Am J Nurs,* **102**, 48–56.

Easterbrook, P. (2001) The changing epidemiology of HIV infection: new challenges for HIV palliative care. *J R Soc Med,* **94**, 442–8.

Greenberg, B., McCorkle, R., Vlahov, D., and Selwyn, P. (2000) Palliative care for HIV disease in the era of highly active antiretroviral therapy. *J Urban Health,* **77**, 150–63.

Meyer, M. (1999) Palliative care and AIDS. 2: Gastrointestinal symptoms. *Int J STD AIDS,* **10**, 495–507.

Peabody, F. (1927) The care of the patient. *JAMA,* **88**, 877–82.

Princeton, D.C. (2003). *Manual of HIV AIDS Therapy.* Laguna Hills, CA: Current Clinical Strategies Publishing.

Chapter 15

Endstage renal disease and discontinuation of dialysis

Susan Chater, Tom Hutchinson, and John F. Seely

Attitude

To enable each student to understand:

- The significant morbidity and reduced life expectancy of patients with endstage renal disease (ESRD).
- The importance of advance care planning in patients with ESRD.
- The important role of palliative care and symptom management in patients with ESRD who discontinue dialysis.

Skill

To enable each student to be able to:

- Provide expert pain and symptom management in patients with ESRD.
- Help with advance care planning for patients who are considering discontinuing dialysis.
- Provide expert end-of-life care to patients discontinuing dialysis.

Knowledge

To enable each student to know:

- The importance of kidney failure in different age groups in the population.
- The high mortality associated with kidney failure even when treated by regular dialysis.
- The major co-morbidity of patients on dialysis that contributes to the desire for discontinuing dialysis.
- The major causes of pain in patients with ESRD.
- The safe pharmacological treatment of pain and other frequent symptoms in patients with ESRD.
- The frequency of discontinuing dialysis and the reasons for such decisions.
- The need for advance care planning in patients with ESRD.
- How to provide expert end-of-life care to patients discontinuing dialysis.
- How to support family members of patients discontinuing dialysis.

A nephrologist asks you to see Mr P.M., a 62-year-old haemodialysis patient, hospitalized for exacerbation of congestive heart failure, stating that the patient is considering discontinuing dialysis. He requests your help in discussing this with the patient and family, and in improving symptom control. You learn that the patient is retired, disabled since age 49, and married with three children. His wife is hearing-impaired and has memory problems. He reports that his life is miserable and that he 'can't take it any more'. In addition to severe functional limitations from his heart disease, he is in constant pain, mainly in his knees, wrists, back, and shoulders, and cannot sleep at night because of pain despite taking acetaminophen (paracetamol) on a regular basis. He tells you that he has not yet decided to stop haemodialysis, but is 'very close'.

In the past 10 years, he has had a myocardial infarct, coronary artery bypass surgery, and frequent admissions to hospital for unstable angina. ESRD was felt to be secondary to hypertension. He has now been on haemodialysis for over 10 years. Several years previously he was considered to be unsuitable for a heart or kidney transplant.

You focus on pain relief for the first visit. Following a detailed history and physical examination, you conclude that the cause of his pain is osteoarthritis. Hydromorphone 0.5 mg orally every 4 h on an as-needed basis was ordered for pain together with docusate 400 mg daily and senna 2–4 tablets at bedtime. You choose to avoid non-steroidal anti-inflammatory drugs (NSAIDs) because of concern about gastrointestinal toxicity. Four days later the patient tells you that he was previously in pain '99 per cent of the time' but is now pain-free '75 per cent of the time'. Over the next few days his hydromorphone is titrated up based on as-needed usage and he is discharged on hydromorphine sustained release 3 mg orally every 12 h, and 1 mg orally every 2 h as needed for breakthrough pain. His mood has improved and his desire for withdrawal has significantly diminished.

Question 1. How frequent a problem is kidney failure in the population?

We are witnessing a virtual epidemic of patients undergoing chronic dialysis in industrialized countries which is largely attributable to two factors. There has been an increasing rate of diagnosis and acceptance of dialysis treatment, particularly for older patients with ESRD. At the same time, the prevalence of patients on treatment at any one time is rising owing to increased survival of patients with renal failure since the introduction of chronic dialysis therapy in the 1960s. This has resulted in an accumulation of patients that is not expected to reach a steady state for some years.[1] In Canada, the prevalence of ESRD rose from 223 to 774 per million between 1981 and 1999.[2] The effect on the utilization of health care resources and the need for palliative care when these patients reach the end of their lives is enormous and increasing.

Question 2. What is the expected survival of this 62-year-old man on dialysis for ESRD?

It is a common misperception that adequate dialysis treatment fully replaces kidney function and returns the expected survival of a patient with ESRD to that of the general population. Current peritoneal or haemodialysis treatment replaces approximately 10 per cent of normal renal function[3] and the survival of patients approximates that of some common cancers. For instance, males aged 35–64 years with ESRD have an expected 10-year survival of 40 per cent, which is slightly worse than patients of the same age with prostate cancer and only slightly better than similar patients with colon cancer, compared with a 90 per cent survival for members of the general population of the same age.[2] Although it is difficult to give an exact prognosis for this

62-year-old patient with ESRD, coronary heart disease, and presumed congestive heart failure, a best guess based on published data would be approximately 1 year.[4]

Question 3. What are common causes of pain in patients with ESRD?

Pain is common in patients with ESRD, and is present in close to 50 per cent of patients who withdraw from dialysis.[5,6] Pain is often multifactorial and tends to be progressive. Common causes of musculoskeletal pain include osteoarthritis, renal osteodystrophy (bone and joint pain), and multiple myeloma (diffuse bone pain and fractures). Patients with coronary artery disease may be even more prone to angina because of hypotension during or after dialysis. Peripheral vascular disease is associated with significant morbidity due to painful ischaemic limbs and a high rate of amputation, as bypass surgery is often technically difficult. Mesenteric angina and ischaemic bowel disease can also occur.

Painful neuropathy is also very troublesome; it is usually secondary to diabetes, but may also be due to uraemic or ischaemic neuropathy. Coexistent ischaemic and neuropathic pain in the extremities is not uncommon. Other causes of pain may be related to procedures such as creation or revision of vascular access for haemodialysis. Leg cramps and headache commonly occur during haemodialysis, and an uncommon, but extremely painful condition is calciphylaxis, a disease associated with calcific deposits and progressive necrosis of skin.

Question 4. How would you manage ischaemic limb pain when surgery is not an option? What if you thought the pain was neuropathic in origin?

When patients are too ill to tolerate bypass surgery or amputation, they are usually suffering considerable ischaemic pain, even at rest. Your best resort at this point is a palliative approach. Opioids are usually quite effective in the management of ischaemic limb pain. Start with oral dosing of either hydromorphone or oxycodone every 4 h as needed to assess the total 24-h opioid requirement. After several days of use, when an average daily requirement has been established, the patient can be switched to a sustained release hydromorphone or oxycodone preparation, while continuing to use a short-acting preparation for breakthrough pain. The rationale for initial as-needed use is to allow for the variable sensitivity to opioids in this population. If there is concern about poor oral absorption (e.g. diabetic gastroparesis or ischaemic gut), parenteral dosing may be necessary. If the patient has good relief but develops opioid toxicity (e.g. excess sedation, confusion, or myoclonus), a switch to transdermal fentanyl in equivalent analgesic doses would be appropriate, with the previous immediate-acting opioid continued for breakthrough pain. As with all patients on opioids, particular attention to, and anticipation of side effects is essential (e.g. constipation needs regular stool softeners and stimulant laxatives, nausea may need regular antiemetics).

The treatment of neuropathic pain is often more difficult and may require several drugs for control. Tricyclic antidepressants (TCAs) (e.g. amitriptyline or nortriptyline) are a reasonable first choice, starting in doses of 10–20 mg at bedtime and slowly titrating by 10-mg increments every few days. Full antidepressant doses are not usually required. If the patient does not tolerate the TCA or relief is inadequate, gabapentin can be substituted or added as it has been found to be quite effective in management of neuropathic pain.[7] The half-life of this drug is prolonged in renal failure and the recommended dose range is 100–300 mg given orally after dialysis.[8]

If sleep is particularly disturbed because of the pain, clonazepam 0.5–1 mg orally at bedtime may help. Occasionally, troublesome neuropathic pain unresponsive to the above therapy can be managed with methadone, although this drug requires close monitoring for dose and side effects.

Question 5. How does ESRD interfere with analgesic prescribing/handling? Would it affect your choice of analgesics?

Although the major analgesic groups such as acetaminophen, aspirin, NSAIDs (including COX-2 inhibitors), and opioids are metabolized by the liver, other considerations are important in the choice of drug. Acetaminophen is generally a safe and useful standby for mild pain and the dose does not need to be changed in dialysis patients. Aspirin directly potentiates the platelet dysfunction of uraemia in dialysis patients and should be avoided as an analgesic. NSAIDs can potentiate platelet dysfunction and cause gastric erosion in dialysis patients; if used, they should be given with a cytoprotective agent.

Active opioid metabolites, which are normally excreted by the kidney, may accumulate in dialysis patients and contribute to enhanced sensitivity to the effects of some opioids.[9,10] The best example of this is the metabolite normeperidine which accumulates in renal failure and may cause seizures; for this reason, meperidine should be avoided in dialysis patients. Morphine-6-glucuronide, one of the metabolites of morphine, is also active and accumulates in renal failure and may lead to opioid toxicity.[10,11] For this reason, as well as the accumulation of the inactive metabolite morphine-3-glucuronide, which interferes with opioid action, morphine should always be used with caution, if at all, in patients on dialysis. Hydromorphone-3-glucuronide, a metabolite of hydromorphone, also accumulates in renal failure[12] and may contribute to toxicity. Oxycodone has an active metabolite, oxymorphone, of uncertain significance in renal failure. If opioid toxicity develops in patients taking these drugs, opioid rotation should be performed. A safer choice in these circumstances would be fentanyl since its metabolites are largely inactive.[10,11] We do not have good information on the removal of opioids or their metabolites by dialysis; however, current recommendations are not to adjust the dose of opioids to account for any possible removal by dialysis therapy but, instead, to titrate to effect.[13]

Two months later, P.M.'s pain is much worse. He is using up to six breakthrough doses per day with relief. He still feels low at times and from time to time has considered stopping dialysis, but is not yet ready to do so. You increase his sustained release hydromorphone to 6 mg orally every 12 h, and a week later he reports that the pain is much better.

Unfortunately, 2 weeks later he is readmitted to the hospital coronary care unit with unstable angina. Despite maximal therapy, he continues to have cardiac pain. To control his pain better, you rotate his opioid treatment to a transdermal fentanyl patch 25 μg/h, applied every 72 h. At the same time you start him on an s.c. infusion of fentanyl 25 μg every 30 min (concentration 50 μg/ml) as needed by patient-controlled analgesia (PCA) for breakthrough angina pain.

Question 6. Why was fentanyl used on this occasion and why these doses and routes?

When ESRD patients require long-term opioids, transdermal fentanyl is a good choice as there is minimal renal clearance; the liver is the primary site of fentanyl metabolism.[14,15] The fentanyl patch was used for the chronic background pain [the 25 μg/h dose is an approximate equianalgesic dose for P.M.'s hydromorphone (12 mg/day)] plus breakthrough doses. The fentanyl infusion was chosen for the intractable angina because the subcutaneous route provides pain relief within minutes. Fentanyl also tends to preserve cardiac stability and is less likely to cause tachycardia or hypotension, in part because histamine release occurs only rarely.[15] The dose of 25 μg per hour is a reasonable starting dose in the acute pain setting, being approximately equivalent to a total oral dose of 45–134 mg *per day*.

You also note during this admission that P.M.'s mood is very low and you suspect depression. He tells you that he wonders if it is worth going on but he would not contemplate suicide. He is frightened of becoming a burden on his family. You discover that because of his increasing disability, they have had to move into a senior's residence. He feels that he does not relate to other seniors, he cannot talk to his wife because of her poor memory and loss of hearing, and he feels 'just worn down'. You learn that his father committed suicide and, although this happened many years ago, it continues to haunt him. He feels that to stop dialysis would be a form of suicide, and he does not want his children to suffer as he did with his father's death. Although the circumstances are very different, it feels the same to him. At this point the primary team consult a psychiatrist who starts him on sertraline and provides supportive counselling.

Question 7. How common is depression in dialysis patients?

Many of the physical symptoms of chronic renal failure are also common to depression (e.g. fatigue, anorexia, and sleep disorders), making the diagnosis difficult at times. By DSM III criteria, the prevalence of depression in haemodialysis patients is low (~5 per cent).[16] In a prospective study by Cohen *et al.*,[17] 10 of 11 patients who elected to stop dialysis were neither clinically depressed nor had a history of depression, suggesting that depression is not a common factor in the decision to withdraw therapy. Where there is significant doubt about whether depression is present in a patient considering discontinuing dialysis, a psychiatric consultation should be obtained.[18] If pharmacotherapy is used, no dose adjustment is required for tricyclic antidepressants or for commonly used selective serotonin reuptake inhibitors (fluvoxamine, fluoxetine, and sertraline).[9]

Question 8. How would you describe the difference between suicide and discontinuing dialysis to a patient?

The most important thing the physician can do is to listen carefully and ask open-ended questions to obtain as clear a picture as possible of what would restrict the patient's ability to make a free choice about stopping or continuing dialysis. For patients such as P.M. where there is a family history, suicide may play a large role in their thoughts and feelings about discontinuing dialysis. It is also important to question patients about their religious beliefs which may also have an important influence on their thinking. If the equation of suicide with stopping dialysis is an important consideration for the patient (or the physician), the following points may be helpful.

- Discontinuing dialysis is relatively common and accounts for approximately 20–25 per cent of all deaths on dialysis.[19]
- Most patients who withdraw from dialysis are not clinically depressed, in marked contrast to the situation with suicide.
- Discontinuing dialysis is not a signal to end medical therapy but the start of more intense palliative measures to prevent and relieve suffering.

Although the resolution of such issues may be possible in one interview, it usually takes a series of discussions over time for a satisfactory conclusion to the discussion.

> The patient was discharged home on a pain pump (PCA) for intractable angina with a fentanyl patch and sertraline, and over the next year or so things remained relatively stable. Eighteen months later, P.M. was admitted to the surgical service with ischaemia of the small bowel and resection and ileostomy was performed. After 4 days in the intensive care unit, he was discharged to the surgical floor and appeared to be doing well.
>
> He asked to speak to his nephrologist and you about his decision to stop dialysis and receive palliative care. He said that he had been thinking about this for 2 years and felt that what lay ahead of him were more complications of his diseases. He was calm and clear about the decision. He had spoken individually to his children, and made arrangements for his wife's best friend to be present when he spoke to her. He then discussed his funeral arrangements and last wishes, and how best his wife could be supported. He also wanted to say his goodbyes to the dialysis nurses and the volunteer coffee lady in the dialysis unit.

Question 9. Why is advance care planning important in such patients?

Many patients on dialysis have rarely considered discontinuing dialysis, nor have they discussed with their nephrologist the circumstances under which they would withdraw treatment.[18,20–22] Actual advance directives are infrequently written; when patients do discuss their wishes regarding treatment in the event of permanent coma (such as cardiopulmonary resuscitation or tube feeding), discussion of the possibility of discontinuing dialysis is not often considered. However, when specifically asked, most patients agree that in planning future medical treatment, it is important to include the option of withdrawing dialysis.[21]

Therefore advance care planning is especially important in dialysis patients, given their reduced life expectancy, high comorbidity, and the short period of time that they survive after discontinuing dialysis.[23–25] Studies of patients dying of cancer have shown that open discussion and honesty regarding their disease is generally well handled by patients and families, and helps them participate in the decision-making around treatment and care.[26,27] Advance care planning helps ensure that the patient's wishes are known and respected, that any outstanding physical, emotional, or spiritual concerns are dealt with, and that someone who knows the wishes of the patient is designated with power of attorney in case of incapacity.[28] This takes time, as well as sufficient cognitive function on the part of the patient. It is important that the immediate family be involved in these discussions to help them prepare for the eventuality of discontinuing dialysis should that become the patient's decision.[29] It is particularly regrettable when patients on haemodialysis become mentally incompetent without the family or team knowing under what circumstances they would wish to discontinue dialysis, and they do not have sufficient cognitive function to engage meaningfully with staff and family about end-of-life concerns.

The American Society of Nephrology and Renal Physicians Association have recently published extensive guidelines to help physicians with regard to withholding and withdrawing dialysis.[30,31]

Question 10. What are the major end-of-life concerns in patients on dialysis?

Surveys of dialysis patients have served to highlight the most prevalent concerns regarding the end of life.[24,25,32] The single most common concern expressed was that of having life inappropriately prolonged at a time when they could no longer enjoy it. Other common issues were wanting to strengthen relationships with loved ones, not to be a burden on their family, to have their wishes respected and to retain control as long as possible, and last but not least to have adequate pain and symptom management. These studies have shown that patients generally would wish to continue with dialysis in only 25 per cent of cases after a severe irreversible stroke; these numbers drop further to 15 per cent in the case of severe dementia and 10 per cent in the case of permanent coma.

> P.M.'s pain was managed with intravenous fentanyl, with options for frequent boluses if dyspnoea or angina became troublesome. Midazolam 2 mg s.c. on an as-needed basis was ordered for possible twitching and myoclonus. He remained lucid until the last 24 h of life, having survived 10 days after withdrawal of dialysis. His dying was remarkably peaceful. The family and dialysis staff fully supported him in his decision.

Question 11. What factors contribute to the decision to discontinue dialysis?

Decisions to discontinue dialysis have been associated with older age, divorced or widowed status, female gender, Caucasian ethnicity, and significant comorbidity.[5,19,33–35] Common comorbid conditions in patients discontinuing dialysis include atherosclerotic vascular disease and its complications (peripheral vascular disease, coronary heart disease, and stroke), congestive heart failure, diabetes and its complications (atherosclerosis, neuropathy, and retinopathy), cancer, cachexia, and dementia.

Question 12. What is the average survival and quality of life after dialysis withdrawal?

The average survival after discontinuing dialysis is about 7 days; 75 per cent of deaths occur in 10 days or less. Cohen *et al.*[5,6] have prospectively studied the quality of death after discontinuing dialysis and concluded that the majority of patients had a 'good' or 'very good' death, while only 15 per cent were classified as having had a 'bad' death. These authors characterized a 'good' death (based on patient and family interviews) as 'pain free, peaceful, and brief', yet many patients in this study (47 per cent) had pain during the last 24 h of life and 30 per cent were agitated. The majority of patients who withdrew from dialysis in this study were unable to participate in interviews because of incompetence or frailty. Earlier involvement of palliative care teams could help improve symptom control, achieve higher rates of advance care planning, and relieve unaddressed emotional, existential, and spiritual suffering.[6,23,36]

Question 13. How would you manage the common symptoms that you might expect after withdrawal of dialysis?

After discontinuing dialysis there is a spectrum of symptoms which become more prevalent and severe the longer the patient survives. The most common are confusion or agitation, pain, dyspnoea, nausea, myoclonus, and pruritus.[6,36] Pain will usually predate discontinuing dialysis, but this is not always the case; for example, an acute ischaemic event may precipitate the decision to withdraw dialysis. Most symptoms can be managed with palliative techniques.

If pain is problematic and the patient is already on opioids, switching to the parenteral route should be considered in anticipation of increased nausea due to progressive uraemia. If the patient needs more than 12 mg hydromorphone orally per day, or equivalent, switching to fentanyl is appropriate in order to reduce the potential for opioid toxicity and preserve mental clarity. Confusion or agitation is best managed with a combination of a neuroleptic (e.g. haloperidol 0.5–2 mg s.c. every 4 h as needed) and a benzodiazepine (e.g. midazolam 2 mg s.c. hourly as needed, or lorazepam 1–2 mg every 4 h as needed). If twitching, myoclonus, or seizure activity is noted, larger doses of midazolam may be needed (e.g. 5 mg hourly as needed by s.c. injection or continuous infusion). Nausea can usually be managed with haloperidol (0.5–1 mg s.c. twice daily) or metoclopramide (10 mg s.c. every 4 h as needed). Dyspnoea may require oxygen, and can usually be managed with opioids. If acidotic (rapid, regular, and deep) respirations are distressing to the family, midazolam added to the opioid will decrease respiratory effort and lessen dyspnoea. Rarely, pulmonary oedema may require ultrafiltration where excess fluid can be removed rapidly without dialysis. Parenteral antihistamines may be necessary for persistent pruritus; failing this, ondansetron (4–8 mg i.v. or orally two or three times daily) can be tried.[37] Because the patient may decline rapidly it is important that appropriate nursing supports are available and anticipatory prescribing done, particularly if the patient is returning home to die.

Future research directions

Clearly, more research is needed to be able to understand better the needs of patients with ESRD, especially those considering discontinuing dialysis. Specifically, there is a need for better pharmacological treatments for pain (particularly that associated with neuropathy and ischaemia) and other symptoms, given the impact of renal failure on the metabolism of many drugs, as well as a better understanding of the multiple causes of pain in the patient with ESRD. More qualitative and epidemiological studies are needed to understand better the reasons behind the decision to withdraw dialysis, and to know how best to respond to the physical, emotional, existential, and spiritual suffering experienced by these patients. Finally, we also need to be know how to better engage dialysis staff, patients, and families in advance care planning, and how best to incorporate the knowledge, skills, and attitudes of palliative care teams in dialysis units.

References

1. **Schaubel, D.E., Morrison, H.I., Desmeules, M., Parsons, D.A., and Fenton, S.S.** (1999) End-stage renal disease in Canada: prevalence projection to 2005. *Can Med Assoc J*, **160**, 1557–63.
2. **Canadian Institute for Health Information** (2001) *Canadian Organ Replacement Register. Annual Report 2001.* Vol. 1: *Dialysis and Renal Transplantation.* Ottawa: Canadian Organ Replacement Register.
3. **National Kidney Foundation** (1997) Dialysis *Outcomes Quality Initiative (DOQI) Executive Summaries of the NKF–DOQI Clinical Practice Guidelines.* National Kidney Foundation. New York
4. **Foley, R.N., Parfrey, P.S., Hefferton, D., Singh, I., Simms, A., and Barrett, B.J.** (1994) Advance prediction of early death in patients starting maintenance dialysis. *Am J Kidney Dis*, **23**, 836–45.
5. **Cohen, L.M., Germain, M.J., Poppel, D.M., Woods, A.L., Pekow, P.S., and Kjellstrand, C.M.** (2000) Dying well after discontinuing the life-support treatment of dialysis. *Arch Intern Med*, **160**, 2513–18.
6. **Cohen, L.M., Germain, M., Poppel, D.M., Woods, A., and Kjellstrand, C.M.** (2000) Dialysis discontinuation and palliative care. *Am J Kidney Dis*, **36**, 140–4.
7. **Backonja, M., Beydoun, A., Edwards, K., *et al.*** (1998) Gabapentin for the symptomatic treatment of painful neuropathy in patients with diabetes. *JAMA*, **280**, 1831–6.
8. **Blum, R.A., Comstock, T.J., Sica, D.A., *et al.*** (1994) Pharmacokinetics of gabapentin in patients with various degrees of renal function. *Clin Pharmacol Ther*, **56**, 154–9.

9. **Aronoff, G.R., Berns, J.S., Brier, M.E., *et al.***(1999) *Drug Prescribing in Renal Failure: Dosing Guidelines for Adults* (4th edn). Philadelphia, PA: American College of Physicians. Available online at: http://www.kdp-baptist.louisville.edu/renalbook/
10. **Davies, G., Kingswood, C., and Street, M.** (1996) Pharmacokinetics of opioids in renal dysfunction. *Clin Pharmacokinet,* **31**, 410–22.
11. **Twycross, R., Wilcock, A., Charlesworth, S., and Dickman, A.** (2002) *Palliative Care Formulary* (2nd edn). Abingdon, UK: Radcliffe Medical Press.
12. **Babul, N., Darke, A.C., and Hagen, N.** (1995) Hydromorphone metabolite accumulation in renal failure. *J Pain Symptom Manage,* **10**, 184–6.
13. **Swan, K.S., and Bennett, W.M.** (2001) Use of drugs in patients with renal failure. In: Schrier RW (ed.) *Diseases of the Kidney and Urinary Tract* (7th edn). Philadelphia, PA: Lippincott–Williams and Wilkins, 3139–86.
14. **Jeal, W., and Benfield, P.** (1997) Transdermal fentanyl: a review of its pharmacological properties andtherapeutic efficacy in pain control. *Drugs,* **53**, 109–38.
15. **Hill, E.M., Marjomacki, D., Wang, R.I.H. and Drugdex Editorial Staff** (2003) Fentanyl (drug evaluation). In: Hutchison TA, Shahan DR (eds) *DRUGDEX r System.* Greenwood Village, CO: MICROMEDEX (Vol. 116).
16. **Churchill, D.N.** (1995) Psychosocial adaptation of dialysis patients. In: Nissenson, A.R., Fine, R.N., Gentile, D.E. (eds) *Clinical Dialysis* (3rd edn). Norwalk, Ct: Appleton and Lange, 827–38.
17. **Cohen, L.M., McCue, J.D., Germain, M., and Kjellstrand, C.M.** (1995) Dialysis discontinuation. A good death? *Arch Intern Med,* **155**, 42–7.
18. **Cohen, L.M., McCue, J.D., Germain, M., and Woods, A.** (1997) Denying the dying. Advance directives and dialysis discontinuation. *Psychosomatics,* **38**, 27–34.
19. **Leggat, J.E. Jr., Bleombergen, W.E., Levine, G., Hulbert-Shearon, T.E., and Port, F.K.** (1997) An analysis of risk factors for withdrawal from dialysis before death. *J Am Soc Nephrol,* **11**, 1755–63.
20. **Holley, J.L., Finucane, T.E., and Moss, A.H.** (1989) Dialysis patients' attitudes about cardiopulmonary resuscitation and stopping dialysis. *Am J Nephrol,* **9**, 245–51.
21. **Holley, J.L., Hines, S.C., Glover, J.J., Babrow, A.S., Badzek, L.A., and Moss, A.H.** (1999) Failure of advance care planning to elicit patients' preferences for withdrawal from dialysis. *Am J Kidney Dis,* **33**, 688–93.
22. **Perry, E., Swartz, R., Smith-Wheelock, L., Westbrook, J., and Buck, C.** (1996) Why is it difficult for staff to discuss advance directives with chronic dialysis patients? *J Am Soc Nephrol,* **7**, 2160–8.
23. **Cohen, L.M., Germain, M.J., and Poppel, D.M.** (2003) Practical considerations in dialysis withdrawal. 'To have that option is a blessing'. *JAMA,* **289**, 2113–19.
24. **Singer, P.A.** (1999) Advance care planning in dialysis. *Am J Kidney Dis,* **33**, 980–91.
25. **Singer, P.A., Thiel, E.C., Naylor, C.D., *et al.*** (1995) Life-sustaining treatment preferences of hemodialysis patients: implications for advance directives. *J Am Soc Nephrol,* **6**, 1410–17.
26. **Curtis, J.R., Wenrich, M.D., Carline, J.D., Shannon, S.E., Ambrozy, D.M., and Ramsey, P.G.** (2001) Understanding physician's skills at providing end-of-life care: perspectives of patients, families and health care workers. *J Gen Intern Med,* **16**, 41–9.
27. **Wenrich, M.D., Curtis, J.R., Ambrozy, D.A., Carline, J.D., Shannon, S.E., and Ramsey, P.G.** (2003) Dying patients' need for emotional support and personalized care from physicians: perspectives of patients with terminal illness, families, and health care providers. *J Pain Symptom Manage,* **25**, 236–46.
28. **Lynn, J., and Goldstein, N.E.** (2003) Advance care planning for fatal chronic illness: avoiding commonplace errors and unwarranted suffering. *Ann Intern Med,* **138**, 812–18.
29. **Hines, S.C., Glover, J.J., Holley, J.L., Babrow, A.S., Badzek, L.A., and Moss, A.H.** (1999) Dialysis patients' preferences for family-based advance care planning. *Ann Intern Med,* **130**, 825–8.

30. **National Kidney Foundation** (1996) *Initiation or Withdrawal of Dialysis in End Stage Renal Disease: Guidelines for the Health Care Team.* New York; National Kidney Foundation.
31. **Moss, A.H. for the RPA and ASN Working Group** (2000) A new clinical practice guideline on initiation and withdrawal of dialysis that makes explicit the role of palliative medicine. *J Palliat Med,* **3**, 253–60.
32. **Singer, P.A., Martin, D.K., and Kelner, M.** (1999) Quality end-of-life care: patients' perspectives. *JAMA,* **281**, 163–8.
33. **Bajwa, K., Szabo, E., and Kjellstrand, C.M.** (1996) A prospective study of risk factors and decision making in discontinuation of dialysis. *Arch Intern Med,* **156**, 2571–7.
34. **Neu, H., and Kjellstrand, C.M.** (1986) Stopping long-term dialysis. An empirical study of withdrawal of life-supporting treatment. *N Engl J Med,* **314**, 14–20.
35. **Port, F.K., Wolfe, R.A., Hawthorne, V.M., and Ferguson, C.W.** (1989) Discontinuation of dialysis therapy as a cause of death. *Am J Nephrol,* **9**, 145–9.
36. **Rich, A., Ellershaw, J., and Ahmad, R.** (2001) Palliative care involvement in patients stopping haemodialysis. *Palliat Med,* **15**, 513–14.
37. **Balaskas, E.V., Bamihas, G.I., Karamouzis, M., *et al.*** (1998) Histamine and serotonin in uremic pruritus: effect of ondansetron in CAPD-pruritic patients. *Nephron,* **78**, 395–402.

Chapter 16

Cardiac disease

Romayne Gallagher

Attitude

To enable each student to:

- Demonstrate an understanding of the suffering of individuals with advanced heart disease and that it is an illness requiring palliative care.
- Understand the complexity of discussing end-of-life issues with a variable prognosis.
- Demonstrate the steps to prevent physical, psychosocial, and emotional problems.
- Have an understanding of the complexity of achieving quality of life without prolonging the dying process.

Skill

To enable each student to:

- Be able to open the discussion around end-of-life issues with patients who have advanced cardiac disease.
- Be able to use appropriate medications to control symptoms of advanced heart disease and to know when to initiate palliative therapies.
- Be able to use opioids, which are helpful in combating the sensation of dyspnoea, as you would for dyspnoea secondary to lung cancer or other lung diseases (see Chapter 12).
- Be able to treat refractory angina pain.

Knowledge

To enable each student to:

- Describe the pathophysiology of heart failure and refractory angina.
- Describe the mechanisms of death in advanced cardiac disease.
- Describe the medications used in heart failure and have an understanding of their effect on quality of life versus quantity of life.
- Describe the effect of opioids in heart failure and intractable angina and how they assist in symptom relief.

Case 1. Congestive heart failure

Advanced cardiac disease is the most common cause of death in many countries. Its incidence and prevalence rises dramatically after age 75. The age-related mortality of acute cardiac disease, such as myocardial infarction, is falling because of therapies that prolong life. With the ageing of the population; the number of people living with advanced cardiac disease will grow dramatically over the next few decades. In the over-65 age group, heart failure accounts for more hospital admissions than any other condition.

M.C. is an 83-year-old widow who was diagnosed with congestive heart failure 3 years ago. She had a history of hypertension for many years and had a myocardial infarction 4 years ago. She has been admitted to hospital with increasing pedal oedema, dyspnoea, insomnia, and chest pain for the past week. On examination in emergency, she has a New York Heart Association (NYHA) class IV degree of failure (Table 16.1) with evidence of shortness of breath at rest. Her echocardiogram shows a left ventricle ejection fraction of 24 per cent (normal is >55 per cent) with a dilated left ventricle, and her chest rediograph shows pulmonary oedema with bilateral small pulmonary effusions. Current medications include furosemide 80 mg orally daily, atenolol 12.5 mg orally twice a day, captopril 6.25 mg orally three times a day and ASA 81 mg orally daily.

M.C. is treated with intravenous diuretics and her ACE inhibitor and β-blocker are adjusted. She has a diuresis of several litres of fluid over the subsequent 2 days, is relieved of her shortness of breath at rest, and is able to resume walking slowly over the next week. She is gradually mobilized and sent home 15 days after admission. At a family meeting prior to discharge, a neighbour attends, as M.C. has no children. She is told that she will be receiving home care nursing to help manage her heart failure. She is instructed to weigh herself daily and report changes to the nurse. A follow-up appointment is arranged with her family physician. Her admitting physician sees her prior to discharge and says she is doing very well.

Question 1. What steps have been taken to help the patient manage her illness that will be helpful?

The natural history of chronic heart failure is one of a slow progressive decline in function punctuated by episodes of rapid decompensation. Thus the patient may feel that he or she is facing the possibility of death only to be 'pulled out of the fire'. Many patients will be in NYHA class IV failure (dyspnoeic at rest) when they are first admitted to hospital with heart failure. Effective diuresis can improve patient symptoms dramatically. Medical therapy of chronic heart failure includes the identification and treatment of correctable causes such as atrial fibrillation, NSAID-induced fluid retention and renal failure, and titrating medications such as ACE inhibitors and β-blockers to target doses to achieve the maximal benefit. The goal of medical therapy is to reduce the work load on the heart by improving either ventricular function or ventricular filling.

Table 16.1 Functional classification of heart disease (New York Heart Association)

NYHA class	Description	One-year mortality (%)
I	Asymptomatic with low left ventricular ejection fraction	5–10
II	Symptoms with vigorous activity (able to walk three blocks)	15–30
III	Symptoms with mild exertion	15–30
IV	Symptoms at rest	50–60

The major symptoms of heart failure are oedema, fatigue, and breathlessness with exertion. These symptoms result in reduced physical activity and loss of mobility and function, resulting in deconditioning and further loss of function. Chemicals are released by both the myocardium and at the periphery in order to adapt to the reduced heart function. These substances, such as cytokines, natriuretic proteins, sympathetic stimulants, and products of renin–angiotensin–aldosterone system activation can induce or sustain cachexia. As the disease progresses, fluid retention occurs, resulting in peripheral oedema, ascites, and pleural effusions. With advanced disease there is breathlessness at rest, difficulty in sleeping lying down, anorexia, cachexia, nausea, severe fatigue, and pain.

Many heart failure patients have psychological issues and psychiatric comorbidities that complicate their illness. Social isolation and depression are known to lead to worse outcomes with cardiac failure. Lack of social support has correlated with increased hospital readmission, lack of compliance with therapy, increased morbidity, and increased cost of therapy. Depression is common in patients with chronic illness of any kind, particularly those with prolonged disability and ongoing symptoms such as those found in chronic heart failure. One study found a significantly higher rate of depression in those with congestive heart failure and severe functional impairment compared with those who were able to remain more independent.[1] Unfortunately, the depression was unrecognized in the majority of patients and many of them remained depressed for a year or more.

M.C.'s discharge meeting focused on involving routine visits by the community nurse, who would work with the family physician to keep symptoms controlled and avoid hospitalization. A systematic review of multidisciplinary heart failure management programmes revealed reduced hospitalization due to heart failure and cost-effectivness.[2] Some of the studies have shown improved compliance with diet and medications, quality of life, patient satisfaction, and function. The programmes included home-based programmes that focused on routine visits by nurses to monitor symptoms and weight and to encourage compliance with diet and medications. Having a plan to intensify the diuretics, should the daily weight rise, is an example of preventing suffering by acting in advance of severe symptoms. These studies, including the randomized controlled trials, involve selected patients who were willing to enter them. Further work needs to be done on larger more heterogeneous populations that are broadly representative of the heart failure population.

Question 2. What is missing in the discharge discussion of this patient?

What is missing from the discharge planning for M.C. is a discussion on end-of-life issues and a plan for future care that includes the goals of the patient (Table 16.2). Studies with heart failure patients have revealed that this group of patients finds it hard to retain information provided by health care providers and may not have an understanding of the relevance of the information.[3] Caregivers of patients who have died of heart failure reported that although their loved ones believed they were dying, few had been told this by their physicians or had discussed it.

Difficulty in predicting prognosis is one of the key reasons cited for the lack of palliative care involvement in non-cancer diseases such as cardiac disease. Many patients do not receive palliative care because the physicians are not sure when to initiate it and what it might have to offer. The predictive accuracy of many prognostic variables, including serum markers, echocardiography variables, and functional capacity, has been studied. In NYHA class IV patients a persistently low sodium level, resting tachycardia, and hypotension complicating diuresis are poor prognostic signs. Functional capacity measured by NYHA class and left

Table 16.2 Comprehensive care of heart failure

	NYHA class			
	I	II	III	IV
Disease/symptom management	Treat hypertension, diabetes, lipid disorders →			
	ACE inhibitors →			
		β-Blockers →		
		Diuretics →		
			Aldosterone antagonists →	
			Opioids →	
			Multidisciplinary team management →	
	Formal exercise programme →			
Psychosocial care			Monitor for depression →	
			Monitor for social isolation →	
			Loss of independence →	
Spiritual care	Meaning of illness, suffering →			
		Life closure →		
Practical care			Non-pharmacological management of dyspnoea (e.g. energy conservation) →	
			Assistance with ADL →	
End-of-life planning		Advance care planning →		
			DNR →	
Patient and family education	Life style changes (smoking cessation, exercise, diet) →			
		Sodium restriction →		

ventricular dilatation by echocardiography is helpful in assigning risk of mortality but not in establishing a clear time prognosis. Brain or B-type natriuretic protein (BNP), produced in the ventricular myocardium in response to dysfunction, will be a useful factor in predicting prognosis as it becomes more readily available as a routine test.[4] Having a variable prognosis should not prevent discussion of end-of-life issues with patients.[5] Some health care providers have found it easier to discuss 'advanced disease' planning rather than 'endstage disease' planning as the end is very unpredictable. Studies of patients with endstage heart and lung disease have shown that people want to know what is happening and welcome the chance to discuss their goals of care and what may transpire, even if the subject makes them anxious.

M.C. does well at home for several months with regular visits from the home care nurse and from you, her family physician. However, she is gradually becoming less active and has lost 10 pounds in weight over the last 4 months. Decreasing her diuretic resulted in greater shortness of breath and so it was resumed at the previous dose. Dietary supplements have not been successful and she is becoming emaciated. Over a holiday weekend, M.C. develops an upper respiratory tract infection, becomes acutely short of breath, and comes into hospital. On admission she is hypoxic and tachycardic, and is in great distress with dyspnoea and chest pain. ECG changes confirm ischaemia in the lateral leads. Troponin serum levels suggest that she has sustained a small myocardial infarct. She is again managed with intravenous diuretics, ACE inhibitors and a small increase in β-blockers. She is started on a potassium-sparing diuretic, spironolactone, in addition to the furosemide. Despite 2 weeks of therapy she remains short of breath at rest and extremely fatigued. When her attending physician visits, she expresses frustration with the management of her heart failure and is angry with the medical team because they are unable to improve her condition.

Question 3. What is happening to M.C.?

M.C. has now reached a very advanced stage of her illness. While the principles of palliative care should be applied throughout the course of chronic heart failure, specific palliative efforts now become the primary focus of therapy.

Key trials of pharmaceuticals such as ACE inhibitors have shown impressive reductions in mortality rates at 6 months and 1 year (CONSENSUS and SOLVD trials), but the mean increase in life expectancy—clearly of the most interest to the patient—is only 260 days.[6] In fact, the prognosis for advanced cardiac disease is worse than many metastatic cancers. Mortality figures using the NYHA Classification show that 1-year mortality rate in stages II and III heart failure is 15–30 per cent, and in stage IV it is 50–60 per cent. Those who die with less severe heart failure often die suddenly, due to an arrhythmia, making prediction and preparation difficult for the patient, family, and health care providers. Those who die with advanced heart failure may not die suddenly; rather, death is often the result of cachexia and the more prolonged process of multi-organ failure due to low cardiac output.

The SUPPORT study was one of the first large studies to establish that the symptoms of advanced cardiac disease were frequent and burdensome.[7] Dyspnoea was reported by 65 per cent and pain by 42 per cent of 263 patients with heart failure in the last 3 days of their life. A survey of patients with moderate to severe heart failure attending an outpatient heart failure clinic reported breathlessness, pain/angina, tiredness, difficulty in walking, and loss of independence as their most troublesome problems. Caregivers of these patients observed pain, breathlessness, and mental disturbance such as low mood, insomnia, and anxiety as the most common symptoms in the last few weeks of life. These same witnesses reported that hospitalization provided suboptimal or negligible symptom relief in 60–75 per cent of patients and that the management plans ignored patient wishes in one-third of the cases.[8]

Chronic heart failure is best thought of as a systemic disease.[9] While cardiac failure begins with a loss of pump function, the progression of the disease is dominated by the involvement of the peripheral organs and tissues. The homeostatic mechanisms of the peripheral tissues and organs are helpful in maintaining cardiac output in acute situations, but in the chronic state they cause further deterioration of cardiac function. Reducing the peripheral resistance through medications such as ACE inhibitors and β-blockers has led to significant improvements in the management of heart failure. The addition of spironolactone, an aldosterone antagonist, counteracts the fluid-retaining actions of aldosterone and in combination with loop diuretics (furosemide) may provide effective diuresis in advanced heart failure.[10] Patients with advanced heart failure symptoms, left ventricular ejection fraction <35 per cent, and a left bundle branch block on ECG may benefit from cardiac resynchronization therapy that uses a pacing system to regulate contraction of the atria and ventricles, increasing the efficiency of the heart. The addition of cardiac defibrillators with a pacing system may reduce mortality even further but it is extremely costly and there is a need for long term randomized trials comparing it with medical therapy.

Question 4. M.C. retains fluid, yet is losing weight. What is happening?

The most difficult aspect of the systemic syndrome may be cardiac cachexia, which is found in >35 per cent of patients with advanced cardiac disease.[11] It appears to be an independent poor prognostic factor and cannot be directly correlated with heart function measures such as ejection fraction or left ventricular dilatation. Cardiac cachexia is defined as a weight loss of

>7.5 per cent of the previous normal weight over a period of <6 months, excluding other cachectic states such as cancer and thyroid or liver disease.[12]

Neurohormonal and immune mechanisms appear to play a central role in the pathogenesis of cardiac cachexia. Neurohormonal activation, mediated by epinephrine and norepinephrine, contribute to heart rate irregularities and an increased metabolic resting rate. Tumour necrosis factor-α (TNF-α) and other cytokines are commonly produced in excess, contributing to anorexia and weight loss. These metabolic effects result in muscle loss weakness and fatigue, resulting in severe exercise intolerance and dyspnoea at low exercise workloads. Respiratory muscle atrophy secondary to the cachexia may be a major contributing factor to dyspnoea in cardiac failure. Patients with cardiac cachexia may have adequate left ventricular ejection fraction, but have severe fatigue and shortness of breath primarily due to the cachexia. Their prognosis relates to their symptoms of heart failure, cachexia, and degree of functional capacity rather than the parameters of heart function.[13]

Management of cardiac cachexia is in its infancy. It is clearly a multifactorial disorder that will not be controlled by any single agent. Inadequate nutritional intake prior to the onset of cardiac failure may predispose the patient to cardiac cachexia. Attention to nutrition may help cachexia in the early stages. Exercise rehabilitation training can reduce the peripheral resistance and improve symptoms of dyspnoea and fatigue in those who are not in advanced stages of heart failure. Exercise seems to retard the progression of cachexia.[14] ACE inhibitors and angiotensin receptor blockers such as candesartan are inhibitors of both immune and neurohormonal factors through their reduction of angiotensin II.[15] Agents that will reduce cachexia-related cytokines are under investigation.

Question 5. Why is M.C. angry and how would you deal with this?

While it is clear to the health care providers that M.C. has advanced heart disease, it may not be clear to her. Thus she may feel that her heart failure is inadequately managed and she may be angry with her caregivers. She feels that she has not been given adequate information about her illness and what is happening to her.

> The attending physician and you schedule a meeting with M.C. and, with M.C.'s permission; a neighbour is also present to listen. She is given information about the nature of heart failure and that she has advanced disease. She tells you that she had been thinking that herself, but wanted to believe that maybe some adjustment in medications could make her well again. When you ask about symptoms, she tells you that she is extremely fatigued and short of breath most of the day and often sleeps sitting up due to dyspnoea. Her chest is uncomfortable and tight, especially when she is short of breath. Her legs are now grossly swollen with oedema, in sharp contrast to her spindly wasted arms. When she tells you about her symptoms she seems fearful and worried.

Question 6. What medications can you use to control her symptoms?

In a patient with advanced heart failure, who remains in NYHA class IV failure despite the best balance of cardiac medications, the addition of opioids can provide significant relief of the dyspnoea and pain often experienced. A systematic review of opioids used in advanced disease of any kind showed significant relief from dyspnoea with the use of oral or parenteral opioids.[16] Inhaled opioids did not show a significant benefit. The mechanism of action of opioids is thought to be through several actions:

- Reduction of cardiac venous return by depression of sympathetic reflexes and histamine release. This results in venodilation.

- Suppression of the CO_2-sensitive respiratory centre in the medulla, resulting in a reduction of the perceived breathlessness.
- A central effect of relaxation that relieves the distress of dyspnoea.
- Blocking airway irritant receptors resulting in less bronchospasm.

The choice of opioid is important as many patients with advanced heart failure will also have comorbid renal failure and hypoxia and will be sensitive to the toxic effects of the active metabolites of opioids. While morphine and hydromorphone share the same metabolite profile, hydromorphone has a shorter half-life and the metabolites are cleared faster, which may result in fewer side effects.[17] It is important to start with very low doses in those who are opioid naive and to titrate slowly until dyspnoea is relieved with as few side effects as possible. Doses as low as 0.5–1 mg of oral hydromorphone every 4 h can be started in outpatients, provided that there is a caregiver to monitor the patient for the first 24–48 h after the opioid is started or the dose is increased. Once a stable dose is reached, the short-acting opioid can be converted to a long-acting formulation to improve compliance. Oxycodone's long-acting form comes in a convenient starting dose (e.g. oxycodone CR 10 mg every 12 h).

The dose of opioid is titrated according to the patient's symptoms. It is the relief achieved rather than the actual dosage that is the key to achieving successful management of dyspnoea and pain. If the patient is on oral medications and is unable to swallow in the last days of life, subcutaneous opioids can be used to provide relief of pain and dyspnoea.

In advanced heart failure, it is important to continue the diuresis even in the last few days to prevent the patient being symptomatic with pulmonary oedema in their last hours. Although research evidence is lacking, furosemide can be given subcutaneously in addition to opioids. Bronchodilators may be helpful in certain patients, although their cardiostimulatory role must be kept in mind. ACE inhibitors and β-blockers should be maintained until the patient can no longer swallow oral medications, titrated relative to hypotensive effects.

The role of oxygen in advanced heart failure is not well researched. Only a few level 4 studies have been done on oxygen in patients with advanced non-cancer disease. Oxygen may be helpful in those with hypoxia, but it is cumbersome for those who choose to stay at home with their illness. It is important not to measure pulse oximetry in those who are in their final days with heart failure, as it does not relate to the degree of dyspnoea. If oxygen is dutifully titrated to keep the oxygen saturation >90 per cent, patients will die with masks blowing 10 l/min on their faces, unable to communicate with their families and with no guarantee that their dyspnoea will be relieved.

Question 7. What can you do to address M.C.'s fear and anxiety?

Empathy for the patient will do a great deal to help him or her feel well looked after and may reduce anxiety. Most patients fear the dying process more than death itself, and you will greatly relieve their concern if you address this issue. Opening lines such as 'Many people worry about what the end will be like' or 'Many people in your situation are frightened of becoming short of breath as they get sicker', are helpful in introducing this discussion. It is rare for a patient to initiate this conversation, and so you should take the opportunity to raise the issue when you sense the patient is fearful. Reassuring the patient of how you are able to control shortness of breath or pain will help them feel comfortable, but you must also demonstrate that you are able to do this by attending to their current symptoms and working with them to maximize their quality of life.

M.C. is helped by the use of opioids. Her dyspnoea is relieved with small doses of short-acting hydromorphone, which you switch to a controlled release formulation once her dyspnoea and chest discomfort are adequately controlled. M.C. wants to be in her own home and live there until she dies. Her neighbours are willing to arrange a schedule of times to be with her, in addition to community resources such as home-making and nursing. She does not wish to return to hospital again.

Question 8. What do you need to put in place for M.C. to remain at home?

Since M.C. wants to be at home and not return to hospital, strategies will have to be in place to deal with exacerbations of dyspnoea or pain. These strategies would focus on increasing the opioid dose to control dyspnoea, having adjuvant medications available for the management of dyspnoea, and having alternate formulations of opioids, diuretics, and adjuvants for when she is no longer able to swallow pills. Home oxygen should be arranged if this proves helpful for her shortness of breath. This plan should be communicated to all the team members—the family physician, home nursing, home-making, neighbours—and any concerns or problems should be resolved. The team needs to know that this plan is in keeping with M.C.'s wishes.

In addition, a do not resuscitate order (DNR) will have to be written and communicated to the team. By having a DNR order the ambulance paramedics may attend and assist in management of the patient's symptoms, but they are not obliged to resuscitate her if she should die.

M.C. goes home with home-making support, home care nursing, and strategies in place for her exacerbations. You visit her regularly. You manage several of her episodes of shortness of breath with increased opioid doses and small doses (1.25–5.0 mg) of methotrimeprazine on a regular basis. (see Chapter 12 for more information on adjuvant medications for dyspnoea). Four weeks after discharge, M.C. wakes up one night feeling very short of breath. Within a few minutes of awakening her level of consciousness begins to decline and she dies a few minutes later.

The majority of patients with heart failure will die quite suddenly with an arrhythmia that results in cardiac output that cannot sustain life.

The same issues and therapies for heart failure will also apply to those with congenital heart disease and cardiomyopathies that may develop advanced disease. Many of these patients may be eligible for a heart transplant and the goal may be to keep them alive as long as possible, hoping that a suitable donor may become available. These patients may opt for more aggressive therapy such as inotropes or ventricular assist devices to 'bridge' them to a transplant. However, many patients will die waiting for transplants, and so the patient must be prepared for this outcome as well.

Case 2. Refractory angina

F.H. is a 69-year-old man who has had diabetes mellitus for the past 16 years. Over the years he developed a moderate degree of renal failure and coronary artery disease secondary to the diabetes. He has been managed with oral hypoglycaemics and insulin-sensitizing agents but developed progressively worse hyperglycaemia and eventually required regular insulin. Eight years ago he underwent three-vessel coronary artery bypass surgery for unstable angina. Unstable angina is defined as an acute coronary syndrome presenting as either severe new onset angina, increasing angina, or prolonged angina at rest. His renal failure worsened as a result of the surgery, but the angina resolved. Unfortunately, his angina recurred 2 years ago and a coronary angiogram revealed patent bypass grafts but high-grade obstruction in the distal small vessels. His angina has been managed with multiple medications including a β-blocker, a calcium-channel blocker, nitrate, an ACE inhibitor, a lipid-lowering agent and aspirin. Despite all this therapy, F.H. has been admitted to the hospital with severe angina again. He has been forced to reduce his activity dramatically over the past few months to try to prevent angina attacks. He is housebound and relies on his wife for much of his daily care. As well as daily episodes of angina, he also has dizziness, unsteadiness on his feet, and fatigue. His wife is worried about his mood, as he has become very irritable and withdrawn over the last months. On examination he has a mildly elevated jugular venous pressure (JVP), crackles in both lung bases, and mild pedal oedema. He is in sinus rhythm at 56 beats/min with occasional premature ventricular contractions (PVCs). His blood pressure is 85/55 mmHg.

Question 1. What is the cause of F.H.'s symptoms?

F.H. has refractory angina. This is defined as the presence of stable angina due to advanced coronary artery disease (CAD) that is not controlled by a combination of maximal anti-anginal medication in a patient who is not suitable for coronary revascularization.[19]

CAD is a common disease in our society. One-third of patients with CAD will die suddenly, and the rest may develop either an ischaemic cardiomyopathy and heart failure or a chronic angina syndrome over the ensuing years. The prognosis for patients with chronic angina syndrome depends on many factors, but the prognosis is worse with comorbid illnesses, a history of multiple myocardial infarctions, multi-vessel CAD, unstable angina, poor left ventricular function, and symptoms of congestive heart failure. F.H. has been managed with multiple anti-anginal therapies but many of his symptoms (dizziness, fatigue, and irritability) may be due to hypotension and bradycardia resulting from the medication.

Question 2. What other diagnoses might you suspect on hearing this history?

F.H. may have dizziness due to low blood pressure. With advanced cardiac disease it is often a fine balance between controlling the cardiac symptoms and maintaining an adequate blood pressure. F.H. may also be symptomatic from his chronic renal failure, accounting for fatigue, dizziness, and perhaps some of his irritability. However, with his long history of multiple chronic illnesses and the loss of his independence, he may have developed concurrent depression. While there are no specific screening tools for depression in advanced cardiac disease, a review of depression screening tests found the single question 'Are you depressed' to be the tool with the highest sensitivity and specificity and positive predictive value in palliative patients.[20]

Laboratory results for F.H. reveal moderate renal failure with a creatinine of 330 μmol/l (normal range, 60–120 μmol/l). Troponin is slightly elevated, suggesting slight myocardial damage. An ECG shows ischaemia in the lateral leads, poor R wave progression, and evidence of an old inferior myocardial infarct. His blood sugar is 17.3 mmol/l (normal range, 3.9–6.7 mmol/l). Thus the other diagnosis is chronic renal failure and poorly controlled diabetes, both of which can be contributing to his symptoms.

F.H. wants to know what you can do to resolve the angina. He is scared that he is going to die with each episode. His wife is exhausted and worried that she can no longer care for him at home.

Question 3. Would an angiogram and possible angioplasty be indicated in this patient?

An angiogram 2 years ago showed distal vessel obstruction in the coronary arteries. Angioplasty is not successful in these patients and is very risky. In addition, he has diffuse disease and so angioplasty would be unsuccessful.

Question 4. Would dialysis improve F.H.'s symptoms?

Offering this man dialysis would not improve his quality of life and would probably prolong the dying process. Since F.H. is at high risk for a myocardial infarction in the future months, dialysis may not extend his life. The risks and benefits of dialysis would have to be discussed with F.H. and his wife.

Question 5. How would you treat the angina and other symptoms?

The goals of therapy at this point are to relieve F.H.'s angina and improve his quality of life. Pain relief in refractory angina despite maximal medical therapy can be achieved with the addition of opioids.[21] Since F.H. is in renal failure, morphine would not be a good choice as it has active metabolites that accumulate in renal failure. While hydromorphone has lower levels of active metabolites, accumulation of metabolites can still occur. Opioids with no or less consequential active metabolites, such as oxycodone or fentanyl, may be the best choice. Small regular doses can be initiated and titrated to the most effective dose. Opioids help to relieve the angina by providing analgesia and decreasing cardiac workload, thus reducing oxygen demand by the myocardium. Oxygen may be helpful for some patients with refractory angina. Small case studies have shown relief from refractory angina with a stellate ganglion block, spinal cord stimulation, or the use of epidural opioids and local anaesthetics. [22,23] However, these options are invasive and have complications that may outweigh the benefits.

Question 6. What other issues would you need to address with F.H. and his wife?

F.H. and his wife would appreciate information about several key issues that they must face. Every patient with angina has been taught to seek immediate medical intervention with angina as it is a potential myocardial infarction. Many patients will be concerned that the opioid will mask their pain and that they will be harming themselves by being active and controlling the pain. They need reassurance that the medication is not only relieving the pain but also reducing the workload on the heart. There is a great need for larger studies on the use of opioids for the management of refractory angina. The few studies that do exist do not indicate a higher risk of dying from a myocardial infarction as a result of normal activity.

In addition, F.H. and his wife would benefit from referral to home-care nursing in their community. F.H.'s wife may also appreciate someone to be with her husband to give her regular respite from her caregiving duties. Setting up a roster of friends, family, volunteers, or paid home support workers will help her to cope with the demands of caregiving.

Future trends in palliative care of cardiac disease

The future for advanced heart disease would be much brighter if heart failure could be prevented. Essential strategies for prevention would be comprehensive management of diseases that lead to heart failure, such as hypertension, atherosclerosis, and diabetes. The next step would be to identify those with asymptomatic heart failure who would benefit from early intervention to prevent progression to advanced disease. Natriuretic peptide and other neurohormonal agents will be helpful in early detection and optimizing therapy. Patients, families, and health care providers would welcome better prognostic accuracy. Upon identifying patients in the early stages, medications to prevent progression may be helpful.

Reforming the current health care system to manage chronic disease by multidisciplinary teams will undoubtedly help patients with heart failure maintain wellness longer and prevent frequent hospital admissions.

There will be increasing debates over the use of 'bridging to transplantation' therapies, such as inotropes and ventricular assist devices, in advanced heart disease.[24] Studies with inotropes have shown symptomatic improvement but a deleterious effect on mortality. Left ventricle reduction surgeries have been done to improve cardiac output in dilated left ventricles. Implantable defibrillators, now in greater use, are being associated with anxiety and other psychiatric disorders, as well as raising ethical questions around withdrawal of therapy. For refractory angina, a transendocardial laser has been used to improve vascular supply to ischaemic heart muscle.[25]

Management of symptoms in advanced heart failure will be improved with further research into cachexia, as many mechanisms are probably common across disease entities, including cancer cachexia. In addition, large studies looking at the use of opioids in the management of heart failure may help to define when opioids should be started for maximum relief of dyspnoea and pain, and which are preferable in advanced heart disease.

More research into the needs and desires of patients with advanced heart failure is needed to improve understanding of the importance of quality versus quantity of life. Research into the experience of those coping with uncertain prognosis and chronic illness will help in the design of advance planning for those living with an illness where their prognosis is so uncertain.

Bibliography

Anderson, H., Ward, C., Eardley, A., *et al.* (2001) The concerns of patients under palliative care and a heart failure clinic are not being met. *Palliat Med,* **15**, 279–86.

Gibbs, J.S.R., McCoy, A.S.M, Gibbs, L.M.E., Rogers, A.E., and Addington-Hall, J.M. (2002) Living with and dying from heart failure: the role of palliative care. *Heart,* **88** (Suppl II), ii36–9.

Taylor, G.J. (2003) Heart disease. In: Taylor GJ, Kurent JE (eds) *A Clinician's Guide to Palliative Care.* Boston, MA: Blackwell, 47–75.

References

1. **Koenig, H.G.** (1998) Depression in hospitalized older patients with congestive heart failure. *Gen Hosp Psychiatry,* **20**, 29–43.
2. **Rich, M.W.** (1999) Heart failure disease management: a critical review. *J Card Fail,* **5**, 64–75.
3. **Rogers, A.E., Addington-Hall, J.M., Abery, A.J., *et al.*** (2000) Knowledge and communication difficulties for patients with chronic heart failure: qualitative study. *BMJ,* **321**, 605–7.

4. **Jessup, M., and Brozena, S.** (2003) Medical progress: heart failure. *N Engl J Med,* **348**, 2007–18.
5. **Lynn, J.** (1997) An 88-year-old woman facing the end-of-life. *JAMA,* **277**, 1633–40.
6. **Ward, C.** (2002) The need for palliative care in the management of heart failure. *Heart,* **87**, 294–8.
7. **Levenson, J.W., McCarthy, E.P., Lynn, J., Davis, R.P., and Phillips, R.S,** (2000) The last six months of life for patients with congestive heart failure. *J Am Geriatr Soc,* **48**, S101–9.
8. **McCarthy, M., Addington-Hall, J., and Ley, M.** (1997) Communication and choice in dying from heart disease. *J R Soc Med,* **90**, 128–31.
9. **Kleber, F.X., and Petersen, S.** (1998) The peripheral syndrome of heart failure: the overlooked aspects. *Eur Heart J,* **19**(Suppl L), L10–14.
10. **Brater, D.C.** (1998) Diuretic therapy. *N Engl J Med,* **339**, 387–95.
11. **Anker, S., Negassa, A., Coats, A., Poole-Wilson, P., and Yusuf, S.** (1999) Weight loss in chronic heart failure (CHF) and the impact of treatment with ACE inhibitors—results from the SOLVD treatment trial. *Circulation,* **100**, I-781 (abstr).
12. **Anker, S.D., and Sharma, R.** (2002) The syndrome of cardiac cachexia. *Int J Cardiol,* **85**, 51–66.
13. **Cowburn, P.J., Cleland, J.G.F., Coats, A.J.S., and Komajda, M.** (1998) Risk stratification in chronic heart failure. *Eur Heart J,* **19**, 696–710.
14. **Coats, A.J., Adamopoulos, S., Meyer, T.E., Conway, J., and Sleight, P.** (1990) Effects of physical training in chronic heart failure. *Lancet,* **335**, 63–66.
15. **Lui, L., and Zhao, S.P.** (1999) The changes in circulating tumor necrosis factor levels in patients with congestive heart failure influenced by therapy. *Int J Cardiol,* **69**, 77–82.
16. **Jennings, A.L., Davies, A., Higgins, J.P.T., and Broadley, K.** (2001) Opioids for the palliation of breathlessness in terminal illness (Cochrane Review). In: *The Cochrane Library*, Issue 4. Oxford: Update Software.
17. **Gourlay, G.K.** (1999) Clinical pharmacology of the treatment of chronic non-cancer pain. In: Max M (ed) *Pain 1999—an Updated Review.* Seattle, WA: International Association for the Study of Pain Press, Seattle, 443–52.
18. **Levy, M.H.** (2001) Advancement of opioid analgesia with controlled-release oxycodone. *Eur J Pain,* **5** (Suppl A), 113–16.
19. **Chester, M.R.** (1999) UK National Refractory Angina Centre. Available online at: www.angina.org
20. **Lloyd-Williams, M., Spiller, J., and Ward, J.** (2003) Which depression screening tools should be used in palliative care? *Palliat Med,* **17**, 40–3.
21. **Mouallem, M., Schwartz, E., and Farfel, Z.** (2000) Prolonged oral morphine therapy for severe angina pectoris. *J Pain Symptom Manage,* **19**, 393–6.
22. **Andersen, C., and Hole, P.** (1998) Long-term home treatment with epidural analgesia does not affect later spinal cord stimulation in patients with otherwise intractable angina pectoris. *Clin J Pain,* **14**, 315–19.
23. **Lieberman, I., Wilmshurst, S., Krysiak, Y., and Makin, R.** (2003) Chronic refractory angina management for under $5 a day: one year follow up results of the Greater Manchester Refractory Angina Service, UK. *The J Pain,* **4** (2), 529.
24. **Mehra, M.R., and Uber, P.A.** (2001) The dilemma of late stage heart failure: rationale for chronic parenteral inotropic support. *Cardiol Clin,* **19**, 627–35.
25. **Guleserian, K.J., Maniar, H.S., Camillo, C.J., Bailey, M.S., Damiano, R.J., and Mo, M.R.** (2003) Quality of life and survival after transmyocardial laser revascularization with the holmium:YAG laser. *Ann Thorac Surg,* **75**, 1842–7.

Chapter 17

Nausea and vomiting

Ingrid de Kock

Attitude

To enable each student to:

- Recognize the impact of nausea and vomiting on a person's quality of life and daily care as well as the potentially devastating effects on the family.
- Recognize that the aim of treatment is the patient's comfort and that this can be achieved even if full control of nausea and vomiting is not possible.
- Appreciate the complexity of the concerns that may face the person with advanced illness, and that nausea interrelates with other symptoms, emotions, and fears and cannot be dealt with in isolation.

Skill

To enable each student to:

- Develop a logical approach to identification of the specific causes of nausea and vomiting for each patient.
- Design a treatment plan for each patient based on the specific triggers for nausea, the receptor(s) and neurotransmitter(s) involved, and the targeting antiemetic medications.
- Integrate non-pharmacological modalities into the treatment plan.
- Discuss the causes and treatment options appropriately with the patient and his or her family.

Knowledge

To enable each student to:

- Discuss the pathophysiology of nausea and vomiting.
- Discuss the different groups of antiemetic medications and their indications, as well as give examples from each group with the main side effects and contraindications.

Case 1

Mrs L. is a 62-year-old woman who was diagnosed with breast cancer 2 years ago. She had chemotherapy and is now using tamoxifen. She fell 6 days ago and sustained a pathological fracture of her right humerus. Because of extensive bone loss the orthopaedic surgeon was not able to pin the humerus, but did apply a splint to the arm. She was given a prescription for morphine 5 mg orally every 4 h, which has effectively relieved her pain. She presents to your office with nausea that she rates as 7/10 on a visual analogue scale (0 = no nausea; 10 = worst possible nausea); her last bowel movement was 5 days ago. She has not vomited. She is very distraught and tearful; she had experienced severe refractory nausea and vomiting during and after chemotherapy and is very worried that this might be as difficult to control.

Question 1. What are the more common causes of nausea and vomiting in palliative care patients?

Nausea and vomiting occur in 50–70 per cent of advanced cancer patients.[1,2] Causes include the following:

- Pharyngeal irritation:
  - oral/oesophageal candidiasis
  - tenacious sputum/persistent cough
- Gastric irritation:
  - peptic ulcer disease (PUD)/gastritis
- Gastric stasis:
  - opioids/anticholinergics
  - hepatomegaly/mechanical gastric outlet obstruction
  - autonomic dysfunction (may be associated with anorexia/cachexia syndrome)
- Stretch/distortion of gastrointestinal tract:
  - constipation (common in patients with advanced cancer)
  - intestinal obstruction
  - mesenteric metastases
- Infections of the gastrointestinal tract:
  - fungal, bacterial, parasitic (common in AIDS/HIV)
- Medications:
  - opioids (introduction/increase in opioids cause emesis in about 30 per cent of patients)[3]
  - cytotoxics
  - selective serotonin-reuptake inhibitors (SSRIs)
  - antivirals
  - antibiotics
  - idiosyncratic response to virtually any drug may occur
- Metabolic:
  - hypercalcaemia

  - renal failure
  - liver failure
  - related to diabetes
- Raised intracranial pressure:
  - primary brain tumour/brain metastases
  - cerebral infections (e.g. AIDS)
- Movement induced:
  - vestibular disorders (rare in advanced cancer)
  - traction on tumour-involved mesenterium/viscera
- Psychosomatic:
  - anxiety/emotions
  - pain
  - anticipatory nausea (occasionally seen with chemotherapy)
- Tumour induced:
  - autonomic dysfunction (not well studied)
  - cytokines and other tumour factors (not well studied)

Question 2. How do you narrow down the differential diagnosis?

The history should include a complete list of medications, as well as a full review of systems and past history (PUD, gastritis). Enquire about the meaning of the nausea and vomiting to Mrs L. and her family; it can be a source of great anxiety about disease progression and prognosis. Identify any specific triggers or alleviating factors. Ask about the frequency of nausea and vomiting, as it can lead to inadequate fluid intake, subsequent dehydration, and opioid toxicity. The nature of the vomitus can provide clues to the cause: feculent vomitus might signify a more distal bowel obstruction; haematemesis might be due to severe gastric irritation, but can also be a sign of the more ominous condition of oesophageal varices associated with portal hypertension. Vomiting without nausea may be a sign of proximal bowel obstruction or raised intracranial pressure. Question Mrs L. about any neurological or cognitive changes that might indicate central tumour involvement. This is also an important point when managing nausea and vomiting in a patient with HIV/AIDS, as it may signal central nervous system infections or degenerative conditions. You have already asked Mrs L. to rate the nausea on a visual analogue scale (0 = no nausea; 10 = worst possible nausea); repeat this at each assessment to monitor treatment effect. During the physical examination assess for dehydration, any abnormalities of the gastrointestinal tract including signs of obstruction, constipation, and hepatomegaly, and signs of raised intracranial pressure or central nervous system infection in HIV/AIDS patients.

Laboratory investigations should be individualized: exclude renal impairment (urea and creatinine), hypercalcaemia, hyponatraemia, hypomagnesaemia, liver failure, and changes in blood sugar. An abdominal radiograph (supine view) may be useful to assess for constipation. If an obstruction is suspected, request three views of the abdomen.

Frequently reassess her until the nausea has subsided to a level at which she is comfortable.

Question 3. What are the most likely causes of nausea in the case of Mrs L.?

She was recently started on opioid medication and was not prescribed an antiemetic to prevent/treat nausea. She did not receive instructions on the use of laxatives to prevent constipation. The most likely diagnoses include opioid-induced nausea, opioid-induced constipation, and hypercalcaemia (in her case possibly associated with bone metastases), and the situation could be aggravated by anxiety.

Question 4. How do you decide on the appropriate treatment for her nausea?

Understanding the pathophysiology enables you to choose the most appropriate antiemetic. Nausea is an unpleasant expression of autonomic stimulation, sometimes accompanied by pallor, cold sweat, and salivation. Retching and vomiting are expressions of a complex process requiring coordinated activities of the gastrointestinal tract, diaphragm, and abdominal muscles.[4]

Anatomy, pathways and receptors

The chemoreceptor trigger zone (CRTZ) is a functional entity located in the area postrema, the floor of the fourth ventricle. Since it is outside the blood–brain barrier and is 'bathed' by the systemic circulation, dopamine type 2 (D_2) receptors in the area postrema can be stimulated by high plasma concentrations of emetogenic substances such as calcium ions, opioids, and urea. The area postrema also receives input from the vagus nerve and the vestibular apparatus and contains opioid and cannabinoid receptors (Fig. 17.1).

The vomiting centre is not a specific anatomical entity, but rather a diffuse network which acts as central pattern generator for the vomiting reflex.[5]

Using the knowledge about the neurotransmitters and pathways allows you to target specific stimuli of nausea and vomiting. Identifying specific triggers and tailoring the antiemetic have been shown to be effective in 93 per cent of patients.[6] The best choice in a specific group depends on the side effects. Antiemetics can be classified according to their receptor activity and site of action (Table 17.1).

Question 5. Which antiemetic do you choose for Mrs L.?

Mrs L. is probably experiencing nausea from stimulation of the CRTZ by morphine. D_2 receptors are one of the main receptor-types in this area and it would be appropriate to use one of the dopamine antagonists. Palliative Care centres have different preferences for first-line antiemetics. The dopamine blocker metoclopramide has the added benefit of promoting gastric and duodenal motility, which is impaired by opioid use. For refractory nausea it can be administered as continuous subcutaneous infusion. Other reasonable choices include prochlorperazine and haloperidol, the most widely used butyrophenone. Dosages and routes of administration are shown in Table 17.2.

Antihistamines are avoided in some centres because of their sedative effects and a tendency to increase constipation. Many patients complain of feeling 'drugged' when using the antihistamines. It is more appropriate to target the CRTZ directly if nausea is due to medications or metabolic disturbances.

Serotonin receptors are present in both the vomiting centre and the CRTZ. Serotonin antagonists are used for nausea associated with chemotherapy and radiotherapy, but their benefit in palliative care has not been clearly established yet. Their use is limited further by high cost.

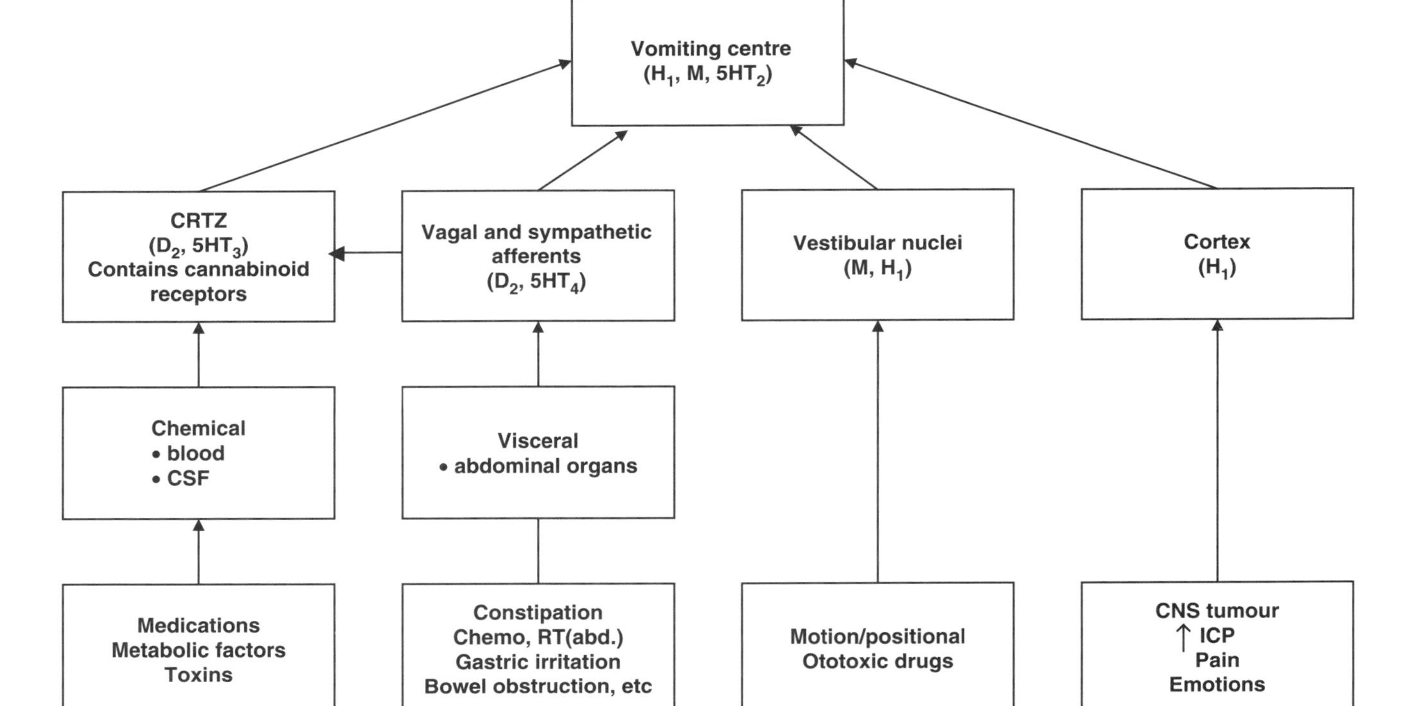

Fig. 17.1 Receptor pathways and neurotransmitters (D_2, dopamine; 5HT, serotonin; H_1, histamine; M, muscarine/acetylcholine). Chemo, chemotherapy; RT, radiotherapy; abd, abdominal; CRTZ, chemoreceptor trigger zone; CSF, cerebrospinal fluid; CNS, central nervous system; ICP, intracranial pressure. Adapted from Lichter, I. (1993) Which antiemetic? *J Palliat Care,* **9**, 42–50.

Table 17.1 Antiemetic medications

Site of action	Class/receptor antagonism	Example	Side effects/comments
Vomiting centre	Antihistamine-anticholinergics	Antihistamines: cyclizine, diphenhydramine, dimenhydrinate Phenothiazines: prochlorpromazine, methotrimeprazine	Drowsiness, dry mouth, constipation extra pyramidal symptoms (EPS), sedation, hypotension
	Anticholinergics	Hyoscine hydrobromide (scopolamine)	Sedation, dry mouth, constipation, confusion, increased intra-ocular pressure, urinary retention
	Serotonin antagonists	Ondansetron, tropisetron, granisetron	Expensive, mostly used for chemotherapy-induced nausea and refractory nausea
		Metoclopramide (at high doses)	Drowsiness (10 per cent),[7] EPS
CRTZ	Dopamine (D_2) antagonists	Butyrophenones: haloperidol	EPS
		Phenothiazines: prochlorperazine, methotrimeprazine	EPS, sedation, hypotension
		Prokinetics: metoclopramide, domperidone	Metoclopramide—drowsiness (10 per cent),[7] EPS Domperidone—does not cross BBB (no central effect at usual doses)
	Serotonin antagonists	Ondansetron, tropisetron, granisetron	Expensive, mostly used for chemotherapy-induced nausea and for refractory nausea and vomiting
		Metoclopramide (at high doses)	EPS
	Cannabinoids	Dronabinol, nabilone	Euphoria, dysphoria, anxiety, mania, tachycardia, dry mouth, appetite stimulation, later drowsiness
Gut receptors and vagus nerve	Dopamine (D_2) antagonists	Butyrophenones: haloperidol	EPS
		Phenothiazines: prochlorperazine, methotrimeprazine	EPS, sedation, hypotension
		Prokinetics: metoclopramide, domperidone	EPS Domperidone does not cross BBB (no central effect at usual doses)
	Serotonin antagonists	Ondansetron etc.	Expensive, mostly used for chemotherapy-induced nausea and for refractory nausea and vomiting
		Metoclopramide (at high doses)	EPS

Table 17.1 (continued) Antiemetic medications

Site of action	Class/receptor antagonism	Example	Side effects/comments
Vestibular nuclei	Anticholinergic	Scopolamine (hyoscine hydrobromide not hyoscine butylbromide)	Sedation, dry mouth, constipation, confusion, increased intra-ocular pressure, urinary retention
	Antihistamine-anticholinergics	Antihistamines: cyclizine, diphenhydramine, dimenhydrinate	Drowsiness, dry mouth, constipation
		Phenothiazines: prochlorpromazine, methotrimeprazine	EPS, sedation, hypotension
Cortex	Antihistamine-anticholinergics	Antihistamines: cyclizine, diphenhydramine, dimenhydrinate	Drowsiness, dry mouth, constipation
		Phenothiazines: prochlorpromazine, methotrimeprazine	EPS, sedation, hypotension
	Anxiolytics	Benzodiazepines: lorazepam	Drowsiness, lethargy, confusion (increased risk if on opioids)
	Cannabinoids	Dronabinol, nabilone	Euphoria, dysphoria, anxiety, mania, tachycardia, dry mouth, appetite stimulation, later drowsiness
	Corticosteroids (mechanism of action not clearly understood)	Dexamethasone	Confusion, euphoria, insomnia, psychosis, fluid retention, gastric irritation, increased blood sugar

EPS, extrapyramidal syndromes; CRTZ, chemoreceptor trigger zone; BBB, blood–brain barrier

Question 6. Which other issues do you need to address?

Mrs L. is also suffering from constipation due to morphine use and this can be a major contributing factor in nausea. This needs to be addressed by relieving the present constipation followed by regular maintenance laxatives, usually a stool softener and a stimulant laxative (for a discussion of the management of constipation in palliative care, see Chapter 18). Her blood calcium levels are normal.

Sit down with Mrs L. and provide a clear direct explanation of the causes of her nausea and the best treatment options in order to allay her anxiety. Reassure her that there are many choices available to improve her level of comfort, but it is advisable not to guarantee or promise total control of her symptoms as this can not always be achieved.

Question 7. Which other non-pharmacological approaches will you suggest?

- Avoidance of the sight or smell of food or other odours (e.g. perfumes) that may trigger nausea.
- Small frequent bland meals.
- Good oral hygiene.

Table 17.2 Dosage and routes of administration of commonly used antiemetics

	Dose	Frequency of administration	Route of administration
Metoclopramide	10 mg/day; may increase to 120 mg/day if nausea refractory	Every 4 h around the clock and hourly as needed	Oral, s.c., i.v.
Haloperidol	0.5–5 mg/day in two divided doses	At bedtime or twice a day and hourly as needed	Oral, s.c.
Prochlorperazine	5 or 10 mg orally 10 or 20 mg rectally	Every 4 h or 6 h and hourly as needed	Oral, rectal
Domperidone	10 mg	Every 4 h or 6 h	Oral
Cyclizine	25 to 50 mg	Every 8 h	Oral, s.c., rectal

- Fresh air, calm environment, distraction.
- Sitting upright after a meal.
- Acupressure/acupuncture are less often recommended, but may be considered if nausea is refractory. There is some research evidence to support the use of acupuncture;[7] acupressure is less well studied, but wrist/pressure bands may be helpful in some cases.

Over the next three days, Mrs L. has several large bowel movements and her nausea is well controlled by metoclopramide taken every 4 h with the morphine. She receives radiotherapy to the right humerus with good pain control. She is switched to long-acting morphine and asks you if she has to continue using metoclopramide every 4 h, as she finds it difficult to remember to take it on time.

Question 8. What do you tell her?

You expect that she will have developed tolerance to the emetic effect of the opioid after 5–7 days and therefore you advise her to use the metoclopramide only as needed or 30 min before meals if she experiences nausea regularly after eating.

Several months go by, and then you are called to see Mrs L. at home by her home care nurse. She is much weaker, has continuous nausea, and vomits several times a day. She resumed taking regular metoclopramide, but is occasionally too nauseated to take the medication; at other times she has emesis after taking it. She has been using more breakthrough doses of morphine, although she is not always able to retain it. She is again constipated, with hard stool in the rectum on examination. When you screen her cognition, you detect subtle deterioration which raises your suspicions about an early delirium. She has experienced visual hallucinations during the past 2 days, but no myoclonus. A bone scan 3 weeks previously had demonstrated widespread bone metastases.

Question 9. What is the most likely cause of her present condition?

Hypercalcaemia is probably the main cause of her nausea, constipation, and delirium, aggravated by dehydration causing early opioid toxicity (visual hallucinations, cognitive changes). Hypercalcaemia occurs in 10–40 per cent of cancer patients and is most commonly associated with myeloma and breast, lung, and renal cancers.[8] It is usually seen with metastatic disease and is an indicator of poor prognosis. Bone metastases are not always present. The clinical presentation may include nausea and vomiting, constipation, weakness, somnolence, confusion, agitation, and anorexia.

Serum calcium is affected by serum albumin and thus the measured calcium has to be corrected according to the serum albumin level. The formula is as follows:

$$\textit{corrected serum calcium (mmol/l)} = \textit{measured serum calcium (mmol/l)} + [40 - \textit{measured serum albumin (g/l)}] \times 0.02].$$

Normal corrected serum calcium is <2.65 mmol/l. (Values may vary in different laboratories.)

An ionized calcium level is the most accurate laboratory investigation, but is not widely available and is more expensive. It is the preferred test in myeloma patients because of the potential calcium-binding effects of myeloma paraproteins.

> Mrs L.'s serum calcium level is 2.6 mmol/l and her albumin level is 20 g/l. Using the above formula, her corrected serum calcium level is 2.6 + [(40–20) × 0.02] = 3.0 mmol/l. Her urea is 12.6 g/l and the creatinine level is normal.

Question 10. How do you manage this situation?

The decision to treat hypercalcaemia is based on the severity of symptoms, the corrected calcium level, the prognosis, and the patient's wishes. The treatment consists of rehydration (subcutaneous administration is a less invasive alternative to intravenous administration in the palliative care population) and usually administration of a bisphosphonate after assessing renal function. A few patients with mildly elevated calcium levels will have normocalcaemia after rehydration only. The bisphosphonates can aggravate renal impairment, including pre-renal failure due to associated dehydration. The commonly used bisphosphonates are shown in Table 17.3.

Clodronate is less expensive than pamidronate and is the only bisphosphonate indicated for subcutaneous administration. In our programme we use clodronate as first-line therapy, as we prefer the subcutaneous route of administration, and only use pamidronate if clodronate therapy fails to control hypercalcaemia within 3 days. Other centres prefer pamidronate as first choice. Zoledronic acid is usually used as third-line treatment in refractory hypercalcaemia.

Table 17.3 Commonly used bisphosphonates

	Dose	Route of administration	Infusion period	Usual expected duration of effect
Clodronate	1500 mg in 250 or 500 ml NS 900 mg if serum creatinine >150 mmol/l	s.c. or i.v.	Over 4 h	2 weeks
Pamidronate	60 mg in 250 ml NS or 90 mg in 500 ml NS	i.v.	Over 2.5–4 h	3–4 weeks
Zoledronic acid	4 mg in 100 ml NS	Slow i.v.	Over 15 min	4–6 weeks

NS, normal saline.

Repeat calcium, albumin, creatinine, urea, and electrolyte levels on the third day after bisphosphonate administration if symptoms persist. Calcium levels will usually show an improvement 3 days after treatment correlated with clinical improvement. Symptomatic hypocalcaemia is rare following bisphosphonate use. If a patient has a highly elevated calcium level and is very symptomatic, consider using calcitonin as a temporary measure to reduce the calcium levels rapidly. The effects of calcitonin are not sustained and most patients will still need a bisphosphonate after correction of prerenal failure. The usual dose for calcitonin is 100 U s.c. three times a day for 1–2 days.

The regular administration of bisphosphonates has been shown to decrease the incidence of skeletal events (e.g. pathological fractures) as well as preventing recurrent hypercalcaemia.[9,10] When bisphosphonates are used on a regular basis, the patient should be monitored for dehydration and renal impairment before administration. If clinically dehydrated or with a previous history of renal problems, obtain serum electrolytes, urea, and creatinine. If the creatinine level is >150–160 mmol/l decrease the dose of the bisphosphonate.

The nausea should be dealt with by using a drug that targets the CRTZ. First-line choices include metoclopramide, haloperidol, or a phenothiazine (more sedating which is useful if the patient is restless). Mrs L. has not been able to retain oral metoclopramide and needs subcutaneous administration of the antiemetic as well as the opioid. She is showing signs of early opioid toxicity with decreased pain control, and should be rotated to another opioid (see Chapter 2).

You arrange with home care to administer normal saline subcutaneously ('hypodermoclysis' or 'clysis') at a rate of 90 ml/h and you order clodronate 1500 mg in 250 ml of normal saline to be infused subcutaneously over 4 h. You start her on subcutaneous metoclopramide 10 mg every 4 h around the clock with 10 mg hourly as required and rotate her to hydromorphone s.c. every 4 h around the clock. Her sister looks after her now and is taught do do subcutaneous injections. You ask her home care nurse to do a fleet enema, followed by an oil retention enema with a soap suds or saline enema the next morning. She responds well to the treatments and you arrange for clodronate infusions every 2 weeks with the support of home care. Once the nausea settles, you resume oral administration of medications.

Mrs L. is maintained at home for 2 months with the help of her family and home care but then presents to the hospital with severe nausea (rated as 9/10) not responding to metoclopramide. She vomits after eating and drinking more than a sip of fluid, with slight improvement of the nausea. She is cachectic and has almost no appetite (loss of appetite rated at 8/10) as well as early satiety for the past month. This worries her family, as they think that she will starve to death if she does not eat. She is very weak. Her pain is well controlled and she has soft bowel movements every second day. Mrs L. feels that she is a burden to her family, adding to her suffering. On gentle questioning she expresses fear of dying, but denies fear of death. Her family members are stressed, exhausted, and unable to continue her care at home. On examination you detect hepatomegaly with a large medial lobe, ascites, tachycardia, and a low blood pressure. An ultrasound examination of the abdomen confirms multiple liver metastases and moderate amounts of ascites. Her liver functions are high normal. Her electrolytes and renal functions are normal.

Question 11. Which possible causes of nausea and vomiting come to mind?

She is probably experiencing gastric outlet compression due to hepatomegaly. The low blood pressure, tachycardia, and nausea suggest autonomic dysfunction as part of an anorexia–cachexia syndrome seen in advanced cancer[11] (see Chapter 7). Large volumes of ascitic fluid may contribute to slowed gastric emptying, with aggravation of nausea and vomiting. She might have refractory nausea, although her metoclopramide use has not been optimal due to inability to tolerate/retain the oral medication consistently.

Question 12. How do you manage her present situation?

There are several issues to be considered: nausea and vomiting, anorexia–cachexia, weakness, moderate ascites, psychosocial concerns, and caregiver exhaustion. This illustrates the complexity of the concerns that may confront the person with advanced illness.

You suggest admission to hospital to stabilize her condition. Mrs L. and her family are very relieved. You decide to optimize the metoclopramide, as its prokinetic effect may help to alleviate gastric stasis caused by gastric outlet compression. You prescribe a dose of 10 mg every 4 hours to be given subcutaneously, with the same amount for breakthrough nausea given hourly as needed. You also add dexamethasone 8 mg divided in two doses given subcutaneously in the morning (administration earlier in the day may prevent insomnia) to help relieve the gastric compression caused by the hepatomegaly as well as for its central antiemetic effect. She receives 2/3–1/3 solution via clysis at a rate of 80 ml/h. You conclude that the ascites is not contributing in any significant degree to her present symptoms and continue to monitor it.

A day later her nausea has slightly decreased (7/10). She finds the breakthrough doses effective for a short period only. You change the metoclopramide to a continuous subcutaneous infusion of 120 mg/day, with the same breakthrough doses as the previous day. She has further improvement in the nausea and finds that she is able to tolerate sips of water. Her anxiety is lessening and her family are more relaxed. You use this opportunity to spend some time exploring her emotions regarding the loss of independence, increased care needs, and the perceived impact on her family. With the help of the unit's social worker and chaplain, her fears regarding the dying process are addressed. You meet her and her family to discuss anorexia–cachexia and help them come to terms with her deteriorating condition. This opens up a very emotional and meaningful dialogue within her family. She is transferred to a nearby hospice, where she dies peacefully a week later. Her family members express their relief and gratitude that she died with dignity, free of distressing symptoms.

Case 2

Mr W., aged 78 years, presents to the Emergency Department with progressive nausea (7/10) over the past week and copious vomiting for the past 3 days. He had been diagnosed with an adenocarcinoma of the colon at the level of the splenic flexure 6 months ago and subsequently had a hemicolectomy and primary anastomosis. At the time of surgery, he had localized disease with no distant metastases. His postoperative course was complicated by a myocardial infarction and subsequent congestive heart failure. His cardiac performance status is markedly impaired. He has not needed an opioid, but is now experiencing intermittent cramping central abdominal pain which he rates at 8/10. He has been increasingly constipated over the past few weeks and has noticed a decline in his appetite and a weight loss of 10 kg over the past month. On examination he appears dehydrated and exhausted. He has mild tenderness around the umbilicus with fullness, but no definite masses. His bowel sounds are increased. His rectal examination reveals an empty rectum.

Question 1. Which are the two most likely causes of his nausea and vomiting?

Mr W. probably has a bowel obstruction due to recurrent tumour or adhesions, but severe or complete constipation (obstipation) needs to be ruled out. Impacted stool can cause a functional bowel obstruction as well as obstruct a lumen already narrowed by postoperative stricture or compression from a tumour mass.

Erect and supine abdominal radiographs show very little faecal load in the transverse colon, but multiple air–fluid levels and dilated loops of small bowel confirm your diagnosis of a bowel obstruction. Serum electrolyte determination reveals hypokalaemia. His urea and creatinine are both mildly elevated.

Question 2. What is your management plan?

His impaired cardiac status precludes further surgery, which necessitates medical management of the bowel obstruction. This includes rehydration, correction of hypokalaemia and possibly hyoscine butylbromide (Buscopan®) to relieve the cramping abdominal pain. A trial of dexamethasone 8 mg given subcutaneously twice in the morning may alleviate the obstruction.[12] Some palliative care physicians would not use hyoscine butylbromide at this stage, but would use octreotide, a somatostatin analogue, to reduce intestinal fluid secretion and thereby reduce the amount of emesis[13] (see Question 3 below).

To control the nausea and vomiting associated with the bowel obstruction, choose a medication that will target the vagal and sympathetic afferent pathway with its dopamine and serotonin neurotransmitters. Metoclopramide is best avoided in a patient with a complete bowel obstruction or when there is colicky pain, as it can increase abdominal cramping. You choose haloperidol 2 mg s.c. twice a day with breakthrough doses of 1 mg every hour as needed. You discuss the situation with Mr W. and his wife. They seem overwhelmed and you suggest a short admission to hospital, with a goal of a discharge home once his symptoms are controlled. (For a detailed discussion of bowel obstruction, see Chapter 19.)

Mr W.'s nausea improves to 1–2/10 and he tolerates oral sips. He still vomits moderate volumes twice or three times a day. He is not very concerned by the emesis, but his wife is very upset every time he vomits and this increases his anxiety. His wife asks you if a nasogastric tube will benefit him. She wants to care for him at home, but is worried that she could not cope with the repeated emesis.

Question 3. How do you respond and what are your suggestions?

Mr and Mrs W. need a gentle explanation that the vomiting is a way for the bowel to empty, as it cannot empty its contents through the rectum because of the obstruction. You explain to them that this kind of vomiting is not detrimental to him and you support Mr W. when he states that since the nausea has been relieved, the vomiting does not bother him much. You reassure them that there are medications available to reduce the vomiting. You explain that a nasogastric tube is a very short-term solution because of discomfort, and that it is only used when surgery is planned or when the nausea is due to a reversible factor like severe obstipation.

You suggest a trial of octreotide. His bowel obstruction is not relieved by a trial of dexamethasone and you discontinue it after 5 days. It is our experience that dexamethasone can safely be discontinued without tapering if used for less than a week.

Mr W. vomits only once over the next 3 days and after careful discharge planning with home care and teaching by the nursing staff on the unit, he returns home. He continues to enjoy small amounts of fluids, including his usual bedtime glass of port. He eats a few bites of soft food occasionally, to the delight of his wife. Mr W. dies peacefully at home 2 months later. His wife has a comforting sense of achievement that she was able to care for him until his death.

Useful points in the management of nausea and vomiting:

- Nausea can be a severely distressing symptom with far-reaching implications for the patient and family and needs to be addressed urgently. Many patients state that they find it equally as distressing as pain.
- The causes of nausea can be multifactorial, but it is important to identify the causes to be able to target the specific trigger with the appropriate antiemetic medication.
- The most widely used dopamine antagonists are metoclopramide (also prokinetic effect), haloperidol, and prochlorperazine. The most commonly used antihistamine (often limited by sedation, dry mouth, and constipation) is cyclizine, but should be used only if control of nausea and vomiting at the CRTZ fails or for conditions involving the vestibular nuclei.
- Patients may not be able to tolerate oral medications when nauseated or vomiting, and thus administration should be by alternative routes. Subcutaneous injections and infusions are commonly used. Try to avoid the pain of an intramuscular injection in a palliative patient.
- A multidisciplinary team approach is often very effective in the management of nausea and its accompanying concerns.
- There is a very limited role for a nasogastric tube in the management of nausea and vomiting in the terminally ill population. It can be helpful in mechanical upper gastrointestinal obstruction if medical (conservative) management fails.
- Always check for constipation in the nauseated patient.
- Do not use a prokinetic and an anticholinergic (e.g. Buscopan®) at the same time, as the anticholinergic will interfere with the prokinesis.

Future directions

Trials are needed to compare serotonin blockers with the other commonly used antiemetics to define their role in the control of nausea and vomiting in palliative patients. New cannabinoids with better side-effect profiles are under development and might open up useful therapeutic options. The new atypical antipsychotics such as olanzapine are potentially useful as antiemetics.[14] Trials are ongoing.

Substance P may be an important factor in the emetogenic pathway. Its biological actions are mediated through the neurokinin-1 receptor. A new group of non-peptide compounds, the neurokinin-1 receptor blockers, are showing great promise in controlling emesis from a wide spectrum of emetogenic substances.[15] Trials are under way to examine their antiemetic activity in patients undergoing chemotherapy.

Bibliography

Herndon, C., Jackson., K., and Hallin, P. (2002) Management of opioid-induced gastrointestinal effects in patients receiving palliative care. *Pharmacotherapy,* **22**, 240–50.

Mannix, K. (2004) Palliation of nausea and vomiting. In: Doyle D, Hanks G, Cherny N, Calman K (eds) *Oxford Textbook of Palliative Medicine* (3rd edn). Oxford: Oxford University Press, 459.

Micromedex® Healthcare Series, Vol. 116, 2003. www.micromedex.com

Reuben, D., and Mor, V. (1983) Nausea and vomiting in terminal cancer patients. *Arch Intern Med,* **146,** 2021–3.

Twycross, R., and Lack, S. (1990) Nausea and vomiting. In: Twycross R, Lack S (eds) *Therapeutics in Terminal Cancer.* New York: Churchill Livingstone, 57–62.

References

1. **Grond, S., Zech, D., Diefenbach, C., and Bischoff, A.** (1994) Prevalence and pattern of symptoms in patients with cancer pain: a prospective evaluation of 1635 cancer patients referred to a pain clinic. *J Pain Symptom Manage,* **9**, 372–82.
2. **Fainsinger, R., Miller, M., Bruera, E., Hanson, J., and Maceachern, T.** (1991) Symptom control during the last week of life on a palliative care unit. *J Palliat Care,* **7**, 5–11.
3. **Compora, E., Merlini, L., Pance, M.,** ***et al.*** (1991) The incidence of narcotic-induced emesis. *J Pain Symptom Manage,* **6**, 428–30.
4. **Twycross, R., and Back, I.** (1998) Nausea and vomiting in advanced cancer. *Eur J Palliat Care,* **5**, 39–45.
5. **Naylor, R., and Rudd, J.A.** (1994) Emesis and anti-emesis. In: Hanks GWC, ed. *Cancer Surveys,* Vol 21. *Palliative Medicine: Problem Areas in Pain and Symptom Managemen.* Cold Spring Harbor, NY: Cold Spring Harbor Laboratory Press, 117–35.
6. **Lichter, I.** (1993) Which antiemetic? *J Palliat Care,* **9**, 42–50.
7. **Weightman, W., Zacharias, M., and Herbison, P.** (1987) Traditional Chinese acupuncture as an antiemetic. *BMJ,* **295**, 1379.
8. **Ralston, S.H.** (1994) Management of cancer-associated hypercalcemia. *Eur J Palliat Care,* **1**, 170–4.
9. **Fleisch, H.** (1991) Bisphosphonates: pharmacology and use in the treatment of tumour-induced hypercalcemia and metastatic bone disease. *Drugs,* **42**, 919–44.
10. **Singer, F.** (1991) The efficacy of bisphosphonates for the treatment of hypercalcemia. *Endocrinologist,* **1**, 149–54.
11. **Bruera, E., Catz, Z., Hooper, R., Lentle, B., and MacDonald, R.N.,** (1987)Chronic nausea and anorexia in patients with advanced cancer: a possible role for autonomic dysfunction. *J Pain Symptom Manage,* **2**, 19–21.
12. **Ripamonti, C., De Conno, F., Ventafridda V, Rossi, B., and Baines, M.** (1993) Management of bowel obstruction in advanced and terminal cancer patients. *Ann Oncol,* **13**, 44–9.
13. **Khoo, D., Hall, E., Motson, R., Riley, J., Denman, K., and Waxman, J.** (1994) Palliation of malignant intestinal obstruction using octreotide. *Eur J Cancer,* **30a**, 28–30.
14. **Passik, S.D., Lundenberg, J., and Kirsh, K.L.** ***et al.*** (2002) A pilot exploration of the antiemetic activity of olazepine for the relief of nausea in patients with advanced cancer and pain. *J Pain Symptom Manage,* **23**, 526–32.
15. **De Wit, R.** (2003) Current position of $5HT_3$ antagonists and the additional value of NK_1 antagonists; a new class of antiemetics. *Br J Cancer,* **88**, 1823–7.

Chapter 18

Constipation

Paul Daeninck and Garnet Crawford

We ha' only twa things to keep in meend, and they'll serve us for here and herea'ter; one is always to have the fear of the Laird before our ees, that'll do for herea'ter; and the t'other is to keep your booels open, and that will do for here.

Quoted by Sir Astley Cooper[1]

Attitude

To enable each student to:

- Recognize that assessment of bowel function is a physician's duty, which can be shared with nurses, patients, and family.
- Recognize that the hand that writes the opioid order should, unless there is a contraindication, write the laxative order.
- Adopt the habit of regularly checking the rectum as part of the original assessment in patients who are constipated.

Skill

To enable each student to:

- Classify commonly used laxatives and enemas and apply a protocol for the use of these agents in patients who are receiving opioid analgesics or are otherwise constipated.
- Describe the approach to patients with constipation, including assessment, investigations, and an orderly programme of treatment.

Knowledge

To enable each student to:

- Describe the pathophysiology of altered bowel motility with emphasis on the effect of drugs on the bowel and presence of an altered state of motility in patients with advanced cancer and other terminal illnesses.
- Describe the signs and symptoms of severe constipation and faecal impaction.

76-year-old Mrs D.C., a widow with oestrogen receptor negative carcinoma of the breast and cutaneous metastases to the right lateral chest, presents to the emergency department of her local hospital complaining of increasing pain and foul-smelling discharge from her open skin lesion. She has been using acetaminophen–codeine tablets (325 mg–8 mg) as well as ibuprofen, but these have been poorly effective for her pain. She denies fever or chills. Up until the present, she has been managing at home by herself. Her appetite has been reasonably good. Bowel movements have been hard in consistency, and two to three times per week. She states that this has been her pattern for 3 or 4 years now. Her medications include the aforementioned pain relievers (which she has been taking for several years for osteoarthritis) and daily psyllium fibre.

The emergency medical officer on duty notes the tender raw area on her lateral right chest and swabs it for culture. Mrs C. is well hydrated and has a normal white blood count. While she is in the emergency department, the pain is brought under control with morphine sulphate 5 mg orally every 4 h and she is sent home on long-acting morphine 15 mg twice a day, with 5 mg every 4 h as needed for breakthrough pain, and a 10-day course of ciprofloxacin. She returns home feeling much more comfortable with instructions to follow up with her family doctor in a week.

Question 1. Discuss risk factors for constipation. Does Mrs C. have chronic constipation?

Constipation is a frequent but underestimated problem in the elderly, those with chronic illnesses, and certainly a large proportion of oncology and palliative patients. It can be functionally defined as difficult passage of hard and/or infrequent stools, or a decrease in stooling frequency to twice or less per week. A more formal definition, the Rome Definition[2] (Table 18.1), may not apply to those patients who have advanced illness and are taking opioids. Factors which predispose to constipation are many and include the following.

- diet poor in fluid or bulk
- malnutrition
- decreased mobility
- environmental factors (e.g. change of setting, lack of privacy, inconvenient facilities)
- medications [diuretics, chemotherapeutics (especially the vinca alkaloids), opioids, sedatives, anticholinergics, non-sterodal anti-inflammatory drugs, antihistamines, phenothiazines, iron, serotonin antagonists (e.g. ondansetron)]
- metabolic disorders (dehydration, hypercalcaemia, hyponatraemia, uraemia, hypothyroidism)
- advanced age, depression, and chronic illness or malignancy (especially affecting bowel or spinal cord)
- altered attention to rectal fullness in the elderly.

Table 18.1 The Rome definition of constipation

Two or more of the following symptoms lasting for at least 12 months while not taking laxatives and provided that irritable bowel syndrome has been excluded
◆ Straining during >25 per cent of bowel movements
◆ Sensation of incomplete evacuations on >25 per cent of bowel movements
◆ Hard or pelletted stools on >25 per cent of bowel movements
◆ Less than three stools passed per week

This list is by no means definitive. For example, aberrations in autonomic function are thought to contribute to fatigue and gastric stasis. If this is a systemic effect, abnormal autonomic control could also influence bowel function.

Mrs C. has had what may be considered mild chronic constipation for several years, perhaps due to a combination of her age, decreased activity (from arthritic disease), and use of ibuprofen and codeine. It would be easy to assume that, since she does not complain of any change in bowel habits over the past years, she cannot be constipated. Diagnosis of constipation often requires a high index of suspicion. An accurate history, detailing medication, laxative use, frequency and consistency of stools, diet, mobility, and associated symptoms, should be obtained, especially prior to starting or increasing an opioid analgesic.

Question 2. Describe the pathophysiology underlying constipation in patients with advanced illness?

Normal bowel function requires coordination of gut motility, molecular transport across the bowel wall, and reflexes of defecation. Motility is mediated by the autonomic nervous system as well as by hormones active in the gut. Adrenergic, muscarinic, dopaminergic and opioid receptors all have a role in modifying gut motility and transit time. Fluid and electrolyte transport across mucosal surfaces is a complex phenomenon whose elucidation is incomplete. We know that opioids prolong intestinal transit time in both the small and large intestine. Prolonged bowel transit results in increased fluid absorption. Moreover, opioids increase rectal sphincter tone and reduce awareness of rectal filling. As both increased fluid absorption and prolonged transit are present in constipated patients, laxative therapies will usually combine laxatives maintaining hydration of bowel contents with those stimulating bowel transit (see below).

At her follow-up appointment, Mrs C. reports that she has not moved her bowels for 5 days and is beginning to complain of mildly decreased appetite and abdominal bloating. Her physician, having read the emergency department report from the previous week, realizes with some annoyance that Mrs C. was not prescribed a laxative concurrently with her opioid and rectifies this by recommending one to two senna tablets (elemental sennosides, 8.6 mg per tablet) daily as needed. The culture report from her wound swab is positive for *Pseudomonas aeruginosa*, and since clinically the area is improving with treatment, he advises her to complete her prescribed course of antibiotic. No further follow-up is arranged.

Question 3. To his credit, Mrs C.'s physician has recognized the inadequacy of her initial bowel management. Do you think his subsequent management was appropriate? Why, or why not?

It cannot be overstressed that **all** patients when commencing an opioid should, unless there is a contraindication, concurrently be prescribed a prophylactic bowel regimen. If opioids are taken regularly, then a laxative should be as well. Prescription of laxatives as needed has little place in the prophylaxis of opioid-induced constipation. They only serve to cause 'seesawing' between stooling which is alternately hard and infrequent, and that which is loose and diarrhoea like. Neither of these extremes is pleasant, and the frustration they engender contributes to non-compliance with both analgesics and laxatives. Laxative dosing should be on a regular schedule, and should be titrated according to response rather than by the opioid dose (since the constipating effects of opioids are not necessarily dose dependent). In the case of normal bowel function despite opioids (and this does occur, though rarely), laxatives can be decreased to as needed or discontinued. Vigilance is demanded.

Mrs C.'s physician has recommended a stimulant laxative (Table 18.2) but has omitted a stool softener. Both of these should be prescribed initially in sufficient daily doses, especially since the patient has a history of constipation. It may also be prudent at this point to advise Mrs C. to discontinue use of daily psyllium fibre if her fluid intake is declining as disease progresses. Dietary fibre is important to proper bowel function, but can contribute to constipation if there is insufficient fluid to provide soft bulky stools. Finally, there is no plan to stop Mrs C.'s strong opioid analgesic if her pain decreases with treatment of the causative infective agent. Although opioids are a mainstay of treatment for cancer patients with pain, their periodic review and re-evaluation is often overlooked.

Since her infection is clearing up and she has no pain from the area of skin metastasis, Mrs C. telephones her physician and receives permission to stop her morphine and go back to her previous analgesics for osteoarthritic pain.

Over the next several months, Mrs C. begins to have more problems with episodic constipation despite taking her senna tablets every second day and her psyllium fibre daily. She is losing weight and her appetite is decreasing. She begins to have mild to moderate mid-back pain, a new symptom for which she increases her dose of ibuprofen and acetaminophen–codeine to the maximum recommended on the packages. When this is not effective she switches back to the long-acting morphine (with her physician's permission). Bowel movements become less frequent despite daily senna and psyllium, and soon she begins to complain of soiling herself with liquid stool. After several days of daily liquid stool passage and increasing nausea, she goes to a community clinic and is advised that she has 'a touch of flu'.

Question 4. Discuss the management outlined in the above scenario. How do we adequately conduct an assessment for constipation?

The proper approach to a constipated patient is, in general, similar to that of any patient presenting with symptoms. A thorough history is paramount, followed by a directed physical examination.

The **history** should include questions about the present bowel movement pattern, the quantity and consistency of the stool, difficulties encountered during defecation (pain due to hard stool or burning due to diarrhoea-like stool), and the patient's normal pattern of movements prior to the illness or change in medication. Recall that normal bowel patterns range from once every 3 days to as much as three times a day. Questions regarding the colour or odour may be important if the patient notices a change (e.g. black tarry foul-smelling stools may indicate a gastrointestinal bleed). A complete list of medications taken is necessary. Assessment of accompanying symptoms (appetite, nausea, vomiting, abdominal pain, cramping, fullness) is also required. Fever, chills or rigors, abdominal pain, and change in cognition may indicate a surgical abdomen (obstruction, infection, perforation), and requires hospital admission and further investigation.

The **physical examination** should include inspection and auscultation of the abdomen, including all four quadrants. Normal bowel sounds do not rule out constipation, but low-pitched and infrequent sounds are more consistent. High-pitched sounds with a protuberant and tympanic abdomen may indicate obstruction or obstipation. Palpation of the abdomen may reveal a distended bladder, which commonly accompanies severe constipation. Inspection of the anal area may reveal areas of excoriation, erythema, or breaks in the skin (anal fissures, tears, fistulae). These problems and consequent discomfort when defecating may cause patients to resist the urge to pass stool.

A **rectal examination** is essential for the proper assessment of constipation, and should be performed on all patients except those with severe neutropenia and/or active septicaemia. One of three findings will be present: an empty and collapsed rectum (no rectal impaction), an empty but ballooned rectum (faecal mass obstructing beyond the reach of the examining finger), or a loaded rectum indicative of faecal impaction.

Imaging of the abdomen can help in the diagnosis and continued assessment of severe constipation. A flat and upright abdominal radiograph can reveal the extent of the faecal load. Large amounts of stool can appear as lumps of rounded masses associated with entrapped gas, often with varying degrees of dilated bowel. A simple scoring system to quantify the problem has been developed.[3] Each area of the colon is identified (ascending, transverse, descending, and rectosigmoid) and the amount of stool versus air is noted. A numerical value is assigned (0, no stool; 1, stool occupying <50 per cent of the lumen of the colon; 2, stool occupying >50 per cent of the lumen; 3, 100 per cent occupation of the lumen by stool) to each quadrant, and a total out of 12 is calculated. Any value greater than 7 out of 12 requires intervention.

In Mrs C.'s case, the physician did not take a full history or a drug history, both of which would have provided major clues as to the aetiology of her symptoms. He did not examine the patient and did not perform a rectal examination. No investigations were ordered and the physician failed to identify the phenomenon of rectal stool impaction with overflow diarrhoea, mislabelling the patient as having 'the flu', rather than recognizing her progressive constipation.

> Mrs C. returns home and the following day begins to have abdominal pain and nausea so severe that she again presents to the emergency department, where she is found to be dehydrated and confused. Her abdomen is generally tender with no peritoneal signs. A soft indentable mass is palpable in the left lower quadrant and a rectal examination reveals hard stool in the rectum. A plain radiograph of her abdomen shows large amounts of stool in the transverse and descending colon. She is admitted for intravenous fluid hydration, receives metoclopramide regularly (both for nausea and as a prokinetic agent) and several doses of lactulose, bisacodyl and glycerin suppositories are administered, and finally a high-saline enema is given, after which she passes a large amount of stool over the next 2 days.

Question 5. Explain the rationale behind this choice of medication regimen

Comprehensive management of constipation focuses on prevention as the primary goal. Failing this, we must eliminate or reverse causative factors and judiciously apply laxative therapy. Advice on the importance of maintaining a good fluid intake and physical activity within comfortable limits should always accompany laxative counselling. Most patients will benefit from advice on a nutritional high-fibre diet.

Medical agents used in the treatment of constipation can be categorized as follows (see Table 18.2):

- bulk-forming agents
- faecal softeners
- lubricants

Table 18.2 Agents for treatment of constipation

Type	Onset of action	Side effects	Mechanism of action and comments
Bulk agents Bran Psyllium Methylcellulose Polycarbophil	12–24 h	Bloating; flatulence	↑Stool bulk; ↓ transit time; ↑gastrointestinal motility
Stool softener			
Docusate	12–72 h	Well tolerated	Detergent activity; avoid mineral oil concurrently
Hyperosmolar agents			
Lactulose	24–48 h	Very sweet; abdominal cramps and flatulence	Non-absorbable molecules draw fluid into intestinal lumen
Sorbitol	24–48 h		
Polyethylene glycol	30 min–1 h		As for lactulose/sorbitol
Stimulants			
Anthraquinones (senna; cascara; danthron) Bisacodyl	6–12 h	Dependence with prolonged use; may cause cramping or electrolyte disturbances	Myenteric plexus stimulation; ↑motility; ↓absorption of fluid and electrolytes
Castor oil	2–6 h		Seldom used in clinical setting
Lubricant			
Mineral oil	6–8 h	Malabsorption of fat-soluble vitamins; risk of lipid pneumonia	Lubricates and softens stool
Saline laxatives			
Magnesium (citrate; hydroxide; sulphate) Sodium phosphate	1–3 h	Electrolyte disturbances; avoid in renal insufficiency	Osmotically active particles draw fluid into colonic lumen
Suppositories			
Glycerin	15 min–1 h	Rectal irritation	Induces defecation by distention of rectum
Bisacodyl			Similar to senna
Enemas			
Saline	5–15 min	Rectal irritation	Large volume; useful in impaction
Phosphate	5–15 min	Hypocalcaemia	
Oil retention	6–8 h		Softens impacted stool
Prokinetic agents			
Domperidone	30–60 min	Extrapyramidal effects	D_2 antagonist
Metoclopramide		Confusion; extrapyramidal effects	D_2 antagonist and cholinergic agonist
Opioid antagonists			
Naloxone Naltrexone	1–3	Opioid withdrawal and loss of pain control	Orally administered; limited use; competitive central and peripheral opioid receptor antagonists
Methylnaltrexone			Acts peripherally only; not yet commercially available

- prokinetic agents
- stimulant and saline laxatives
- hyperosmolar agents.

Opioid receptor antagonists, specifically for use in opioid bowel dysfunction, are a topic under investigation and will be covered later in the chapter.

Bulk producers work with the natural processes of the bowels to retain fluid, softening stool and increasing its size, thereby enhancing gastrointestinal motility and ease of passage. They are usually unsuitable for debilitated persons. If sufficient fluid is not consumed concurrent with their use, they can exacerbate constipation. Bulk or fibre laxatives should be avoided in cases of suspected bowel obstruction.

Stool softeners promote faecal water retention by surfactant activity. Generally well tolerated, they are also ineffective if overall hydration is poor. They are rarely used alone; a common clinical regimen is a stool softener combined with a stimulant laxative (e.g. senna or bisacodyl), especially when starting an opioid.

Stimulant laxatives produce peristalsis by directly stimulating the myenteric plexus in the intestine, making them a reasonable choice to combat opioid-induced bowel dysfunction. They will reduce electrolyte absorption in the colon. Onset of action is between 6 and 12 h, making bedtime dosing most logical. However, divided dosing (twice daily) may reduce abdominal cramping.

Lubricants such as mineral oil lubricate the intestinal mucosa and stool surfaces, thus easing passage through the bowel lumen. Prolonged administration may interfere with absorption of fat-soluble vitamins (resulting in a nutritional deficiency), as well as leading to unpleasant faecal leaking or dangerous lung aspiration. Use of lubricant laxatives is not recommended, although when combined in a preparation with magnesium hydroxide (25 per cent oil), adverse effects are said to be unlikely. Mineral oil enemas may also be used (see below).

The osmotically active molecules of saline laxatives such as magnesium hydroxide (Milk of Magnesia®) or sodium phosphate (Fleet Phospho-soda®) draw water into the bowel lumen, which alters stool consistency and size, and promotes reflex peristalsis by gut distension. These agents differ from the hyperosmolar agents in that they are capable of systemic absorption across the bowel mucosa and therefore can complicate pre-existing conditions such as congestive heart failure, hypertension, or renal failure. Lactulose, sorbitol, and polyethylene glycol (PEG or Golytely®) are indigestible synthetic molecules that work on a similar principle to the saline laxatives. Their onset of action is more delayed and their sweet taste (i.e. lactulose and sorbitol) or large volumes (PEG) are not generally appreciated by patients. However, they are very potent and are often used as second-line agents when patients do not adequately respond to a stimulant and/or softener. It is wise to increase fluid intake when giving any osmotic laxative. In Europe, PEG-based laxatives (e.g. macrogol) have recently been proposed as first-line therapy for functional constipation and faecal impaction,[4] and may provide long-term benefit in these patients.[5]

Prokinetic agents work to increase the peristaltic movements through the stomach and small bowel, reducing transit times. These effects are mediated through cholinergic activity and are blocked by anticholinergic drugs. Metoclopramide and domperidone are the two most common agents used, and they can also play a role in nausea relief (see Chapter 17) due to this activity as well as their role as dopamine receptor (D_2) antagonists. It is useful to combine these agents with the laxatives active on the large bowel to achieve benefits throughout the entire gut. These are best used to prevent constipation rather than to treat established severe constipation.

Rectal laxatives can be administered as either enemas or suppositories and generally work in a similar fashion to the orally administered forms. Some patients resist their use, but they are often necessary when oral laxatives cannot be used, and may be helpful in stimulating anocolonic defecation reflexes. A combination of glycerin (to soften) and bisacodyl (to stimulate) suppositories is often effective for hard stool low in the rectum. This may obviate the need for an undignified and unpleasant manual disimpaction.

Question 6. From time to time you and your nursing colleague concur that enemas are required. Which types of enema will you consider?

Fleet enema

This enema consists of 150 ml sodium phosphate. It presumably acts by stimulating colonic peristalsis and providing additional volume to stimulate a rectal colic reflex. It may be safely used in short intermittent courses. Prolonged use of a phosphate preparation can result in hypocalcaemia and rectal irritation, particularly in patients with haemorrhoids. Fleet enemas must be used as part of an overall bowel regime.

Saline enema

This term is often applied to the somewhat cumbersome use of higher volumes of warmed saline. They are safe but awkward. Saline enemas may need to be used in patients with impaction, as the patients usually have a long column of backed up stool.

Tapwater and soapsuds enema

These enemas are not recommended because of the associated risk of inappropriate changes in blood volume and electrolytes. Moreover, soap is particularly irritating.

Mineral oil enema

This is most commonly employed in the clinical setting as a high enema given overnight to be retained in the colon for the purpose of softening and lubricating hard-packed stool which is resistant to passage using other less invasive means. Of course, its use is depends on the recipient's ability to retain the fluid for a prolonged period. To facilitate this, the enema can be administered high in the descending colon with a Foley catheter and the balloon can be inflated for 10–15 min to minimize initial returns. A mineral oil retention enema is generally followed by a high saline enema to produce laxation. An oil retention enema can be helpful in patients with a large quantity of stool in the sigmoid colon and rectum either before faecal disimpaction, or immediately after, to assist with further removal of stool caught in the sigmoid colon.

As Mrs C.'s back pain has also become more severe and her overall condition has deteriorated, she undergoes further investigations and is found to have extensive spinal metastases and a serum calcium (corrected) of 3.05 mmol/l. She receives a dose of i.v. pamidronate and a course of palliative radiation to her thoracic spine. These interventions result in normalization of her serum calcium, resolution of her delirium, and significant improvement of her pain. She is discharged home with daily home care services in place. Mrs C. is now taking long-acting morphine 30 mg twice daily, two to four senna tablets at bedtime, and docusate sodium 200 mg each morning. She is instructed to take lactulose 15–30 ml twice a day if she does not move her bowels for 3–4 days. Her ibuprofen and psyllium are stopped. A discussion is carried out with the home care nursing team who agree to monitor Mrs C's bowel habits on a daily basis, perform rectal checks when appropriate, and consider an enema if there is no bowel movement in 4 days. The importance of the relationship of the nursing staff to Mrs C. in the monitoring and prevention of further episodes of constipation cannot be overemphasized.

Question 7. What other laboratory data would have been helpful in treating this patient's constipation?

Several metabolic abnormalities can contribute to the picture of delirium and constipation we see in Mrs C. In addition to the serum calcium level, electrolytes (hyponatraemia, hypothyroidism), renal indices (dehydration, uraemia), and liver enzyme tests would be helpful in determining the cause of her problems.

Mrs C. has spent another 2 months at home during which she has been receiving i.v. pamidronate every 4 weeks on an outpatient basis. However, over the past week her mid-back pain has again become severe and is accompanied by bilateral leg pain. Both legs have become profoundly weak. She is again admitted to hospital and found to have a spinal cord compression at the previously irradiated site which does not improve with high-dose steroids. Her opioid dose requires escalation and she is now taking morphine sulphate 40 mg orally every 4 h to control her pain.

Over the next few days she again becomes confused. Her confusion is accompanied by nausea and emesis. Bowel movements are duly noted each day in the hospital chart. An opioid rotation (to hydromorphone 3 mg subcutaneously every 4 h) is performed because of suspected opioid neurotoxicity. Blood tests are unhelpful in diagnosing any other cause of the confusion and an endstage delirium with agitation is assumed. A student nurse performs a rectal examination on the patient which reveals a large amount of very hard-packed stool. Radiographs show stool completely filling the bowel lumen but no air–fluid levels. Mrs C. undergoes manual disimpaction followed by a high sodium phosphate enema and (to her family's delight) after evacuating her colon of a substantial amount of faeces, she feels more comfortable and consequently becomes far less agitated. Her cognition returns to normal a few days later, the delirium apparently having been a result of opioid neurotoxicity exacerbated by the discomfort of severe constipation.

Question 8. How can we improve the patient's bowel function given her present neurological problems?

Bowel management is especially problematic and unfortunately a common problem in patients with spinal cord compression or cauda equina syndrome. A combination of loss of rectal sensation, loss of voluntary control, poor anal tone, immobility, and pain may result in constipation with overflow 'diarrhoea' accompanied by abdominal distension, nausea, and vomiting. A cauda equina lesion will abolish the anocolonic reflex, but a higher spinal cord lesion leaves this reflex intact. In the latter, rectal simulation by suppositories or by digit will stimulate the reflex and colonic contraction will aid evacuation.

The aim in managing spinal cord compression or cauda equina syndrome is to attain a 'controlled' or 'scheduled' continence. This means administering a combination of daily oral laxatives with suppositories (or enemas) every 2–3 days to achieve rectal evacuation.

The intention is to avoid incontinence as well as repeated and uncomfortable manual disimpaction in these patients with loss of rectal sensation.[6]

Question 9. What are the other options for pain control that may optimize her bowel function?

There are several options available for pain control, including opioids, which may improve Mrs C's constipation. A series of reports have shown that the use of the transdermal fentanyl patch is associated with decreased constipation compared with morphine.[7,8] This transdermal action appears to reduce the gastrointestinal concentration, and thus the direct action of the opioid upon the receptors in the gut. Methadone has also been reported to reduce constipation and laxative requirements in terminally ill patients. Rotation (or changing) of the opioid to methadone usually results in a decrease in the total morphine-equivalent dose, which may allow less overall activity on opioid receptors in the gut, similar to fentanyl.[9]

For the last 4 weeks of her life, Mrs C. remains in her hospital bed. Her physician orders daily senna and docusate (in a combination format) together with glycerin and bisacodyl suppositories every 2 days to maintain regularity. Despite her deteriorating condition and poor oral intake, her symptoms remain well controlled during her remaining time. She passes away peacefully with no further bowel concerns.

Future directions

Although the subject of constipation may not necessarily excite the mind in the way that some other fields of research do, nonetheless new agents and ideas are currently under investigation. Opioid receptor antagonists, while well known for their ability to reverse potentially life-threatening opioid toxicity quickly, are now being studied for their role in the management of opioid adverse effects (gastrointestinal, as well as pruritis, respiratory depression, etc.).[10,11] Opioid receptors exist peripherally as well as in the central nervous system, and opioid action on the bowels seems to be mediated primarily by receptors located in the gastrointestinal tract. Non-selective opioid antagonists (such as naloxone and naltrexone) have been used both parenterally and orally to treat constipation. Of course, the risk in using these agents is that of precipitating opioid withdrawal or a pain crisis, especially with parenteral use (orally administered naloxone has approximately 3 per cent systemic bioavailability and also carries the risk of withdrawal or pain, although less so).[11] Methylnaltrexone[12] and ADL 8–2698[13] are two peripherally selective opioid receptor antagonists currently under investigation for use in the treatment of opioid-related constipation. These two agents offer the advantage of targeted action on the gut, thereby maintaining analgesia. At the time of writing, methylnaltrexone is undergoing phase III trials in North America. Results are promising, as a treatment for both opioid-related constipation and other opioid side effects.[12]

Conclusion

We would again emphasize the importance of this topic, and the facile manner in which practitioners commonly ignore it. Despite the overwhelming prevalence of constipation and its resultant morbidity, especially in the elderly and those with advanced or chronic illness, its treatment often remains either neglected or delegated to nurses, medical students, family members, or the patients themselves. It is not pleasant to have constipation or to treat it, but remember that it is the duty of all health care providers to make the comfort and well-being of our patients a primary goal. To this end, management of constipation must be a shared responsibility that all members of the team take seriously.

References

1. **Cooper, A.P.** (1831) *The Lectures of Sir Astley Cooper.* Boston, MA: Lilly and Wait, 56. Quoted in Whorton J (2000) Civilisation and the colon: constipation as the 'disease of diseases'. *BMJ,* **321**, 1586–9.
2. **Lamparelli, M.J., and Kumar, D.** (2002) Investigation and management of constipation. *Clin Med J R Coll Physicians Lond,* **2**, 415–20.
3. **Starreveld, J.S., Pols, M.A., Van Wijk, H.J., Bogaard, J.W., Poen, H., and Smont, A.J.P.M.** (1990) The plain abdominal radiograph in the assessment of constipation 2. *Gastroenterolog,* **28**, 335–8.
4. **Klaschik, E., Nauck, F., and Ostgathe, C.** (2003) Constipation—modern laxative therapy. *Support Care Cancer,* **11**, 679–85.
5. **Kamm, M.A.** (2003) Constipation and its management. *BMJ,* **327**, 459–60.
6. **Fallon, M., and O'Neill, B.** (1997) ABC of palliative care: constipation and diarrhoea. *BMJ,* **315**, 1293–6.
7. **Ahmedzai, S., and Brooks, D.** (1997) Transdermal fentanyl versus sustained release oral morphine in cancer pain: preference, efficacy, and quality of life. *J Pain Symptom Manage,* **13**, 254–61.
8. **Allan, L., Hays, H., Jensen, N-H., *et al.*** (2001) Randomised crossover trial of transdermal fentanyl and sustained release oral morphine for treating chronic non-cancer pain. *BMJ,* **322**, 1–7.
9. **Daeninck, P.J., and Bruera, E.** (1999) Reduction in constipation and laxative requirements following opioid rotation to methadone: a report of four cases. *J Pain Symptom Manage,* **18**, 303–9.
10. **Choi, Y.S., and Billings, J.A,** (2002) Opioid antagonists: a review of their role in palliative care, focusing on use in opioid-related constipation. *J Pain Symptom Manage,* **24**, 71–90.
11. **Liu, M., and Wittbrodt, E.** (2002) Low-dose oral naloxone reverses opioid-induced constipation and analgesia. *J Pain Symptom Manage,* **23**, 48–53.
12. **Foss, J.F.** (2001) A review of the potential role of methylnaltrexone in opioid bowel dysfunction. *Am J Surg,* **182** (Suppl 5A), 19S–26S.
13. **Taguchi, A., Sharma, N., Saleem, R.M., *et al.*** (2001) Selective postoperative inhibition of gastrointestinal opioid receptors. *N Engl J Med,* **345**, 935–40.

Chapter 19

Malignant bowel obstruction

S. Lawrence Librach, A. Nina Horvath, and E. Anne Langlois

Attitude

To enable each student to:

- Recognize the complexity of the management of bowel obstruction with regard to symptom control, prognosis, and informed consent around treatment options.
- Demonstrate an approach that includes educating the patient and caregivers about the mechanisms and natural history of intestinal obstruction.
- Address the goals of care.
- Use a collaborative approach with surgeons and other members of the multidisciplinary health care team.

Skill

To enable each student to:

- Assess the patient with bowel obstruction.
- Address, integrate, and communicate the prognosis and goals of care for patient and family in an effective and multidisciplinary manner.
- Develop a patient-centred management plan.

Knowledge

To enable each student to:

- Describe the pathophysiology of bowel obstruction.
- Describe the natural history of malignant bowel obstruction.
- Describe the prevalence of bowel obstruction in malignant disease.
- Identify symptoms and signs of malignant bowel obstruction and appropriate investigations.
- List the factors associated with surgical outcomes in the context of advanced disease.
- Describe surgical options for treatment and the risks and complications associated with surgery.

- Describe indications and limitations for other options such as decompressive techniques including venting procedures, stents, and nasogastric tubes.
- Describe the medical (pharmacological) management of bowel obstruction symptoms such as nausea, vomiting, and pain (constant or colicky), including examples, routes of administration, and titration.
- Describe any measures to try to prevent or minimize risk of recurrence of bowel obstruction.
- Describe a palliative and supportive approach to patients and their families.

Introduction

Malignant bowel obstruction (MBO) is a common complication seen in cancer patients. Patients often have far advanced disease when MBO presents and options for aggressive surgical management are limited. The management of MBO has changed over recent years with more effective surgical, pharmacological, and interventional techniques. The emphasis is on prevention and early management.

> Patricia is a 58-year old woman with newly diagnosed ovarian cancer. She presented with a history of abdominal pain and abdominal swelling caused by a large tumour of her left ovary. She had a total abdominal hysterectomy and bilateral salpingo-oophorectomy. At surgery, para-aortic lymphadenopathy and a few peritoneal nodules were noted.

Question 1. What is the likelihood that she will develop bowel obstruction at some time during her cancer journey?

Epidemiology

MBO may be the first presentation of an abdominal malignancy. More commonly it occurs in patients with advanced cancer. MBO is most common in gynaecological cancers, particularly in ovarian cancer, and in gastrointestinal cancers. However, any cancer that metastasizes to the abdomen can cause MBO. The three most common neoplasms originating outside the abdominal cavity to be associated with MBO are lung cancer, breast cancer, and malignant melanoma.

The frequency of MBO in cancer patients is not fully characterized. The prevalence figures available in the literature are from retrospective studies and autopsies. MBO occurs in 4–28.4 per cent of patients with gastrointestinal cancer and 5–51 per cent of patients with ovarian cancer.[1,2]

MBO may be partial or complete, and may be single or multiple. The small bowel is more commonly involved than the large bowel (61 vs 33 per cent) and both are involved in over 20 per cent of patients.[3]

MBO in cancer patients may be secondary to non-malignant or malignant causes. Examples of non-malignant causes include post-surgical adhesions, post-radiotherapy bowel damage, and causes unrelated to cancer (inflammatory bowel disease, hernia, etc.). A non-malignant mechanism is more likely in gastrointestinal cancer (48 per cent) and is relatively rare in gynaecological cancer (6 per cent).[1] The prevalence of non-malignant causes decreases in advanced disease.

> Patricia has had 6 months of chemotherapy and has done fairly well. She still has evidence of cancer on CT scan but the nodes have decreased in size. She has lost 3 kg weight in the last 2 months and has had to stop working because of increasing fatigue. She presents in the emergency department with a 1-week history of progressive colicky abdominal pain and vomiting.

Question 2. What is the pathophysiology of MBO?

MBO may be mechanical or functional. Functional obstruction is much less common. In mechanical bowel obstruction, the lumen is occluded. This may happen in three ways:

- extrinsic occlusion of the lumen (progression of the primary tumour, recurrence, mesenteric or omental masses, adhesions, etc.)
- intraluminal occlusion of the lumen (primary or metastatic tumour)
- intramural occlusion of the lumen (intestinal linitis plastica).

In functional bowel obstruction, a motility disorder is present, without occlusion of the lumen. This may occur with tumour infiltration of the mesentery, bowel muscle, and nerves as in carcinomatosis, coeliac plexus involvement, cancer-related neuropathy, decreased motility secondary to medications such as opioids, and bowel motility problems secondary to other illnesses such as diabetes mellitus. Other contributory causes may include inflammatory oedema, faecal impaction, constipating medications, and dehydration.

Question 3. What are the common symptoms of MBO?

Once the bowel is obstructed (mechanically, functionally, partially, or completely), there is a decrease or absence of propulsion of intestinal contents with resultant fluid accumulation proximal to the obstruction. This in turn causes bowel distension with increased gut epithelial surface area, increase in secretion of water and sodium into the lumen, and consequent nausea and vomiting. In mechanical obstruction, the bowel may contract to overcome the obstruction, causing colicky pain. Bowel distension damages the intestinal epithelium, resulting in a bowel inflammatory response with oedema and hyperaemia in the bowel wall and production of prostaglandins, vasoactive intestinal peptides, and nociceptive mediators, resulting in abdominal pain.[1]

Question 4. You suspect that an MBO is present. What other conditions must be considered?

Differential diagnosis

When a cancer patient presents with suspected MBO, all the possible causes of constipation, nausea and vomiting, and abdominal pain have to be considered and ruled out. Two situations deserve special attention: severe constipation and opioid (narcotic) bowel syndrome.

Severe constipation vs MBO

Always rule out constipation as the sole cause or contributing cause of obstructive symptoms. Have a high degree of suspicion when there is a history of increased hardness of faeces, decreased frequency of defecation, use of constipating drugs (opioids, anticholinergics, etc.) without the use of laxatives, inactivity, hypercalcaemia, hypokalaemia, hypothyroidism, and dehydration. On physical examination of the abdomen, there may be faecal masses palpable in the bowel and rectal examination may reveal hard faeces. When the rectal ampulla is empty but distended, there may be obstipation at a higher level in the colon. Plain radiographs may be very helpful to give a more objective assessment of the faecal load.

Opioid (narcotic) bowel syndrome

Opioids produce alterations of gastrointestinal motility through more than one mechanism and at different points of the digestive tract. Up to 4 per cent of cancer patients treated with opioids may develop opioid (narcotic) bowel syndrome,[4] characterized by nausea, vomiting, mild abdominal discomfort, constipation, gaseous abdominal distention, and weight loss. Rapid resolution of these symptoms occurs within days of discontinuation of opioids.

Question 5. What is your assessment approach?

History and physical examination

MBO can develop at any time in the illness trajectory of cancer, but it is more common in the advanced stages. An accurate assessment of the stage of the cancer is needed.

MBO is less likely to have an acute presentation. It is usually slowly progressive and passes through partial obstruction phases before a complete obstruction develops. Partial obstructive episodes may resolve spontaneously early on in the natural history. Consequently, MBO is rarely an emergency event. Intestinal strangulation, ischaemia, and perforation are uncommon in MBO.

A full history detailing every symptom, current medication, stage of the cancer, and patient and family goals of care must be done.

Common symptoms in patients with MBO include the following:

- Nausea and vomiting may be intermittent or continuous. Depending on the level of obstruction, the vomitus may range from undigested stomach contents to feculent material.
- Continuous pain may be due to bowel distension, tumour mass, or hepatomegaly.
- Colicky pain is of variable intensity and localization and occurs only in mechanical obstruction.
- Abdominal distension is variable.
- Constipation may be intermittent or complete with absence of flatus.
- Diarrhoea, as a result of bacterial liquefaction of faecal material blocked in the sigmoid or rectum, may occur initially.
- Other symptoms include dry mouth, acid reflux, bloating, hunger, anorexia, thirst, drowsiness, and dyspnoea.

Common signs of MBO on physical examination may include the following:

- On inspection, there may be abdominal distension, visible loops of distended bowel, or visible peristalsis.
- On palpation, there may be masses, organomegaly, ascites, and tenderness including rebound tenderness.
- Abdominal distension varies. With extensive peritoneal spread, there may be little or no abdominal distension.
- Bowel sounds may be increased or decreased. They will be absent in late obstruction, peritonitis, and functional bowel obstruction. There may be a succussion splash when the stomach is filled with a large amount of fluid, as in gastric outlet obstruction.
- Rectal examination is an essential part of an assessment of a patient with suspected MBO. There may be palpable masses, a rectal shelf, impacted rock-hard stool indicating significant constipation, or a ballooned empty rectal ampulla that may indicate colonic obstruction higher up or high-level constipation.
- Signs of dehydration such as dry membranes, decreased skin turgor, decreased urine output, and a postural drop in blood pressure may be present.

Varying patterns of symptoms and signs may occur with bowel obstruction. The clinical presentation is influenced by the level of obstruction. Therefore, when diagnosing MBO, it is helpful to think in terms of three syndromes.

1. **Gastric outlet and proximal small bowel MBO.** With gastric outlet or duodenal obstruction, nausea and vomiting develops early and is severe, with large amounts of undigested food. Even with no oral intake, the stomach has to clear swallowed saliva (1500 ml/24 h) and gastric juices (at least 1500 ml/24 h). This vomiting is almost odourless. Upper small bowel obstruction vomitus is often bile-stained. There is often epigastric distension and usually no colicky pain. Bowel movements may be present, with the faecal matter being made up of intestinal cellular debris and bacteria.
2. **Distal small bowel MBO.** Nausea and vomiting is moderate to severe. There is moderate generalized abdominal distension present. If the obstruction is mechanical, there will be upper to central abdominal colic. Again, constipation will be present in varying degrees and occasionally diarrhoea as well.
3. **Large bowel MBO.** Nausea and vomiting develops late and in smaller amounts. Vomitus is eventually feculent. Abdominal distension is great, and central to lower abdominal colic may be present in mechanical obstruction. The colicky pain is generally not as severe as in higher obstructions. There is often a preceding history of alternating diarrhoea and constipation before obstruction becomes complete.

Question 6. What investigations will you consider

The diagnosis of MBO is established on clinical grounds through history and physical examination with complementary investigations, including bloodwork and radiological evaluation. Patients with advanced cancer and suspected MBO on clinical grounds should be referred for further investigation only if these will influence the treatment offered.

Haematology and biochemistry are used to assess for major abnormalities such as electrolyte disturbances that may need to be corrected or may be responsible for symptoms.

Plain film radiography is the initial evaluation tool. Findings include dilated loops of bowel, air fluid levels on an upright film proximal to the site of obstruction, and paucity or absence of intraluminal gas distal to the point of obstruction. Plain films will correctly establish the diagnosis of small bowel obstruction in 30–70 per cent of cases.[5] They offer limited information on the cause of the obstruction and are unlikely to show multiple levels of obstruction. They are useful in assessment of constipation, as they provide an objective assessment of faecal load. On plain films, functional obstruction will show a uniform gaseous distension of the stomach, small bowel, colon, and rectum. Free air from perforation would show as well. If there is tumour encasement of the bowel, this would prevent bowel dilatation. In this situation, plain films may be unremarkable. There will not be dilated loops of bowel, even in the presence of bowel obstruction.

Anterograde and retrograde contrast studies are helpful in obtaining information regarding the site and the extent of the obstruction and the presence of multiple levels of obstruction.[6] The accuracy of gastrointestinal contrast studies is in the range 70–100 per cent. If partial bowel obstruction is suspected clinically, water-soluble contrast such as Gastrografin should be used rather than barium. The water content of the barium can be absorbed by the colon and the barium can become inspissated above the partially obstructing lesion, increasing the degree of obstruction.

CT scanning is useful in identifying the cause of the obstruction, staging, and assisting in the choice of invasive treatment such as surgery or stenting. Studies have demonstrated CT to be quite sensitive (78–100 per cent) in identifying small bowel obstruction with specificities >90 per cent.[7] CT is the best diagnostic modality in identifying rare complications of bowel obstruction, such as strangulation or ischaemia.

Management

General issues

Quality of life may be severely affected for all patients with bowel obstruction. Decision-making is necessarily very complex in the patient with advanced disease. Good communication skills and comfort in discussing prognosis, realistic goals of care, and treatment options are essential. A team approach is advisable when formulating a management plan for a patient with the clinical dilemma of MBO in advanced cancer. Non-operative management must be considered and discussed in all MBO presentations, even in cases in which a patient could tolerate and benefit from operative intervention. The consent process should prepare the patient for the possibility that an operation might fail to palliate. Symptom management should always be a prime goal, irrespective of the possibility of surgery. The priority for symptom control should be communicated to both patient and family.

Patricia was assessed in the emergency department. She has had continuous pain for over a week, with frequent episodes of severe colic in the past 2 days. She has been nauseated all the time. She has vomited large amounts of bilious fluid six to eight times a day. She was clinically dehydrated, and no masses or abdominal distension were present. There were air fluid levels present in the distended small bowel on plain radiograph. You make a diagnosis of MBO.

Question 7. A surgical consultation is requested. What are the indications for and the outcome of surgery in patients with malignant bowel obstruction?

Surgery

Patients with progressive cancer presenting with bowel obstruction require an assessment for the possibility of surgery. Surgery may be required for the percentage of patients who have non-malignant obstruction related to previous surgery and radiation.[8] However, even in these patients, surgery may not be an option that is realistic or feasible. Surgery is rarely needed on a very urgent basis in MBO, which is often partial, resolves spontaneously after a few days, and is rarely associated with bowel gangrene, and so there is time to contemplate options for treatment.[9] The possibility of surgery also depends on where the patient is in the trajectory of disease, other indicators of poor outcome, and the goals of care for patient and family.

The median survival in MBO treated surgically is quite variable at 2–11 months.[10] This may reflect the surgical selection process that is often based on non-validated prognostic factors. In several series, the median survival of MBO patients treated surgically or medically was not statistically different.[11,12] Performance status has been correlated with survival in several studies of MBO patients,[8,13] and this parameter may represent a more reliable tool (Table 19.1). Low serum albumin appears to be an independent predictor in many studies in cancer.[14]

Table 19.1 Eastern Cooperative Oncology Group (ECOG) performance scale

ECOG scale[a]	Mean survival time from first MBO episode (months)
0–1	17
2–3	7
4	0.7

[a]0 = fully active; 4 = completely disabled.

Adapted from S. M. Weiss *et al.* (1984) *J Surg Oncol* **25**, 15–17.

There are no prospective randomized trials of surgery for MBO and no universally accepted clear guidelines for patient selection for surgery. Patients with extreme tumour burden, such as bulky abdominal carcinomatosis or parenchymal liver metastases, large amounts of ascites, impairment of vital organs from distant metastases, or multiple sites of obstruction would not be considered good candidates for surgery.[15] Prognostic indicators have been tabulated.[16] In most reviews, operative mortality is significant (5–32 per cent), perioperative morbidity is high (42 per cent), and re-obstruction is frequent (10–50 per cent),[17] so that decision-making is complex. Surgery should be palliative in focus, i.e. focused on relief of symptoms and the quality of the life remaining. Currently, bowel obstruction is managed empirically by surgeons and so practice patterns vary from centre to centre. The role of surgery needs careful evaluation using validated and consistent outcome measures.[18]

Patricia has surgery, and she is found to have multiple peritoneal and omental metastases and a single site of bowel obstruction. She has a resection of a portion of small bowel. After she recovers, she is discharged home.

Three months after this initial bowel obstruction, she presents with another small bowel obstruction with multiple levels. She has lost another 5 kg, her appetite is greatly decreased, and she spends most of her time resting. She has ascites and some peripheral swelling. Her albumin level is 25 g/l. She is not considered to be a surgical candidate.

Question 8. Is she a candidate for an intraluminal stent?

Self-expanding metal stents have been used in a variety of clinical scenarios of MBO. They are often used in patients with single obstructions who are not candidates for surgery or who need further assessment for the possibility of surgery. Endoluminal stents can be placed in the upper and lower bowel with good relief of symptoms. Of course this requires physicians with expertise in these techniques. Lasers may occasionally be used to canalize through tumours to allow stent placement or to maintain stent patency. Stent insertion can be associated with fairly frequent complications such as bowel perforation, stent migration and re-obstruction.[19,20]

Question 9. How can her bowel obstruction be managed medically?

Bowel decompression

Nasogastric suction is frequently used to decompress gas and fluid in the bowel. However, success in relieving symptoms without other medical intervention is often incomplete, especially in patients with advanced disease. Nasogastric suction is often uncomfortable, and long-term use is associated with significant morbidity such as erosion of the nares, nutritional deficiency, and aspiration pneumonia. The use of nasogastric suction may also limit the site of terminal care, making home care less of an option in many areas. If a nasogatric suction tube is required, it should be on a temporary basis before the start of surgical and pharmacological treatment, and perhaps during the first few days after such treatment. The use of antisecretory agents as described later in this chapter may obviate the need for physical decompression in the majority of patients.[3]

Venting procedures such as gastrostomy and enterostomy have been used, but usually when pharmacological management is not effective or for very high gastric outlet or upper small bowel obstruction that cannot be bypassed. A double-lumen tube can sometimes be used in gastric outlet or duodenal obstruction, providing a way of venting secretions while at the same time allowing access for fluids and nutrition. As with other options of care, venting procedures need to be considered in the light of the disease trajectory and the patient's overall condition.

Chemotherapy and radiation therapy

With the usual causes of mechanical bowel obstruction in cancer, there is little evidence that chemotherapy is effective except perhaps in carcinoma of the ovary that is responsive to chemotherapy. Radiation therapy for relief of rectal or gastric outlet obstruction may be effective in some cases.

Pharmacological management

There are a number of basic issues or principles that need to be addressed in managing MBO using medications and supportive care.

Patient and family education about MBO and the medication and care components to be provided must be a continuing process. Patient and family should be provided with clear written instructions.

No single structured approach will guarantee success in managing the symptoms. It sometimes takes time to obtain an appropriate therapeutic response. However, if a partial response is not seen within 24 h, the management plan must be altered. In many cases the management plan must be reviewed every 48 h. Prevention and early intervention with medications is essential. In the home setting, 24-h 7-day-a-week access to skilled health care professionals is desirable. This also requires medications such as antimotility and antisecretory agents to be easily accessible so that pharmacological interventions can begin at the first signs and symptoms of MBO.

Pain relief

Opioids are the mainstay of pain control in MBO. Relief of pain and decrease in abnormal motility causing cramps are the goals. Opioids should be administered parenterally (the subcutaneous route is preferred because of ease of administration and certainty of effect unless a permanent intravenous access exists) either by intermittent injections or by continuous infusion. For crampy pain, some authors recommend oral loperamide or diphenoxylate as antimotility agents.[21] These drugs may also relieve nausea associated with initial bowel hypermotility. Loperamide in a dose of 4 mg every 4 h for the first 24 h and then every 4 h as required may prevent cramps and nausea and avoid hospital admission. The use of antisecretory agents as described later in this chapter may also contribute to the relief of crampy pain.

Antiemetics

There are no clear data favouring one antiemetic over another. Many of the prospective and retrospective trials of pharmacological control of MBO symptoms have used antidopaminergic agents such as phenothiazine derivatives (e.g. prochlorperazine, chlorpromazine) and butyrophenone drugs such as haloperidol. These drugs have been given by intermittent as well as continuous infusion.

Metoclopramide is an antidopaminergic prokinetic agent that can be considered for use in partial small bowel obstruction. It should never be used in complete bowel obstruction or when the patient has abdominal colic that will be worsened by the prokinetic effect. It can be given subcutaneously by infusion or by intermittent injections. Metoclopramide may cause extrapyramidal side effects. Domperidone, another prokinetic agent, does not cross the blood–brain barrier and therefore does not have extrapyramidal side effects. There is no parenteral form of this medication.

Complete relief of the nausea and vomiting of MBO with antiemetics alone is usually not possible because of hypermotility issues initially, and then pooling in the gastrointestinal tract with bowel distension and subsequent nausea.

Antisecretory agents

As a large volume of intestinal secretions contribute to the abdominal distension, pain, and nausea and vomiting of MBO, pharmacological control of secretions is an important part of the medical management of MBO. The effective use of antisecretory agents for symptom management should be seen as first-line therapy even when the patient is being considered for surgery.

Antimuscarinic/anticholinergic drug These drugs are parasympatholytics. Their action on muscarinic receptors decreases gastrointestinal secretions and inhibits ganglionic neural transmission of the bowel wall, with consequent inhibition of bowel tone and peristalsis. However, these drugs also have a number of other effects that could be troublesome, including decreased salivary secretions, effects on heart rate, and effects on the eyes. Some of these drugs can cross the blood–brain barrier, causing a variety of disturbing psychotomimetic effects. Hyoscine butylbromide or glycopyrrolate are preferred to hyoscine hydrobromide as they are less likely to cause side effects, are useful for colicky abdominal pain and are less likely to cross the blood–brain barrier.

Antisecretory hormones: somatostatin analogues Somatostatin has widespread effects in the body, some of which have significant impact on the pathophysiology of MBO. Its clinically useful analogue octreotide inhibits release of gastrin, cholecystokinin, vasoactive intestinal peptide, and pancreatic enzymes, thereby decreasing bowel secretions. Octreotide also decreases neurotransmission in the nerves of the gastrointestinal tract, leading to decreased peristalsis, decreased sphlanchnic blood flow, and increased absorption of fluids. Octreotide has few side effects, especially since its use in MBO generally is short term. Dry mouth may be reported. Long-term use may be associated with mild hyperglycaemia and biliary sludging.

Octreotide has proved to be at least as effective as other antisecretory agents.[22,23] It is usually administered subcutaneously either as intermittent doses or as a continuous subcutaneous or intravenous infusion. The usual dose of octreotide is 300–600 mg daily, although up to 1500 mg daily can be used. The major drawback is its expense, but it may be cost effective when compared with the costs of hospitalization and the previous 'suck and drip' method.

Corticosteroids

Corticosteroids have been widely used in MBO. Their mechanism of action are not known but may include an antiemetic effect, analgesia, and an anti-inflammatory effect that decreases peritumour oedema. A systematic review of the literature[24] showed there was a trend of evidence in randomized trials that intravenous dexamethasone 6–16 mg/day may aid in the resolution of bowel obstruction. Reported side effects were minimal and survival was no different. However, the picture is complicated by the fact that MBO often resolves spontaneously. If the patient does not respond to the corticosteroid within 4 or 5 days, it should be discontinued. If there is a response, the dose should be reduced over time to a minimum effective level to lessen the risk of the usual side effects of corticosteroids.

Management of fistulae

A fistula is an abnormal communication from one internal hollow organ to another or from a hollow organ to the skin surface. Percutaneous fistulae are not uncommon after surgery to repair bowel obstruction and can be extremely distressing and difficult to manage. Symptoms from fistulae include significant skin problems from effluent, skin and other pain, discharge of large quantities of bowel contents, odour, and psychological concerns. The goals of care in managing fistulae include the following.[25]

- Protecting perifistula skin integrity from maceration from mostly alkaline bowel fluids. This requires appropriate ointments for protecting skin and absorptive dressings.
- Managing any skin pain associated with skin damage.
- Containing fluid effluent through effective pouching or suctioning. The most difficult area for fluid containment is in the perineum or vagina.
- Reducing fluid effluent, perhaps through the use of antisecretory agents such as octreotide.
- Managing odour.
- Addressing psychological and educational needs with ongoing support.
- Taking an interdisciplinary approach with involvement of an enterostomal therapist.

Hydration

Intravenous or even subcutaneous hydration may be necessary to correct severe fluid imbalances and serious electrolyte abnormalities. However, once secretions, nausea, and pain are controlled, patients with MBO can often tolerate clear fluids orally until the obstruction resolves. When antisecretory agents are being used, the rate of infusion for hydration should be adjusted downwards.

Nutrition

The issue of total parenteral nutrition (TPN) or nutritional supplementation may be raised in the setting of recurrent episodes of partial obstruction, decreased food intake, progressive weight loss, and asthenia, or in complete unremitting bowel obstruction. The literature reflects that artificial nutrition does not prolong life in advanced cancer.[26,27] There is a small subgroup of patients—young, with slow-growing tumours with involvement of the gastrointestinal tract and sparing of other major organs—who experience weight loss from starvation rather than tumour spread. TPN may be considered in this population[28] (see Chapter 7).

TPN may be indicated only in patients with a true long-term prognosis, but these patients are infrequent in the face of MBO.

> Patricia is discharged home on octreotide 100 μg subcutaneously every 8 h and haloperidol 1 mg orally every 12 h. The octreotide and haloperidol are tapered over 2 weeks and then discontinued. Once again she is passing stool, indicating that her obstruction is not yet complete and irreversible.

Question 10. How will you manage other episodes? Can they be managed at home?

Between obstructive episodes

Re-obstruction occurs frequently. Proactive management of patients between obstructive episodes should include the following.

- Maintain adequate hydration.
- Metoclopramide as a prokinetic drug to keep intestinal content moving through areas of partial obstruction.
- Meticulous attention to maintaining soft bowel movements daily:
    - stool softener (e.g. osmotic laxatives like lactulose and magnesium hydroxide or lubricants such as mineral oil)
    - rectal suppositories as necessary (glycerine and bisacodyl)
    - avoid high enemas.
- Diet alteration using a soft or liquid low residue diet is often advised although the exact efficacy of this has not been proved.
- A treatment plan to prevent or abort further episodes of MBO must be in place. Medications such as antiemetics, antisecretory drugs, antimotility agents and opioids should be kept on hand at home in parenteral and oral forms to be rapidly re-instituted as soon as cramps, distension, nausea or vomiting occur.

Episodes that become more frequent or closely spaced may indicate that complete irreversible bowel obstruction is imminent.

> Patricia has three more episodes of bowel obstruction over the next 2 months, two of which were managed medically at home. Each time she experienced anorexia, bloating, and then nausea and vomiting, progressing over several days. Octreotide and haloperidol were reinstituted subcutaneously. Symptoms rapidly subsided over 12–24 h. During the last episode, her symptoms recurred each time medications were lowered and she has been vomiting small amounts at least once a day. Patricia's husband is not coping well. He feels that she is wasting away and becoming progressively weaker because she cannot eat. He arranges a follow-up visit with her surgeon. Patricia has a complete bowel obstruction that has not resolved. She is in hospital but wants to go home to die.

Question 11. What is the management of complete bowel obstruction at this time? What are the goals of care now?

Management of unremitting total MBO

The prognosis after complete bowel obstruction is quite variable. This turning point in a patient's disease represents an important time to revisit the goals of care.

- Initiate a multidisciplinary meeting with patient and family/caregivers. Allow sufficient time for exchange of knowledge, expectations, fears, needs, hopes, etc. Adopt a sensitive but transparent approach about what is going on and the extent of disease.
- Clarify the medical information, including the limited options for disease treatment, for the patient and for family members or substitute decision-makers. Discuss prognosis and possible outcomes such as sepsis or bowel perforation.
- Assess the patient's functional status in order to plan for resources to support him or her at home or in an institution.
- Establish patient and family wishes about home care.
- Discuss the team's commitment to symptom control and accessibility. It is likely that the patient will vomit occasionally and this must be explained to him or her.
- The issues of hydration and nutrition must be addressed.
- Emerge with a clear management plan that is consistent with the patient's goals of care and agreed upon by all.

Many patients with unremitting bowel obstruction still receive traditional therapy with nasogastric decompression, venting procedures, and intravenous fluids, often requiring hospitalization until death. In recent years, pharmacological therapy, as previously discussed, offers options for a peaceful death, free from distressing and undignified symptoms. This therapy can usually be provided in any setting.

Home care for the patient with terminal bowel obstruction is possible. Components of care that are needed include the following.

- Ensuring adequate and coordinated resources at home including accessibility to physician and visiting nursing services 24 h per day and a plan for options for care if continuing home care is not possible.
- Patient and family counselling support to address psychological and spiritual needs.
- A focus on the goal of eliminating nausea and reducing vomiting to less than twice a day.
- Antisecretory, antiemetic, antimotility, and analgesic drugs in a variety of oral and parenteral forms or via continuous infusion. When doses are stable, many drugs can be combined in the same pump or syringe driver.
- Offer sips or soft foods as tolerated. The fluids may be absorbed proximally. Some patients continue to enjoy certain foods and prefer to vomit after meals as long as there is no significant nausea.
- Meticulous mouth hygiene with hydration of oral membranes is essential.
- Discuss the issue of hydration. Most patients will not opt for hydration. However, parenteral hydration can be provided to patients and families who absolutely insist on it. This can be done via the subcutaneous route (hypodermoclysis) or intravenously. Hydration can be

used in patients who are on morphine and who may experience toxicity because of decreased renal excretion or active metabolite accumulation. Dose reduction should be considered if hydration is not going to be offered.

- Rarely, palliative sedation may be needed for intractable severe distress.

Patricia is discharged home with a continuous subcutaneous infusion of octreotide at 15 μg/h and provision for antiemetics and analgesics to control MBO symptoms. She is able to enjoy small sips of coffee and ice cream. She vomits very occasionally and has no nausea. Her bowels have ceased to function. Pain is stable and well controlled. She becomes increasingly weak and bedridden. During her last few days, she becomes more somnolent and requires parenteral administration of analgesics and antiemetics. She dies peacefully at home 3 weeks after discharge, surrounded by her loved ones.

Summary

Cancer patients with malignant bowel obstruction faces a number of challenging symptoms that add to their suffering. More research and prospective studies are needed to define further the evidence base for our interventions with such patients. New trends such as laparoscopic surgery[30] hold promise for some patients. The use of drugs to control secretions and symptoms has proved to be very effective, and in most patients can replace the need for the traditional 'suck and drip' method of management. A holistic, comprehensive, and collaborative multidisciplinary approach to these patients will relieve much unnecessary suffering.

References

1. **Ripamonti, C., Twycross, R., Baines, M., *et al.*** (2001) Clinical-practice recommendations for the management of bowel obstruction in patients with end-stage cancer. Working Group of the European Association for Palliative Care. *Support Care Cancer,* **9**, 223–33.
2. **Feuer, D., and Broadley, K.E.** (1999) Systematic review and meta-analysis of corticosteroids for the resolution of malignant bowel obstruction in advanced gynaecological and gastrointestinal cancer. *Ann Oncol,* **10**,1035–41.
3. **Baines, M.** (1998) .The pathophysiology and management of malignant intestinal obstruction. In: Doylen D, Hanks, G.W.C, MacDonald, N (eds) *Oxford Textbook of Palliative Medicine.* Oxford: Oxford University Press, 526–34.
4. **Bruera, E., Brenneis, C., Michand, M., and MacDonald, N.** (1987). Continuous subcutaneous infusion of metoclopramide for treatment of narcotic bowel syndrome. *Cancer Treat Rep,* **71**, 1121–2.
5. **Maglinte, D.D., Kelvin, F.M., O'Connor, K., *et al.*** (1996) Current status of small bowel radiography. *Abdom Imaging,* **21**, 247–57.
6. **Anderson, C.A., and Humphrey, W.T.** (1997) Contrast radiography in small bowel obstruction: a prospective randomized trial. *Mil Med,* **162**, 749–52.
7. **Daneshmand, S., Hedley, C.G., and Stain, S.C.** (1999) The utility and reliability of the computed tomography scan in the diagnosis of small bowel obstruction. *Ann Surg,* **65**, 922–6.

8. **Legendre, H., Vahhuyse, E., Caroli-Bosc, F.X., and Pector, J.C.** (2001) Survival and quality of life after palliative surgery for neoplastic gastrointestinal obstruction. *Eur J Surg Oncol*, **27**, 364–7.
9. **Krouse, R.S., McCahill, L.E., Easson, A.M., and Dunn, G.P.** (2002) When the sun can set on an unoperated bowel obstruction: management of malignant bowel obstruction. *J Am Coll Surg*, **195**, 117–28.
10. **Chan, A., and Woodruff, R.K.** (1992) Intestinal obstruction in patients with widespread intraabdominal malignancy . *J Pain Symptom Manage*, **7**, 339–42.
11. **Turnbull, A.D.M., Guerra, J., and Starners, H.F.** (1989) Results of surgery for obstructing carcinomatosis of gastrointestinal, pancreatic or biliary origin. *J Clin Oncol*, **7**, 381–6.
12. **Weiss, S.M., Skibber, J.M., and Rosato, F.E.** (1984) Bowel obstruction in cancer patients: performance status as a predictor of survival. *J Surg Oncol*, **25**, 15–17.
13. **Fernandes, J.R., Seymour, R.J., and Suissa, S.** (1988) Bowel obstruction in patients with ovarian cancer: a search for prognostic factors. *Am J Obstet Gynecol*, **158**, 244–9.
14. **Buccheri, G., and Ferrigno, D.** (2004) Prognostic factors in lung cancer: tables and comments. *Eur Respir J*, **7**, 1350–64.
15. **Rubin, S.C.** (1999) Intestinal obstruction in advanced ovarian cancer: what does the patient want? *Gynecol Oncol*, **75**, 311–12.
16. **Ripamonti, C., and Bruera, E.** (2002) Palliative management of malignant bowel obstruction. *Int J Gynecol Cancer*, **12**, 135–43.
17. **Feuer, D,J., Broadley, K.E., Shepherd, J.H., and Barton, D.P.** (1999) Systematic review of surgery in malignant bowel obstruction in advanced gynecological and gastrointestinal cancer. *Gynecol Oncol*, **75**, 313–22.
18. **Feuer, D. J, and Broadley, K.E.** (2002) Surgery for the resolution of symptoms in malignant bowel obstruction in advanced gynaecological and gastrointestinal cancer. In: *Cochrane Library*, Issue 4. Oxford:Update Software.
19. **Soetikno, R.M., and Carr-Locke, D.L.** (1999) Expandable metal stents for gastric outlet, duodenal, and small intestinal obstruction. *Endosc Clin North Am*, **9**, 447–58.
20. **Khot, U.P., Lang, A.W., Murali, K., and Parker, M.C.** (2002) Systematic review of the efficacy and safety of colorectal stents. *Br J Surg*, **89**, 1096–1102.
21. **Baines, M., Oliver, D.J., and Carter, R.L.** (1985) Medical management of intestinal obstruction in patients with advanced malignant disease: a clinical and pathological study. *Lancet*, ii, 990–3.
22. **Mystakidou, K., Tsilika, E., Kalaidopoulou, O., Chondros, K., Georgaki, S., and Papadimitrou, I.** (2002) Comparison of octreotide administration vs conservative treatment in the management of inoperable bowel obstruction in patients with far advanced cancer: a randomized, double-blind, controlled clinical trial. *Anticancer Res*, **22**, 1187–92.
23. **Ripamonti, C., Mercadante, S., Groff, L., Zecca, E., De Conno, F., and Casuccio, A.** (2000) Role of octreotide, scopolamine butylbromide and hydration in symptom control of patients with inoperable bowel obstruction and nasogastric tubes: a prospective randomized trial. *J Pain Symptom Manage*, **19**, 23–34.
24. **Feuer, D.J., and Broadley, K.E.** (2002) Corticosteroids for the resolution of malignant bowel obstruction in advanced gynaecological and gastrointestinal cancer. In: *Cochrane Library*, Issue 4. Oxford: Update Software.
25. **Barton, P., and Parslow, N.** (1998) *Caring for Oncology Wounds.* Canada: Convatec.
26. **Klein, S., and Koretz, R.L.** (1994) Nutritional support in patients with cancer: what do the data really show. *Nutr Clin Pract*, **9**, 91–100.

27. **Torelli, G.F., Campos, A.C., and Meguid, M.M.** (1999) The use of TPN in terminally-ill cancer patients. *Nutrition,* **17**, 676–7.
28. **Stasser, F.** (2003) Eating related disorders in patients with advanced cancer. *Support Care Cancer,* **11**, 11–20.
29. **Alam, T.A., Baines, M., and Parker, M.C.** (2003) The management of gastric outlet obstruction secondary to inoperable cancer. *Surg Endosc,* **17**, 320–3.

Chapter 20

Spiritual care

Balfour M. Mount

Attitude

To enable each student to:

- Recognize the significance of existential and spiritual issues as modifiers of physical symptoms and quality of life.
- Understand spiritual needs and their interdependence with physical and psychosocial aspects of human experience.
- Understand the significance of personal (caregiver) spiritual issues and counter-transference as determinants of caregiver effectiveness as a healer.
- Recognize humility as a core product of the healer's insight and art.

Skill

To enable each student to:

- Be sensitive to needs arising in the spiritual or existential domain.
- Develop insight into personal spiritual/existential issues.
- Recognize personal comfort or discomfort in responding to patient and family spiritual issues.
- Develop the capacity for presence, empathy, accompaniment and active listening.
- Use open honest communication to enhance the efficacy of the caregiver–patient relationship in spiritual care.

Knowledge

To enable each student to:

- Demonstrate techniques for obtaining a spiritual history.
- Understand a model of healing.
- Understand the potential for realistic hope, healing and a sense of inner peace, integrity, and wholeness that is independent of physical well-being.
- Understand the dynamics involved in empathic care and the process of healing.
- Understand that healing is fostered by awareness of personal (caregiver) limitations rather than through prowess and skill.
- Realize that healing depends on a locus of control that is within the patient.

- Distinguish between spirituality and religion.
- Identify spiritual issues as pertaining to meaning, purpose, suffering, and the relational aspects of experience.

Basic concepts

What does the term 'spiritual care' imply? The traditional classification of our constituent domains as 'body, mind, and spirit' is metaphorical at best, referring as it does to inseparable interdependent aspects of the human condition. Who can distinguish between 'mind' and 'spirit'? In using the term *psyche*, Plato included both. Many find it hard to conceive of a spiritual domain that is not simply a product of human experience and longings, processed by the mind. In that case, is spiritual care merely an aspect of psychological support?

To muddy the waters further, the contemporary use of the term 'spirituality' as separate from 'religion' has a surprisingly short history; thus spirituality is still experienced and expressed by many through conventional religious understanding,[1] yet we now live in a multicultural and largely secular society. Thus Palmer[2] has argued for a clearer distinction:

> We need to shake off the narrow notion that 'spiritual' questions are always about angels or ethers, or must include the word God. Spiritual questions are the kind that (our patients) and we ask every day of our lives as we yearn to connect with the largeness of life: 'Does my life have meaning and purpose?' 'How does one maintain hope?' 'What about death?'

In this chapter I will consider religion to be a system of teachings and practices concerning the living of one's faith and spirituality, the dimension of personhood involved in a personal relationship with ultimate meaning, however conceived by the individual. From this perspective spirituality is an intrinsic domain of personhood. To be human is to be spiritual; it is a potential modifying factor in all human experience.

Case 1

Brad Simpson, a young convicted bank robber and the 'enforcer' of his gang was referred for palliative care unit (PCU) admission from a maximum security penitentiary in another province. He had been one of Canada's 10 'most wanted' men. This formerly muscular six-foot-plus young man was in his early thirties and dying of renal cancer. The referral was suggested in order that he might be near his father, his only surviving family member—not to mention the other members of his gang, who also happened to live in Montreal!

As his admission date drew near, tensions rose on the PCU, particularly among the nurses. He became a focus of concern at staff meetings. We would need extra security. Three of our most experienced and respected nurses refused to care for him, causing our perennially placid quadriplegic psychiatrist to explode. 'How could they?! Surely a dying person is a dying human being after all!' Resentments escalated. An unwarranted tempest in a teapot, I thought. I would have expected more! I, on the other hand, remained calm, benevolent.

As I entered his room for our first meeting, Brad turned from the window where he had been gazing blankly at Mount Royal and strode past me into the bathroom without acknowledging my presence. Moments later he emerged, jostling me with a well placed shoulder as he made his way back to the window. 'Simpson, you ****', I bellowed, 'I don't know what your problem is, but you had better get that chip off your shoulder.' With that, I turned on my heel and left the room. Calm? Benevolent? 'What have I done? I'm a dead man', I groaned, shocked and embarrassed at my unexpected outburst!

As days passed into weeks, three of us on the PCU team grew close to Brad. Were we touched by his life of hardship? Attracted by outlaw bravado? His mother had been released from prison for his birth and then reincarcerated, while Brad was given over to a community of Roman Catholic Sisters to raise. He had spent the majority of the subsequent 30 years in 'the system', graduating from reform school to escalating levels of detention. With all that conditioning, when gang members were in the room he 'got in your face' by adopting a hostile demeanour in both facial and verbal expression. He was a force to be reckoned with, even in his present weakened state.

Anne was Brad's nurse, and Tippy was his volunteer. Although a no-nonsense professional, skilled at establishing limits when dealing with others, Anne never complained despite repeated volleys of verbal abuse as Brad grew weaker. Indeed, she was tireless in her pursuit of comfort in the presence of fluctuating unpredictable symptoms.

Tippy, a diminutive and dynamic long-time PCU volunteer who was pushing 70, quickly established herself as the third team member with whom Brad felt a special bond. When Tippy first entered Brad's room on the evening of his admission, members of Brad's gang were present. 'What do you want?' he snarled. 'I can see you are busy', responded Tippy breezily. 'I'll come back later'. Then, as she made a graceful exit she spun to face him, bent low and squinted at his formerly handsome, now somehow majestic, black features with fixed gaze. 'My God', she erupted, her audience dumbstruck, 'Are you gorgeous, or are you gorgeous?'! Then she was gone—their mouths were gaping. It was Tippy (whom Brad always called 'Tee Pee') who discovered his love of maple icecream, whom in due course he asked to 'tuck him in' at night, and, finally, whom he asked shyly if he could kiss her goodnight. She tentatively bent down, turned her cheek toward him and felt the faintest touch of his lips as he whispered, 'Good night, Tee Pee'.

My friendship with Brad just seemed to grow. We talked easily. 'Bal, we're friends aren't we?' 'Yes Brad, we sure are.' 'But if I was well, we would never have become friends.' He was troubled. 'If I was well, and we had become friends, what could we have done together? What do we have in common?' Tennis, we decided.

I knew that I would feel a keen sense of loss when Brad died and brought my wife to meet him, causing a further uproar on the team. 'You don't bring her to meet other patients! Why him?!' As Linda and I entered the room I commented, 'Brad, do you know what happened today? Rajiv Gandhi was assassinated.' 'Really?!' he exclaimed, with evident interest and amazement, adding, 'Let me see, I guess that would have to be the Tamils.' I was stunned. How would he ever have heard of Rajiv Gandhi, let alone know who his assassins might be? He possessed a towering intellect. He had been playing the game with a very full deck, but had made unwise choices in using the rich hand he had been dealt.

When Brad died I urged Anne and Tippy to come with me to the funeral. Although Brad had admitted that he had 'never been a churchgoer', it was to be held at a local Roman Catholic church. I was uneasy, anticipating a gangland circus with lines of black limousines, Mounties hanging from telephone poles photographing all in attendance, and crowds of shady characters. Instead, we drove past the humble church twice before realizing we had found it. No crowds. No police. None of the gang members' expensive cars that had graced the front door of the Royal Victoria's Ross Pavilion before his death. He was abandoned, forgotten. Anne, Tippy, and I slid into an empty pew, noting two other awkward figures sitting stiffly to one side—gang members from the lower reaches of the pecking order. The dimly lit church was otherwise empty.

The priest looked reassuringly wise and kind. He began to speak, his words tumbling in a staccato of stu…stu…stuttering. I was overcome by a profound sense of grief, anger, and humility. Grief at a wasted life and the loss of a loved friend. Anger that Brad and this gracious priest had been ostracized, thrown together by the rejection earned through a life of crime and the speech-impediment-induced embarrassment of church hierarchy. (What DO you do with a stuttering priest?) Humbled in recognizing the contrast between my friend and me—praise heaped on me for a life that had been rich with blessings and opportunity, scorn heaped on Brad who had never had a chance. But *I* knew his worth, his preciousness, his well-concealed sensitivity, his brilliance, the depth of the fear and emptiness that lay behind the mask, his capacity to love.

Question 1. Why take a spiritual history?

The goal of palliative care is optimal quality of life. The spiritual/existential domain has been shown to be a significant quality of life determinant in cancer patients throughout the disease trajectory.[3,4] Therefore it should be included in both patient assessment and care plan development in all palliative care cases. While at first glance everything about Brad seemed to preclude the significance of spirituality in his life, this proved not to be the case.

Question 2. Would you have assessed Brad's spiritual domain? If so, how and when during the admission? What information is relevant to a spiritual history?

Spiritual assessment can be part of the admission history and physical, or it can be gleaned over time as trust develops. Given Brad's personal history we opted for the latter. Issues of concern in spiritual care include those listed in Table 20.1.[5] The acronym FICA is a useful reminder of relevant aspects of spiritual assessment (Table 20.2): [6]

- Faith, belief, meaning
- Importance and influence
- Community
- Address/action in care.

Question 3. Would you have asked specifically about his religious beliefs?

Brad was raised in infancy by a community of Roman Catholic nuns. Although his comment that he had 'never been a churchgoer' was at face value dismissive, it seemed to refer indirectly to these early ties. As a result we asked the Roman Catholic priest who was part of the hospital pastoral care team to visit Brad. The content of their private discussions was never disclosed to the rest of us on the team. While we left dialogue concerning Brad's religious beliefs to the priest, evidence of his personal spirituality gradually emerged, but *only* during his private interactions with Anne—in showing her a beautifully wrought crucifix that he kept among his few personal effects; in extending his hands silently in a position of prayer, as a gesture of thanks for a kindness Anne had extended to him; in revealing to Anne that he had daily telephone conversations with one of the nuns from his early life. It became clear that this 'hardened criminal' was

Table 20.1 Selected spiritual care issues

1. The life that is lived	10. Concluding relationships
2. Those left behind	11. Saying thank you and goodbye
3. Vulnerability and dependence	12. Loneliness and unresolved past grief
4. Perception of the body	13. Wishes regarding a funeral
5. Fears, mechanism of dying	14. Relationships with health workers
6. Guilt	15. Silence
7. Images of death	16. Boredom
8. Hope, faith and belief	17. How to die
9. Dreams and desires	18. Thoughts regarding an afterlife

Reproduced from M. de Mooij, personal communication, April 2003

Table 20.2 FICA: spiritual assessment

F—Faith, belief, meaning 'Do you consider yourself spiritual or religious?' or 'Do you have spiritual beliefs that help you cope with stress?' IF the patient responds 'No,' the physician might ask, 'What gives your life meaning?' Sometimes patients respond with answers such as family, career, or nature
I—Importance and influence 'What importance does your faith or belief have in your life? Have your beliefs influenced how you take care of yourself in this illness? What role do your beliefs play in regaining your health?'
C—Community 'Are you part of a spiritual or religious community? Is this of support to you and how? Is there a group of people you really love or who are important to you?' Communities such as churches, temples, and mosques, or a group of like-minded friends, can serve as strong support systems for some patients
A—Address/action in care 'How would you like me, your health care provider, to address these issues in your health care?'

Adapted by C. Puchalski with permission from C.M. Puchalski and A.L. Romer (2000) *J Palliat Med,* **3**, 129–37.

on a very private but continual personal spiritual quest. To have ignored this area of need would have been a grave error of omission. Brad gave us a graphic reminder of the importance of never ignoring the spiritual domain.

Question 4. Identify three specific instances of expression of spirituality in this case narrative

Existential anguish as an expression of spirituality

It is safe to assume that questions of meaning, purpose, hope, and death were a preoccupation for Brad, a highly intelligent young man dying of cancer after a life of crime and imprisonment. These issues should be considered in the differential diagnosis of his irritability and the unpredictability of his suffering.

Aggression: a reflection of relational fears

To survive in prison one must develop a mask that projects invincibility. This defence fosters the illusion of control and distances others in the interest of diminishing fear. Brad's habit of 'getting in your face' when gang members were present was evidence of his underlying anxiety. Spirituality is relational in its expression; it is expressed in relationships. Brad reached out to Tippy in a touchingly childlike request for the mothering contact that he had never experienced.

Healing connections

In his relating to me, we both reached across social and cultural barriers with a mutual unqualified acceptance of each other that held meaning for both of us. As death approaches, there may be a loosening of ego defences and an opening to 'healing connections'. Connectedness is at the core of spiritual healing. 'Healing' is understood as a shift toward an experience of integrity and wholeness (Fig. 20.1). This process may be fostered by the establishment of nurturing bonds at

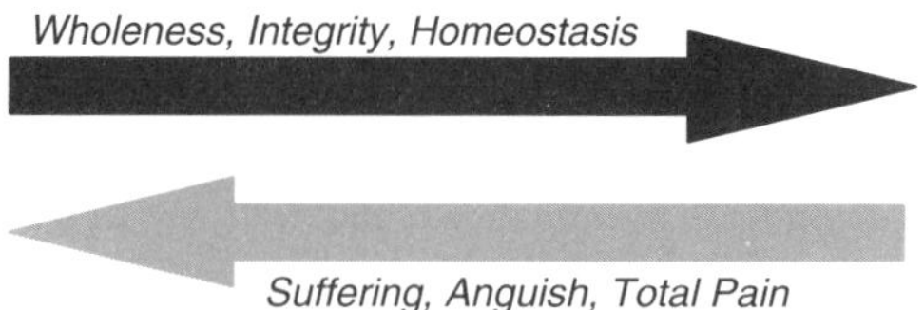

Fig. 20.1 The suffering–wellness dialectic.

any of four levels: **self** (the individuation of Carl Jung[7]), **others**, the **phenomenal world** (nature, music, literature, etc.), and **ultimate meaning** (God, 'the More', however conceived by that person).[8] Such bonds serve to draw the sufferer into a connectedness beyond the ego, and into the present moment where healing occurs. This reality became evident to both Brad and his trio of bonded caregivers. Each of us had an experience of healing.

Question 5. How do we interface with people at a spiritual level?

Spiritual care involves healing interventions that impact on the sufferer's sense of self-esteem, meaning, and connectedness. They do not necessarily involve religious belief, intentional action, or return to physical health. You can die healed. Saunders[9] noted: 'The way care is given can reach the most hidden places and give space for unexpected development'. Through varying combinations of good luck and good management, Anne, Tippy, and I registered our presence to Brad in a way that cut through his wall.

The caregiver assists healing by helping to create a sense of security, accompaniment, and caring presence. Paradoxically, we promote healing through recognition of our own personal vulnerability and limitations rather than by relating from a position of power.[10] Through this realization we enter a deeper level of bonding with the patient—the 'I–thou' relationship described by Martin Buber.[11] As the four of us were to learn, the healing flows both ways across the caregiver–patient bond.

Meaning is a key determinant of quality of life and healing. Supporting the patient's quest for, and experience of, meaning is central to spiritual care. Five avenues to a deeper context of personal meaning are things created and things accomplished, things loved, things believed in, things left as a legacy, and suffering itself.[12]

As trust developed, Brad became able to let down his mask, express feelings, and find a renewed sense of self-worth. Despite all that had been, he discovered that he could still be loved. He could vent his rage at Anne and she would continue to accompany him. Although not *safe* (he was dying), Brad experienced moments of feeling *secure*, perhaps for the first time in his memory. Saunders[13] clarifies the difference when she writes:

> The real presence of another person is a place of security. I recall remarking to two psychiatrists that when patients are in a climate of safety they will come to realize what is happening in their own way and not be afraid. One said: 'How can you speak of a climate of safety when death is the most unsafe thing that can happen?' To which the other replied: 'I think you are using the wrong word. I think it should be "security". A child separated from his mother may be quite safe—but he feels very insecure. A child in his mother's arms during an air raid may be very unsafe indeed—but he feels quite secure.'

In our interactions as caregivers with patients we react emotionally (counter-transference), although we may be unaware of our feelings. Such unrecognized feelings may lead to avoidance (as in the case of three of our nurses), bias (refusal to care for one who ignites intolerable anxiety), and errors of judgement (my unexpected fear-filled angry response on meeting Brad).[14] Cassell[15] reminds us that

> ...the bonding, connectedness of transference of the sick to the healer is not unidirectional. Both the [caregiver] and the sick person become exquisitely sensitive to each other. Thus the sick person is as able to sense anxiety on the part of the [caregiver] as the [caregiver] is on the part of the patient. Indeed, that openness of the flow of feeling back and forth enables the [caregiver] to use [his/her] own feeling in the presence of the patient for therapeutic purposes. What is required is that the [caregiver] be prepared to accept the fact that a feeling within [him or herself] can come from the patient.

Empathic care (including spiritual care) demands emotional engagement.[16] The caregiver's emotions influence even seemingly detached beliefs and decisions, thus the importance of emotional reasoning in medical judgement.[17]

Case 2

Mr L., a 62-year-old bachelor, was admitted for control of pain from metastatic prostate carcinoma. High-dose opioids produced only modest relief. Mr L. underlined 'None' in the 'Religion' section of his hospital admission form and added in the margin the comment 'I do not wish to see a pastoral care person!' His partner noted that he had been bitterly estranged from the Roman Catholic Church in his youth.

Question 1. Would provision of spiritual care be an imposition in this case?

As noted above, spiritual questions, as defined by Palmer,[2] occur on a daily basis and are a documented determinant of quality of life, particularly in palliative care. Attention to spiritual needs is an essential component of whole-person care. However, the patient's request not to see a pastoral care worker should definitely be respected.

Question 2. Are there indicators in this brief vignette that spiritual care is important?

The strength of Mr L's admission form protest suggests unresolved issues in the spiritual domain. Saunders' term 'total pain' suggests that psychological, social, financial, and existential factors may adversely influence the experience of physical pain.[18] Cohen *et al.*[19] have demonstrated in a multicentre trial that competent palliative/hospice care results in enhanced quality of life during the first week following admission, with improvement occurring in all domains measured by the McGill Quality of Life Instrument (MQOL), including the spiritual domain.

Question 3. What would spiritual care involve?

In respecting the patient's request, the pastoral care professional on the palliative care team was asked not to visit. As it happened, the music therapist and the occupational therapist were able to form healing connections with Mr L. These led to natural trusting chats about 'how difficult life is' and 'why bad things happen to good people'. Within a week of admission the patient had been able to express many of his concerns and beliefs. Mr L. seemed more relaxed and his pain control had improved in response to lower opioid doses. The lowered opioid dose needed for improved pain control in Mr L's case is a reminder to think of 'total pain' and the need to assess non-physical dimensions of suffering when response to opioids is less than expected, particularly in the absence of neuropathic pain.

It is often the patient who selects the team member with whom he or she can most easily confide. Mr L. was quick to find two caregivers who quite readily met this need. Although 'spiritual care' was not a conscious aim of their interventions, both therapists were aware of the gift of this opportunity to relate at such a meaningful level with a man who had always found expression of feelings difficult.

Case 3

Alice White was a youthful-looking octogenarian matriarch with an attentive family. An active member of the United Church of Canada for many years, she had had a disagreement with her current minister and had attended church only sporadically in recent years. Prior to death at home with small bowel sarcoma, Mrs White had been symptom free and, although weak, she was able to walk with assistance to the bathroom. Over the ensuing weeks her son began to sense that her condition had changed. Although he could not identify what it was that troubled him, he became certain that she was suffering and argued with the home care nurses for higher analgesic doses (she was taking only an occasional acetaminophen 325 mg tablet, as required). Her physician gave the opinion that she was not in physical distress. Finally, in a chat with the primary care nurse, the son identified the source of his concern. His mother had always been 'other-person-centred'; now she seemed withdrawn and less ready to relate to the family. She consistently lay with her back to the bedroom door. Her son wondered if she were angry, or perhaps depressed. Physical examination and routine bloodwork were normal apart from a mild slightly microcytic anaemia, unchanged over the past 6 weeks. The nursing team felt certain that she was not depressed. The family physician agreed.

Question 1. What is the differential diagnosis? What management do you recommend?

A mild anaemia of chronic disease was diagnosed but deemed stable and irrelevant to her changing affective state. The differential diagnosis included the **demoralization syndrome** described by Kissane *et al.*[20] (the experience of an existential vacuum related to an absence of meaning) that might respond to logotherapy,[21] **decathexis** (physical and emotional withdrawal, perhaps similar to that seen in dying animals and thought to be a protective reaction in response to diminishing physical resources), an important reminder to reassure the family that this is not anger or depression but a normal protective response to illness and that their silent supportive presence may be most helpful to her, and **unresolved emotional or spiritual conflict**, calling for active listening and counselling.

The palliative care team concluded that the latter seemed most likely but that all these issues were possible contributors. A pastoral care professional from her denomination who had not previously known Mrs White was consulted. A number of confidential discussions ensued that addressed old wounds related to unresolved issues arising early in her long marriage. Quiet dialogue, the use of the sacraments and rituals of her faith, and accompaniment by a trained pastoral care professional assisted painful introspection and movement to a place of relative reconciliation and greater peace. The effectiveness of this intervention was a reminder of the efficacy of religious symbols and of involving an experienced professional counsellor.

> **Case 4**
>
> Mrs Weinstein, a widow in her mid-seventies, was admitted to the PCU for poorly controlled pain from metastatic breast cancer. Pharmacological interventions by her physician and the skilled interventions of our attentive palliative care team bore little fruit. As the weeks passed we witnessed the mutual pain caused by her tension-filled relationship with her daughter, and we came to know of the painful events that had marked each chapter of her life. Her glass had always been seen as half empty, at best. The blind alleys of life had left her imprisoned in a personal hell that was ringed by self-pity and bitterness. When asked when she had last felt well, she responded, 'Do you mean physically?' 'No', her doctor replied. 'I mean in yourself'. 'Doctor', she retorted, 'I have never felt well a day in my life'. To which he answered, 'Really! Well if we are body, mind, and spirit, where do you think the problem has been?' Her comment was illuminating: 'I have been sick in mind and spirit every day of my life'.

Question 1. What would you do in this situation?

The strategies outlined in the preceding cases were attempted. Mrs Weinstein became the focus of long discussions during team meetings. In cycles, despite the best intentions, compassion and empathy often gave way to frustration, staff fatigue, irritability, anger, and avoidance—on occasion Mrs Weinstein became last on the list when other patients competed for attention. We never totally succeeded in assisting her to find relief from her suffering. Indeed, Mrs Weinstein's psychological and existential anguish had been well established early in life. It was reinforced by a life script that became cast in iron, and in due course by the challenges of her illness.

We have found several strategies helpful in this situation.

- Develop clear achievable goals as a team; watch for and avoid scapegoating.
- Make the 'problem case' diagnosis early, rather than late, and convene special multidisciplinary team meetings for specific discussion of patient and family needs, team feelings, and the need for limits in expectations, and to create a care plan with specific realistic goals.
- Support family and significant others and ensure that they get sleep and time away from caregiving; listen for relationships in need of reconciliation; use family meetings and ensure that they are run by experienced counsellors.
- Rotate staff (nurses, volunteers, physicians, others) *before* they become demoralized.
- Remind the team that we cannot always make it all better! Indeed, we cannot *ever* make it all better! The most and the least we can do is to accompany the patient at this time in their life journey, while at the same time establishing guidelines such as those listed above that attempt to safeguard our capacity to continue to do so.

Question 2. Are there limits to the responsibilities of caregivers to those who suffer?

Recall the profound truth that only the individual can experience her or his own birth and death, and the quality of each lived moment. As much as loved ones and others may wish to take on the suffering, healing has an internal locus of control. The psychiatrist Averil Stedeford noted,

'When we are with a patient (who is suffering and dying) we should never lose sight of the fact that it is their own death that they are facing and no one else can do this for them'.[22]

What *can* we do? Michael Kearney[23] put it this way:

> The therapeutic use of self by carers is as important as the knowledge and skills they bring to their professional role and of primary importance when it comes to being with another in suffering. ... This involves communicating, encouraging, and especially, *containing*. 'Containing' means psychologically holding the one who suffers even when there is nothing left to do, and no matter what happens. It means recognizing that attending to, thinking about, and working with one's own reactions as a carer facilitates the process of psychological and spiritual healing in the other. The containment of suffering validates the humanity of the patient and the wisdom of his or her own psyche.

References

1. **Larson, D.B., Swyers, J.P., and McCullough, M.E.** (1997) *Scientific Research on Spirituality and Health: A Consensus Report.* Rockville: National Institute for Healthcare Research, 16.
2. **Palmer, P.J.** (1998–1999) Evoking the spirit in public education. *Educ Leadersh,* **56**, 6–11.
3. **Cohen, S.R., Mount, B.M, Tomas, J., and Mount, L.** (1996) Existential well-being is an important determinant of quality of life: evidence from the McGill Quality of Life Questionnaire. *Cancer,* **77**, 576–86.
4. **Cohen, S.R., Mount, B.M., Bruera, E., *et al.*** (1997) Validity of the McGill Quality of Life Questionnaire in the palliative care setting: a multicentre Canadian study demonstrating the importance of the existential domain. *Palliat Med,* **11,** 3–20.
5. **de Mooij, M.** (2003) Adapted from personal communication, Antonius Ijsselmonde, Rotterdam, NL.
6. **Puchalski, C.** (2002) Spirituality and end of life care.In: Berger A, Portenoy R, Weissman D (eds) *Principles and Practice of Palliative Care and Supportive Oncology* (2nd edn) Philadelphia, PA: Lippincott–Williams and Wilkins, 799–812.
7. **Hall, C.S., and Nordby, V.J.** (1973) *A Primer of Jungian Psychology.* Scarborough, ON: New American Library, 81–3.
8. **Mount, B., and Boston, P.** The inner life response to advanced illness: a qualitative study. (unpublished data).
9. **Saunders, C.** (1996) Foreword. In: Kearney M. *Mortally Wounded: Stories of Soul Pain, Death and Healing.* New York: Scribner, 14.
10. **Guggenbuhl-Craig, A.** (1973) *Power in the Helping Professions.* Putnam, CT: Spring Publications, 79–97.
11. **Buber, M.** (1973) *I and Thou* (Smith RG, trans). Edinburgh: T. & T. Clark.
12. **Frankl, V.** (1959) *Man's Search for Meaning.* New York: Simon & Schuster.
13. **Saunders, C.** (1984) *The Management of Terminal Malignant Disease* (2nd edn). London: Edward Arnold, 6.
14. **Halpern, J.** (2001) *From Detached Concern to Empathy: Humanizing Medical Practice.* New York: Oxford University Press, 27.
15. **Cassell, E.J.** (1989) *The Healer's Art.* Cambridge, MA: MIT Press, 138.
16. **Halpern, J.** (2001) *From Detached Concern to Empathy: Humanizing Medical Practice.* New York: Oxford University Press, 26.
17. **Halpern, J.** (2001) *From Detached Concern to Empathy: Humanizing Medical Practice.* New York: Oxford University Press, 34.
18. **Saunders, C.** (1967) *The Management of Terminal Illness.* London: Edward Arnold.

19. **Cohen, S.R., Boston, P., Mount, B.M., and Porterfield, P.** (2001) Changes in quality of life following admission to palliative care units. *Palliat Med,* **15,** 363–71.
20. **Kissane, D.W., Clarke, D.M., and Street, A.F.** (2001) Demoralization syndrome—a relevant psychiatric diagnosis for palliative care. *J Paliatl Care,* **17**, 12–21.
21. **Yalom, I.** (1980) Meaninglessness and psychotherapy. In: *Existential psychotherapy*. New York: Basic Books, 461–83.
22. **Stedeford, A.** (1987) Hospice: a safe place to suffer? *Palliat Med,* **1,** 74.
23. **Kearney, M.** (2000) A Place of Healing: Working with Suffering in Living and Dying. Oxford: Oxford University Press, 208.

Chapter 21

An approach to ethical issues

Elizabeth Latimer and Pauline Lesage

Attitude

To enable each student to:

- Recognize that ethical issues are raised by virtually every clinical decision, and that the main prerequisite for resolving these issues is a high level of moral awareness in the physician.
- Recognize that, while a knowledge of abstract principles is helpful, ethical issues cannot be resolved simply by applying these principles. Each human situation is different, and each presents unique choices between greater or lesser goods or evils. The physician has to make his or her choice in 'fear and trembling', often not knowing in advance whether the decision will prove to be right or wrong.
- Describe the role of moral philosophers (ethicists) in helping the physician to clarify ethical questions in clinical situations and to increase awareness of ethical issues.
- Describe the differing values that patients, families, and caregivers may hold and how these may come into conflict, requiring creative resolutions.

Skill

To enable each student to:

- Demonstrate a strategy for resolving ethical issues.
- Describe how the reality of caregivers, patients, and health professionals with different agendas influences decision-making for patients with advanced illness.
- Apply an ethical frame of reference with respect to the application of therapies, such as the use of nutritional supplementation, sedative medication, the application of potentially life-prolonging measures, and the consideration of the Do Not Resuscitate order for a mortally ill patient.

Knowledge

To enable each student to:

- Elaborate on the practical and clinical application of the cardinal principles of medical ethics.
- Outline the concept and requirements of informed consent, and to recognize its importance in the physician–patient relationship.

- Describe the issues associated with the decision to provide palliative rather than life-prolonging treatment, and to withhold treatment from dying patients.
- Describe the legal, moral, and biological issues raised when active euthanasia is requested or advocated.

Introduction (Elizabeth Latimer)

Biomedical ethics: the four principles and associated moral obligations

Ethics is a generic term for approaches to examining the moral life. Biomedical ethics is a form of applied ethics wherein general moral action guides are applied to biomedicine in an attempt to answer the question: Which action-guides are worthy of moral acceptance and for what reasons?[1] The field of biomedical ethics is large, and the reader is urged to use resource materials to learn more about the principles and rules that govern ethical practice.[1–9]

The principles of beneficence, non-maleficence, justice, and autonomy (defined below) are the foundations of ethical health care delivery. In addition, there are a variety of rules and virtues that are elements of ethical care, such as the moral obligation to tell the truth, to respect the patient, and to exercise fidelity and self-effacement in the professional relationship. The principles are usually balanced and 'weighed' in any particular moral/ethical situation to determine what each of them might bring to bear on the problem. Ethics is thus a balance of science (principles) and context (personhood, communication, uniqueness of the individuals involved and of the physician as a moral and ethical person and professional).[9] In clinical practice, ethical aspects of care can be thought of as falling into two general categories: 'everyday ethics', which comprise the general approach to patient care and professional practice, and 'ethical dilemmas', in which there is an added complexity to a patient's clinical situation in which one 'right' course of action may be difficult to determine with certainty.

The principles[1,2,7–9]

Respect for autonomy recognizes an individual's right and ability to decide for him- or herself according to beliefs, values, and a life plan. Patients' decisions are uniquely their own and may sometimes be opposite to the course that is advised or deemed wise in a given situation. Respect for autonomy is central to the care of dying patients. Gentle truth-telling and exchange of accurate information about status, options, planned care, and future expectations are essential.

Non-maleficence is embodied in the concept 'one ought not to inflict evil or harm'. Causing unnecessary physical or psychological pain to patients, insensitive truth-telling, and denigration of the individual person are examples of violations of the principle of non-maleficence. Continued aggressive life-prolonging or cure-oriented treatment that is not suited to their needs or wishes may be a violation of this principle, as is unnecessary and unwanted sedation or premature unrequested or uninformed withdrawal of treatment.

Beneficence states that 'one ought to prevent or remove evil or harm, and do or promote good'. Beneficence implies positive acts and includes all the strategies that health care professionals employ to support patients and families and reduce suffering. This includes the effective treatment of pain and other symptoms, sensitive interpersonal support, and the acknowledgement of the patient as a unique human being to be respected and valued.

Justice deals with the concept of fairness or what is deserved by people. It describes what individuals are legitimately entitled to and what they can claim. For the individual, justice may serve to limit autonomy; what the individual wishes, chooses, or feels entitled to may not be allowable in the context of the greater good of society.

Clinical skills and practice patterns which will foster ethical decision-making

Certain patterns of practice will facilitate the application of ethics and enhance patient autonomy and participation in the ethical decision-making process. The physician and team are encouraged to consider the following approaches.[9]

- Try to gain a capsule of the patient as a person, in terms of their way of being, values, hopes, and dreams. Ideally, this information comes from patients themselves, but can often be reflected by those closest to them. It is invaluable in formulating treatment and care plans that match the person.
- Be accessible to patients. Practice sitting at the bedside to exchange information, rather than standing; it helps to establish the patient as partner. Ask patients what they understand their situation to be and what information they would like about their illness, treatment plans, and overall status.
- Ask patients what they would like to see happen and what you can do to help them. What goals does the patient have? What are their wishes, hopes, and fears? What is important to them?
- Be knowledgeable about the patient's illness and status, potential options, and likely outcomes. What are the real possibilities and limitations of treatment options?
- Be sure that the patient has the type of information that he or she wants and needs in order to make informed choices. Learn gentle but accurate ways of conveying this. Help patients to think through their options, giving guidance not only about what is possible but also what you as a professional, with knowledge and experience, might recommend. Try to avoid personal bias, but do not present treatment choices as being equal if they are not.
- Do not try to predict certain outcomes where certainty does not exist. Instead, try to address the patient's questions about the future within the context of what is generally known to be likely to happen.
- Balance reality and truth with hope. Emphasize what is possible rather than what is not in order to help patients set goals that are achievable and to enhance their sense of themselves. Use a similar approach when speaking with families. On the occasions that you deem it wise to meet with them apart from the patient, do so with the patient's permission whenever possible.
- Discuss ethical conundrums openly with colleagues of all disciplines. Create a forum where this can occur. Humane practice is more likely to occur when a variety of viewpoints can be heard.

Palliative care is based on a philosophy that acknowledges the inherent worth of each person as a unique individual with his or her own life story, values, and wishes. Patients and their families have a right to respect, compassion, and attentive and skilled physical, psychosocial, and spiritual care. Because of the vulnerability of seriously ill and dying people, the physician's relationship with them is a covenant of trust that he or she will work for the best interests of the patient, seeking always to help and never to harm.[2–4] The physician should strive to exemplify the virtues in medical practice.[5]

Components of ethical care at the end of life include:[6]

- careful physical assessment and diagnosis
- ethical communication
- setting goals of care
- relief of pain and suffering
- use of medications in usual situations
- use of medications in symptom control crisis
- appropriate use of sedation
- decisions regarding cessation and non-initiation of treatments
- ongoing attentive care
- practising with an interdisciplinary team
- practising in a culturally sensitive context.

Case 1 (Elizabeth Latimer)

Mrs D.M., a 54-year-old woman, is referred to the palliative care service of a large teaching hospital for assessment and management of abdominal pain and vomiting. She was admitted through the emergency department the night before, where she was seen by the surgical staff. Rehydration and analgesic interventions were instituted. Her history includes an admission to hospital 4 months ago when she was found to have carcinoma of the colon with metastases to the liver and peritoneum on 'open and close' surgery. You go to see Mrs M. accompanied by the experienced team nurse clinician. As you enter the ward, you are met by nurses and surgical house staff who appear very relieved to see you: 'Palliative care is here now … maybe they can help sort this out'.

The situation is this. Mrs M has never been told her diagnosis and future prognosis. Her family, who accompanied her to the hospital, had met the staff outside her room and insisted that she should not be told how ill she was, stating that this news would destroy her and that she would give up . Since it had been the middle of the night and the attending surgical staff did not know her, nothing much was said to the patient except that she had a blockage in her bowel. She did not inquire further, but her family had been at the bedside throughout the history-taking and examination. Indeed, they continue to be present with her constantly in hospital as though, in the nurses' words, 'they need to protect her from us'.

The health care team is deeply troubled. They think that the family's approach is unethical because it violates the patient's autonomy. In their view, the patient must be told the truth. Besides, there are treatment decisions which need to be made, including decisions about cardiopulmonary resuscitation and other life-prolonging measures which require her informed consent.

Question 1. What are the implications of not telling the truth from an ethical, clinical, and moral viewpoint? How might sociocultural factors influence the relative value placed on each biomedical principle and the concept of truth-telling itself?

Apart from the ethical dilemma surrounding truth-telling, very practical ramifications arise when the patient is deceived. Participation in decisions about treatment and care planning are skewed, because the patient's decisions are not based on reality; she cannot weigh the options available and exercise autonomy of choice.

This may give rise to a conspiracy of silence around a patient, which prevents patient and family from having any meaningful sharing about feelings, worries, and their hopes for the future. The role of the health care team is hampered as the patient cannot accurately convey instructions on treatments or ask relevant questions. Isolated from support, the patient may feel frightened and alone. A sad irony exists because most patients are actually aware of the gravity of their health situation whether or not they are told overtly, and yet they cannot talk about it if not provided with an opportunity.

Truth-telling or disclosure of information is the norm in Western health care practice today. However, the principles of autonomy, non-maleficence, beneficence, and justice will have different meanings and relative values in different cultures. The health care team must be aware of the cultural heritage of the patient and family, and learn sensitive ways of enquiring about the norms and expectations for truth-telling and communication in general within that culture.[10]

Apart from truth-telling, the concept of autonomy, and informed consent, there are many other ways in which culture may influence end-of-life care.[10] Death and dying are life passages deeply influenced by cultural mores and practices. The ethical physician will seek to learn about and respect the cultural values, beliefs, and practices that are held by the patient and family, creating an atmosphere that fosters mutual understanding. It is usually possible to modify practice to adapt to cultural ways while supporting the standards of ethical professional care and the best interests of the patient.

There are a variety of ways of approaching the situation described in the case. The simplest is to involve other members of the interdisciplinary health care team, and to call a family meeting to hear their concerns and to explain why keeping the truth from the patient is not in the best interests of everyone involved. The question 'What do you think your mother knows and understands about her sickness?' can be a good way to begin this dialogue.

The patient's understanding of her situation should be explored. 'What have the doctors told you about your sickness?' and 'Do you have all the information you need about your illness?' are good questions with which to open up this area.

> The team meets with Mrs M.'s family to hear directly about their concerns. They also will establish what Mrs M. knows and what her wishes are for information so that a plan of care and treatment goals can be established and necessary decisions made.
>
> On entering the room, you see a frail cachectic jaundiced woman lying in bed; several family members are by her side. You and the nurse clinician with you identify yourselves as members of the palliative care service, a type of care which you describe as comfort care which will attempt to help Mrs M. and her family through this difficult time. You gently begin to talk about symptoms, comfort, and the general situation. You ask to see Mrs M. alone for a few minutes before chatting further with the family. To your surprise, given what you had heard previously from the team, the family agrees and leaves to go to the coffee shop. You are alone with Mrs M.

Question 2. Where might you begin with your assessment?

Patients suffering from advanced illness require careful detailed assessment of their physical status at various points in the continuum of illness. Such points include the time of initial diagnosis and when significant new problems and change of status arise. The physician systematically assesses changes in health status so that appropriate treatment, often preventive, can be instituted as early as possible. The patient and family are informed of the changing situation. Diagnostic tests may be employed, taking into consideration their burden and their benefit to the patient and the likelihood that they will guide treatment that is consistent with the goals of care of the patient.

> You have examined Mrs M. and reviewed her health record. It is clear that her cancer is advanced. A review of her symptoms reveals that she has some abdominal pain, and nausea and vomiting at intervals. Her only medications include acetaminophen and oral codeine. These do not help the pain and she often vomits after taking them.
>
> Quite spontaneously, Mrs M. begins to talk about how helpful her family have been to her while she has been sick…'they are good kids', who have been very attentive to her. She does not mention her husband, and when asked about him she averts her gaze and looks uncomfortable. She goes on to explain that they are living apart and have done so for several years. Mr M. has a history of alcohol abuse and was abusive to her. She has never spoken of this to her children. As part of assessment, the nurse clinician asks Mrs M. about her thoughts concerning her illness. To your surprise, Mrs M. says that she realizes she is very ill although no one has said anything to her about it. She rather hopes that 'it will not be long'. She would like to be able to talk with her children about the future. She does not want her husband to know how ill she is. She pauses momentarily and then asks 'How much time do you think I have?'

Question 3. Discuss sensitive ways of responding to Mrs M's question

Ethical communication of information has four components:[6]

- it must be timely and desired by the patient
- it must be accurate in content
- it must be provided in words that are understandable to patient and family
- it must be conveyed in a gentle, respectful and compassionate manner.

Communication should be with the patient and, with the consent and the understanding of the patient, with family members. Conveying of information should be ongoing throughout the course of the illness, including initial explanations about the nature of life-threatening illness, with further updates of information on a regular basis and particularly at points of significant physical change.[6]

Communication involves not only sharing information, but also ongoing emotional support and care. The physician and health care team should provide regular opportunities for patient and family to share concerns, thoughts, and feelings, and to seek answers to questions of both practical and philosophical import. The great stress and fatigue that attends the situation of serious life-threatening illness often makes it necessary for families and patients to hear the same information several times so that it can be absorbed and they can feel reassured.

As might have been predicted, Mrs M. is aware of the seriousness of her illness. She also cares deeply for her children and would like to bridge the gap of silence which has developed around her illness. There are a variety of ways to begin to help her. It is paramount to explore her question further before beginning to answer it. What is she really asking? Is there a particular thought, fear, or concern that she has when she asks 'how long?'. When talking about the future, placing the context in terms of days, weeks, or months may be requested; however, remember

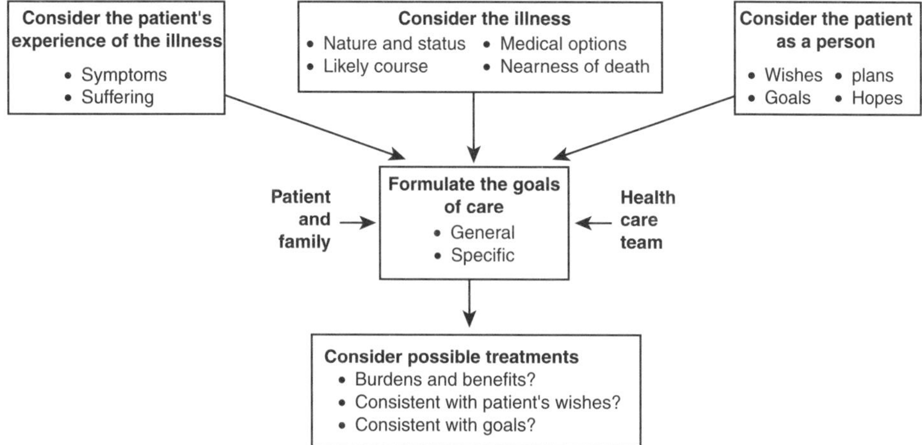

Fig. 21.1 An approach to formulating the goals of care and treatment plans for seriously ill and dying patients. Reproduced with permission from E.J. Latimer (1998) *Can Med Assoc J,* **158**, 1741–7.

(and remind the patient and family) that prognostic time estimates are commonly inaccurate. Ideally, the patient, family, and health care team will all communicate clearly and establish common goals. Figure 21.1 illustrates a way of proceeding.[6]

Prior to family meetings the palliative care team would make sure they were up to date on the key clinical information. This process requires a review of chart notes, test results, consultation with colleagues, and knowledge of the disease process itself and how it usually behaves. Consider current problems, probable future developments, and review possible options for care. What is the recommended or wisest approach to treatment?

Who is this unique person who has the illness? Knowledge about this person will provide the particular context and circumstances in which the illness will be played out.[11,12] What are their values, choices, life circumstances, personal goals, and plans for the time remaining to them? What is possible given the nature of the illness? What is their perception of their illness and experience of it?

Goals of care can then be articulated. The degree to which life prolongation is desired, is possible, and by what means should be gently ascertained. This allows for timely consideration of treatment decisions like the use of hydration, antibiotics, etc. in terms of their benefit and burden to the patient and their potential to enhance the goals of care. It also fosters a consideration of and conversation about the issue of cardiopulmonary resuscitation and other life-support procedures, the burden of which usually far outweighs the benefit to a dying person. Figure 21.2 illustrates a way of thinking about the matter of life prolongation and approaches to care that flow from two paths.[6]

Given information about their illness and a compassionate atmosphere in which to reflect, most patients are able to indicate their wishes for treatment and their goals of care. Where patients are unable to speak for themselves, the process of proxy decision-making is followed using legal and practice parameters. Generally, this will involve family members, powers of attorney for personal care, and following advance directives where these are in place.

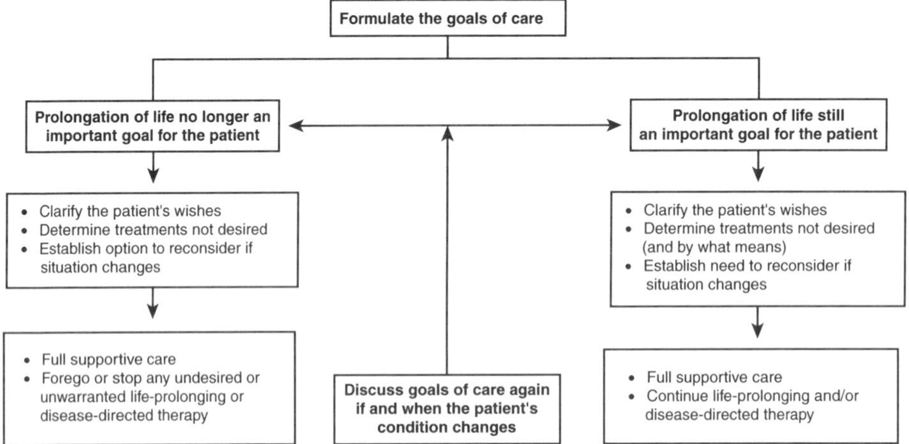

Fig 21.2 Patients' wishes for prolongation of life: an approach to decision-making and care. Reproduced with permission from E.J. Latimer (1998) *Can Med Assoc J,* **158**, 1741–7.

The goals of care, including those treatments to be utilized and those not desired by the patient, must be clearly recorded on the patient's chart and made known to all health care team members. If the patient is at home, a travelling record chart can be utilized to make information about treatment decisions readily available to health professionals in all settings.[13] Goals of care will change as the patient's condition changes.

Question 4. How would you determine how best to treat Mrs M?

Setting goals of care leads to a care plan within which various treatment decisions can be seen as beneficial, futile, or harmful. Transfusion, hydration, antibiotics, thoracentesis, and paracentesis are all examples of interventions that can enhance the quality of life for some patients. Regrettably, patients are not always offered these because of the mistaken belief that care of the dying should be non-interventionist in nature. Dying patients should not be overtreated, but neither should they be denied treatments that may be of help to them. Wherever possible, the patient, with guidance from the physician and team, will be the one to make the decision about procedures and treatments. A trial of therapy may be undertaken and subsequently continued or stopped depending on the patient's experience of its actual benefits and burdens. For example, parenteral hydration is appropriate if Mrs M. has the goal of surviving until her daughter arrives from out of town. It is relatively non-burdensome and would help the patient to meet one of her goals.

It can be ethically sound practice not to undertake certain treatments or to withdraw certain treatments once started. The cessation of treatment should be carried out in a compassionate manner with the use of sedatives and analgesics as required for symptom control and comfort.

The notion of futility of treatment may arise in discussion with your colleagues. Treatments can be considered futile by the health care team if they hold no possibility of helping the patient. However, it can be difficult to say that an intervention holds no possibility of benefit, particularly if the patient or family sees continued life at all costs as being something to be desired—a benefit. The patient has a significant part to play in defining benefit, burden, and futility. The health care team has an obligation to bring to the patient knowledge and experience about expected outcomes of the different potential paths of action (see Case 2 for further discussion of withholding/withdrawing therapy).

Question 5. What would you do if Mrs M.'s husband were to call your office to ask about her illness?

Confidentiality is an essential component of the doctor–patient relationship. Indeed, health professionals should not talk to family members or friends of a patient without the patient's permission. Since Mrs M. has expressly indicated that she does not want her husband to have information about her, it would be wise to discuss with her as to what she would like the response to be should he request information on the telephone or come to visit her in hospital.

Mrs M. should also be advised to consider completing an advance directive and appointing a person of her choice as an enduring power of attorney for her health care decisions. In Canada, because she is married, from a legal perspective, in the absence of such directives her husband would be the person whose consent would be sought if she were not able to speak for herself. In addition to clarifying decision-making, the team might also explore with Mrs M. whether there are any opportunities for healing or forgiveness that would bring her comfort or peace. A similar approach might be taken in asking if she would like to say anything to her children that might bring closure before her death.

Question 6. What about the ethical dimensions of working in teams?

The complex and diverse needs of dying patients and their families make the interdisciplinary team approach the most effective model for care. Colleagues from selected medical specialties, nursing, social work, pastoral care, pharmacy, nutrition services, occupational therapy, physiotherapy, volunteers, and other disciplines have unique skills to bring to care. The team provides a forum where the ethical dilemmas in care can be discussed and input sought. However, team members must be aware of the nature of information shared with other team members and seek the patient's permission before sharing information of a personal or confidential nature. The purpose of sharing information with team members is to help the patient, which is a fundamental ethical goal. Personal information about patients and their families is given to health professionals and teams in trust and faith that we will respect it. Respect for persons and fidelity to trust are two of the virtues which health professionals must espouse.[5]

You and the nurse clinician close your interview with Mrs M. and seek out her family who are now in the family room waiting to talk to you. They are somewhat defensive in talking at the outset. However, when you acknowledge how much you have enjoyed talking to Mrs M. and how hard this illness must be for them, they relax considerably and the daughters begin to cry. As time had gone on, they were less sure about their approach in keeping the nature of Mrs M.'s illness from her. In response to your offers, they would like to have a chance to talk with her about all of this. You will involve the chaplain and social worker of your team to assist with this opportunity for healing.

Question 7. Discuss the positive moral and professional obligations of health care teams to provide pain relief and psychospiritual support to people like Mrs M.

This family illustrates the high degree of distress and sadness which is natural when a loved one is seriously ill. The approach to total family care that is presented is one of the many positive ways in which palliative care can foster the dying process as a time of healing and positive relationships. This is one way in which the ethical principle of beneficence is manifested in clinical care. The team is obligated not only to alleviate suffering and pain as a moral imperative,[2,3] but also to assist patient and family in any positive way on their shared journey towards death, allowing opportunities for forgiveness, laughter, remembrance, and celebration.

The medical profession has a strong moral imperative to do all that can be done to prevent and treat physical symptoms, such as pain, and to work towards the alleviation of suffering. Ethical care requires that patients are provided with methods for symptom control that are in keeping with current standards of practice.[6,14] The physician must be aware of these standards and make the control of pain and other symptoms a top priority in caring for the patient. Unrelieved symptoms must always be seen as an urgent and sometimes emergency problem and dealt with expeditiously by physicians and the health care team.

The skilled treatment of symptoms, such as the effective use of opioid analgesics, is not an option which the physician can decline to employ on the basis of personal bias, misinformation, or lack of knowledge. The ethical physician will actively seek advice and consultation about symptom control from colleagues in medicine and other professional disciplines. The physician will take the initiative in asking patients about their symptoms and create a climate whereby the patient can report pain and be reassured that action will be taken to provide timely relief.

Emotional, psychological, and spiritual suffering should also be addressed. Physicians should ask about the patient's pattern of sleep and any feelings of depression, sadness, fear, and hopelessness. Appropriate treatment should be instituted. This may include reassurance, counselling, medications, consultation, and the involvement of interdisciplinary team colleagues for ongoing support. Skilled and attentive care should be available to patient and family throughout the course of the illness. Patients should be assured of ongoing care and know that they will not be abandoned.

> Mrs M. would like to spend her dying days at home. Her family is willing to try to care for her but will require considerable help in terms of home care resources. There are major gaps in what is possible in the home care programme where she lives. The family expresses to you their concern that Mrs M. may need to remain in hospital or go home with less care than she requires.

Question 8. Discuss the ethical issues involved in resource allocation decisions

Decisions on distribution of resources in the health care system and between the health system and society as a whole present an ethical challenge of the highest order. Resources can refer to money, expertise, staffing, technology, pharmacological agents—essentially anything that is required in the service of health care. Resource allocation decisions are made at the macro (societal) level, at the meso (institutional) level, and at the micro (individual) level. As a rule, matters of resource allocation are best dealt with in discussion and planning at the macro- and mesolevels, rather than in relation to an individual patient's care. However, decisions made at these levels can impact patient care to a great degree. Decisions about allocation are fairest when based on ethical principles and a transparent process reflecting societal values. This is no small task in a pluralistic society of considerable diversity!

Health care systems are seen as increasingly expensive, and in need of downsizing. Within our societies, there is much debate about what proportion of resources should go into 'high-tech' care versus 'low-tech' care like prevention and health promotion, prenatal care, care of the elderly, chronic care, and home care. At present, in most societies, high-tech care consumes a large proportion of health resources, leaving home care underfunded. At the microlevel, this situation serves to limit Mrs M.'s options in terms of whether there are sufficient home care resources to meet her needs.

Question 9. How might you respond to your colleagues who say that dying people consume too many health care resources?

A caring society will develop an effective means for caring for its seriously ill and dying members. Indeed, it has been said that the true measure of a caring society can best be seen in the way it esteems its most frail members. To identify any group of people or patients as 'consuming too many resources' is an implicitly biased mindset, a way of thinking and labelling people that must be resisted. The challenge is to ensure that dying people receive excellent care that is of the type best suited to their needs. Attentive and ethical care of dying people reflects well upon our society, the health care system, and the professions which comprise it.

Mrs M. requires medications for pain and nausea. You plan to order opioid analgesics.

Question 10. What are the ethical principles that guide the use of medications in palliative care?

The purpose of medications is to control symptoms and thereby to enhance quality of life throughout the course of the illness. As death draws near, medications may also be required to allow for peaceful death. Patients should neither be undertreated nor oversedated with medications. In general, the goal should be the relief of symptoms and, where possible, the maintenance of an alert sensorium.

The ethical physician needs to be knowledgeable about approaches to symptom control, will provide for regular assessment of the patient's symptoms, and will not hesitate to order medications with the intention to control symptoms and provide a state of comfort for the patient. The ethical physician will not seek to hasten death by ordering medications in excess of what is required by the patient for control of symptoms.

Question 11. What if Mrs M. develops a symptom control crisis?

Symptom control crisis presents a morally compelling situation for the patient and family and for the health care team. Examples of such a crisis include severe intractable pain out of control, suffocation due to airway obstruction, pleural effusion or massive pulmonary embolus, and severe agitated delirium.

These are very difficult situations to assess and to manage. Often there is fear that medication in the doses required to help may shorten the life of the patient. Such fear may lead to inaction on the part of the physician and team, to the detriment of patient and the great distress of loved ones.

If the possibility of a symptom control crisis can be anticipated, for example in the patient with tumour pressure and airway obstruction from head and neck malignancy or the patient at risk for respiratory crisis from endstage heart failure, emergency symptom control orders should be left on the chart. Orders should include specific detailed instructions about their purpose of the medications and how to use them in a crisis situation.

Such crises require urgent management on the part of the physician. Patients require the physician to be present in active attendance until comfort and a restful state are restored. Families require explanation of the nature of the crisis problem, the steps being taken to alleviate it, and the risk of death if such exists. They and the patient also require comforting and reassurance.

Case 2 (Pauline Lesage)

Ms J.F. is a 48-year-old woman who was in good health until 2 months ago when she noted abdominal swelling and weight gain. Associated symptoms included fatigue, loss of appetite, gastric fullness, nausea, diarrhoea, and intermittent leg swelling. She could not perform her usual activities as a legal secretary and mother of a 19-year-old autistic son. Divorced, she has had a stable relationship with Robert, a teacher, for 5 years.

She is afebrile, anxious, and in obvious discomfort. There is dullness and decreased breath sounds at the left lung base. She has marked abdominal distention with a fluid wave. There is moderate non-localized abdominal tenderness. Rectal and pelvic examination demonstrates a mass in the cul-de-sac. You admit her to hospital for further evaluation and management.

A complete blood cell count, electrolytes, serum calcium, and liver function tests are normal. Serum albumin is decreased. The chest radiograph demonstrates a left pleural effusion. Pelvic ultrasound shows ascites and a normal-sized uterus; the ovaries are not visualized. Retrocrural adenopathy is noted on an abdominal CT scan. Bone scan and gastroscopy are normal. Colonoscopy confirms an extrinsic, compressing mass at 5 cm; a colon tumour is not found. Paracentesis cytology is positive for undifferentiated adenocarcinoma. The tumour marker results are as follows: CA 15.3, normal; CA 125, slightly increased; CA 19l.9, moderately increased; CEA, normal.

During the first week of hospitalization, Ms F. becomes weaker, with increasing diffuse abdominal pain. She is also dyspnoeic and nauseated, and vomits frequently; however, she does not have a bowel obstruction. Control of ascites requires repeated paracenteses. In addition Ms F. receives albumin, morphine, and parenteral metoclopromide.

A multidisciplinary group meets to discuss her care and determine what, if any, limits should be placed regarding further investigations relative to her condition and likely prognosis, i.e. the benefit of identifying the primary site of the adenocarcinoma versus the projected poor outcome and excess burden to the patient.

Question 1. As a member of this group, what would you consider in the decision-making process?

This is a common situation that both physicians and patients face in the clinical practice of medicine. It poses the difficult task of ethical setting of limits.

According to traditional ethical and legal guidelines, a physician should take all the steps necessary to make the most accurate diagnosis possible and apply the best available treatment for that diagnosis. In the present case, one can argue that the sites and source of the pathology must be determined if one is to give the proper treatment; chemotherapy will differ for an ovarian compared with a gastrointestinal carcinoma, the most probable primary sources. Thus some members of staff recommended tumour biopsy and, if need be, a laparotomy.

At first, this plan seems appropriate. However, put in the broader context of this case, i.e. considering the rapid progression of the disease, patient discomfort and condition, and the malignant ascites that reflects advanced and probably incurable cancer, and recognizing that any clinical approach can only be palliative, the group recommended postponement of further investigation and proposed an empirical trial of chemotherapy for the most treatable tumour that may be present, ovarian carcinoma.

Even though one should consider all relevant treatment options, one must also recognize the limits of what is indicated for a particular patient. This means evaluating the benefit and harm of any intervention proposed according to the rule of proportionality.

Question 2. What factors will assist you in determining limits in this case?

One needs to consider the delicate balance of the good and bad effects of therapies or procedures from a medical point of view, and also on a level that considers the values of patients who have the right to choose limits and decide how much they choose to endure. Family input frequently provides us with valuable complementary insight.

As physicians we must be aware of the influences acting upon our reasoning. What guides our decisions? The diagnosis, prognosis, age, quality of life, and, most importantly, the wish of the patient, based on a clear understanding of the situation. A medical decision is never a purely scientific or objective decision; a wide range of values, variables, and biases must be recognized and confronted.

Question 3. How does the issue of futility influence your opinion?

We accept that if treatment is futile, it should not be offered or given. However, the difficulty resides in the definition of futility. One can state that a treatment is futile when it cannot fulfill its intended purpose or when the expectation of success is highly improbable. Obviously, when there is no real chance of achieving a desirable end (whether that end is cure of the patient, patient comfort, or patient dignity) one might conclude that the treatment is futile.[16] An example is cardiopulmonary resuscitation for an endstage cancer patient.

On what does one base decisions on futility? There are at least two different aspects to consider: the quantitative and the qualitative. The quantitative aspect refers to the probability of success and by extension relates to the medical outcome. The qualitative aspect is related to the quality of the result based on the balance of burdens and benefits. Futility is rarely equivocal or absolute: It is always in relation to what and to whom.

> The attending physician proposes to Ms F the option of an empirical chemotherapy trial. He explains to her that the malignancy is widely disseminated, that chemotherapy might slow down the ongoing process, and that she might experience some side effects from the therapy. He is vague regarding the prognosis and potential value of the treatment as he does not want to needlessly alarm the patient or her companion, who is anxious and confused by the rapid progression of her condition. He wants to maintain their 'morale', saying that 'they have enough to deal with at that moment'. The patient consents to chemotherapy.

Question 4. Why is consent a necessary component to therapy?

If at one time it was accepted that the physician decided for the patient by considering his or her best interest (called 'paternalism'); today's society values the principle of self-determination or inviolability of the person (the principle of autonomy). This implies the right to the truth, personal respect, and acknowledgement that decisions concerning the patient need to be made with his or her agreement or that of a proxy (see below). The information provided has to be sufficient for the patient to make the best decision possible under the known circumstances. The patient's decision does not have to be reasonable or 'sound' but informed and well considered, reflecting patient values.

Question 5. What variables can influence consent?

Informed consent depends upon skilful communication—a complex and multifaceted art. From the physician's perspective, there is the translation of technical language, the medical uncertainties, and the concern 'not to worry' the patient. From the patient's perspective, there are the limits of their personal understanding of their disease, along with the influences of culture, personality, and anxieties that often result in 'selective hearing' and contribute to partial understanding.

Patient or family fear and denial of the seriousness of the underlying disease or its likely outcome are commonly present. When a patient who is in denial is confronted by the reality that 'something' will be done versus not done, he or she may choose in favour of the proposed treatment, i.e. chemotherapy, radiotherapy, etc., and may minimize the potential burden or adverse effect of the treatment choice. We make decisions with our reason but also with our emotions and fears.

Question 6. What are the requirements of consent?

In order to be valid, consent must be given by a competent informed person, and be obtained without coercion.

Question 7. How do you evaluate the capacity of the patient?

A physician must be certain that the patient can understand, reason, and evaluate the consequences of a decision. It is important to remember that consent is specific to a particular decision.

The determination of capacity is a matter of clinical judgement; there is no one set of criteria to evaluate it. Because there is no consensus on the bedside basis on which to define capacity, one has to rely on a variety of criteria and make a clinical judgement. Broadly, criteria of patient capacity has five aspects:

- patient expression of a clear choice
- 'reasonable' outcome of choice
- choice based on 'rational' reasons
- ability to understand
- actual understanding.

Although the evaluation of the ability to consent is distinct from the evaluation of mental status, a test such as the Folstein Mini-mental State Examination can nevertheless help the physician to have a broader understanding of the patient's mental status. (The Mini-mental State Examination is a useful test in screening for cognitive deficits. It consists of a series of questions and tasks which assess orientation, registration, attention, calculation, recall, and language.)

Competency may fluctuate with time; it is not a 'steady state'. It may vary according to the amount and quality of information given, the environment, fatigue, medications, etc. This is particularly true in the palliative care setting and is accentuated when patients are on opioids or other drugs which can interfere with cognition. Clearly patients are not automatically incompetent because they are on opioids. Patients on stable doses who are not sedated are not usually cognitively impaired.

Strong denial can also alter the decision process. The patient may be unable to confront reality and thus may distort information.

Considering these factors, a physician should be both thorough and empathic when obtaining consent. If the patient is cognitively impaired, it is necessary to provide information to and obtain consent from a proxy appointed in accordance with local health and legal practices.

Question 8. What information do you need to provide to obtain consent?

There are specific points that need be disclosed including the medical condition and the patient's stage in the evolution of the disease (diagnosis, prognosis), the procedure of treatment proposed, the alternatives, and the benefits and risks in each case.

The first point seems self-explanatory but may present problems in palliative care. The precise diagnosis and extent of disease or prognosis are sometimes difficult to identify. In the case presented here, although the far advanced state of the disease is obvious, the primary source of the adenocarcinoma and the response to the proposed chemotherapy are uncertain.

The physician must propose not only one form of treatment but also possible alternatives, including supportive treatment alone. In each case, one must balance the benefits and harms and describe the risks involved. It is commonly understood that a risk is one that the patient will consider important in the decision-making process—one that will have an impact on his or her decision. Thus to evaluate risks, it is important for the physician to know the patient's background.

Question 9. Do you think that Ms F.'s consent to administer chemotherapy was 'valid' and without influence?

Ms F. had capacity. However, did she make her decision on incomplete information? Should the physician have further emphasized the poor prognosis and proposed comfort measures as an option? What influenced the physician's attitude? Was the patient's anxiety so high as to justify incomplete disclosure or to modify the risk–benefit ratio? Perhaps the patient had a fighting attitude and wanted to try everything possible. The acute onset of the disease and the young age of the patient are other important factors. Could a combination of all these elements have influenced the physician? These questions illustrate the subjective character of the doctor–patient relationship and its impact on informed consent.

Ms F. does not respond to chemotherapy. She is in constant pain despite increasing doses of analgesic medications. Despite corticosteroids and octreotide, nausea and vomiting persist, and ascites continues to accumulate rapidly and requires repeat paracenteses to alleviate pain and dyspnoea. She develops a thrombophlebitis for which she received heparin therapy. At this point, she is fatigued, dyspnoeic, and restless, and must sleep in a sitting position. She reports that low-dose midazolam helps her sleep, but only for short periods because of her physical distress. However, most of the time she remains conscious, alert, and competent.

One morning she speaks to the attending physician. After enquiring about the extent and outcome of her disease and being reassured that everything possible is being done, she asks that all treatments be stopped. She states she is 'at the end of the road' and does not wish to go further. 'I can't bear it any more. Please help me be comfortable. Make me sleep.'

Throughout her illness she is supported by her companion who loves her dearly. He has wanted everything done to restore her health. However, when confronted by her demand, he agrees that the situation is difficult and shares her decision, although very painfully.

Question 10. How would you clarify this request? Is this withholding of treatment?

In this case the patient is making two different demands: the first has to do with 'withholding' or 'withdrawal' of treatment, and the second relates to the relief of pain to the point of sedation.

Before considering these issues one has to clarify the patient's request. Is she seeking better symptom control, allowing her to remain alert, or does she really want to be sedated? Great suffering will alter patients' perceptions and influence their decisions. Indeed, withdrawal or withholding of treatment should occur only after skilful adjustment of symptom control.

Withholding or withdrawal of treatment

The patient has the right to request cessation of therapy or to refuse a treatment. If the patient has capacity, the physician must respect his or her decision. In the case of a patient who lacks capacity, one must consider the best interest of that patient based on the balance of benefits and burdens, and respect previously expressed wishes when they are known.

Obviously, in this case, chemotherapy seems to be more harmful than helpful. The patient is competent and she has a legitimate right to stop anticancer treatment.

'Withdrawal of treatment' can be defined as the cessation of a treatment that is medically futile in promoting an eventual cure or control of the disease. Attempts at prolongation of life are stopped. Death results from causes that seem no longer reasonable or beneficial to fight with medical interventions. Physicians formerly distinguished 'life-sustaining' therapy (e.g. basic nutrition, hydration, symptom control) from 'life-saving' therapy (e.g. chemotherapy, radiotherapy); the distinction depended upon whether one is delaying a death that will happen no matter what is done or whether one is combating an illness to prolong life.

'Life sustaining' measures used to be called 'ordinary', and 'life-saving' therapies used to be termed 'extra-ordinary'. A wiser perspective may be to consider medical interventions of any kind as being 'proportionate' or 'disproportionate'. They are terms which describe the underlying rationale—the proportionality of the treatment, according to the circumstances, referring to the goal of the treatment.

The distinction between 'withdrawal' and 'withholding' of treatment can be confusing. We sometimes act as if a treatment has a life of its own; once started it continues regardless of changing circumstances. This practice has no ethical, medical, or legal basis; it is often in place simply because it is much more difficult to stop a treatment than not to start it. However, the ethical principles governing the futility of initiation or cessation of treatment are the same; the intervention should not be administered if it is not in the best interest of the patient. Once a treatment is deemed futile or burdensome without proportionate benefits, it should be stopped, using the same ethical rationale that you use to decide to not start a futile therapy.

Question 11. Is sedation acceptable treatment for relieving symptoms in a dying patient?

When control of a disease cannot be achieved or when cure is no longer an option, the physician must still relieve pain and other symptoms. The goals of medicine are to 'cure sometimes, relieve often, comfort always'. The relief of pain and other disease-associated symptoms is a moral imperative and overriding goal based on the principle of beneficence.

Despite impeccable palliative care, some physical and psychological problems of the dying may be refractory to current therapies.[19] How does this dilemma reflect on our primary responsibility to relieve pain or symptoms? Does it imply going as far as sedating the patient if requested as in the case of Ms F.? Is doing so an act of assisted suicide or euthanasia?

The physician should take all steps necessary to relieve suffering with all feasible therapies relative to the given circumstances. But if all fail and one is faced with a 'refractory symptom', a symptom that cannot be 'adequately controlled despite aggressive efforts to employ a tolerable therapy that does not compromise consciousness',[19] is it ethical to consider sedation as an option for a patient with only a few days to live?

Given the circumstances, the appropriate treatment is one which considers the will of the patient, the goal pursued, and current medical standards. In this case, when everything has been done and the patient is still not relieved, sedation represents an acceptable and ethically sound alternative. Note that sedation is an 'exceptional measure' that has its own indications. These include intractable dyspnoea, non-reversible agitated delirium, and, less frequently, intractable pain. Sedation should be a group decision with a multidisciplinary approach aimed at clarifying the remaining therapeutic options and the goals of care. The decision should always be made with the consent of the patient, the family, or the surrogate.

Ms F.'s symptoms are not adequately relieved by optimal therapy. Sedation was then considered.

Question 12. What is the ethical rationale of your decision?

You are applying the principle of 'double effect' which holds in situations where there is a difference in the effects of an intended action (alleviating suffering) and the unintended possible consequences of the same action (hastening death). In this case, it is clear that the intent is to relieve symptoms and not to bring about death, which still might occur as a side effect. To be acceptable, the action must comply with the following requirements.

- The treatment proposed must be beneficial or at least neutral (relief of intolerable symptoms).
- The clinician must intend only the good effect (relieving pain or symptoms), although some untoward effects might be foreseen (hastening death or loss of consciousness).
- The untoward effect must not be a means to bring about the good effect.

- The good result (relief of suffering) must outweigh the untoward outcome (hastening death).

The principle's application relies on the integrity of the person and the sincerity of his or her intention. This last point is crucial to the distinction from assisted suicide or euthanasia.

Question 13. How are sedation and withdrawal of treatment different from assisted suicide or euthanasia?

Assisted suicide, often called physician assisted suicide (PAS), and euthanasia are presented by some authors as alternatives to the treatment of uncontrollable pain and suffering. One could either help the patient bring about his or her death (assisted suicide) or act directly oneself to bring about death by compassionate reasons (euthanasia). In both cases, the intent is clear; the control of suffering is achieved through the death of the sufferer.

These two entities contrast with 'withholding of treatment' and 'sedation' for the relief of suffering. Although they might share the same end result, the death of the patient, they are quite different in their intent; death is the unplanned, but foreseen and possible, result in withholding treatment and sedation as opposed to the intended result in PAS and euthanasia. In the case of 'withholding treatment', one stops a treatment that is no longer effective in achieving its goal, thus no longer resisting the process of death-in-progress. One has no obligation to live by technological means. In the 'sedation' case, the best treatment available is chosen to control what is already beyond control by other means.

Unrelieved or unrelievable pain is not the major reason for physician-assisted death requests.[21] The most common underlying issues are:

- depression
- unrelieved psychological distress
- loss of dignity
- loss of control
- other quality-of-life issues.

Question 14. What are the additional factors influencing current ethical thought on euthanasia/physician assisted suicide?

Assisted suicide and euthanasia imply recognition not only of the right to be relieved from suffering but also of the right to die. For many it is seen as the extrapolation of the principle of autonomy: one can choose the moment and means of one's death. Is this really what autonomy is all about? Can persons deliberately use their freedom to end their freedom? Is it not a contradiction to use freedom for self-destruction? If we recognize the right to die, it becomes difficult to set limits on its use. What kinds of limits? Should the choice to die be available only for intractable pain or endstage disease? Why not allow it also for psychological suffering that is often worse than physical pain? How much suffering would be needed? Why limit it only to terminal illness? Are there not other much worse conditions? Besides, suffering can happen at any time during the course of an illness.

Although great advances in the treatment of palliative symptoms have been achieved, cancer pain is still inadequately treated owing to the lack of knowledge by heath care professionals; fear of addiction by physicians, patients, and families, and some restrictions in the health care system.[22] There is much more work to be done to improve the quality of care for suffering patients.

Although euthanasia and assisted suicide are proposed for competent patients only, one cannot dismiss all the subtleties related to consent. In this troubled period of a patient's life, many factors can interfere with the mental process. Is their request consistent? Are they depressed? Do they want to die because of poor symptom control? How do we know that everything possible has been done? Is there a lack of support from family, friends, or even professional staff?

Another consideration is cost control. In a society where this is a priority, may policy-makers or even physicians be tempted to hasten the death of those with incurable disease by legalizing PAS and euthanasia as a means to the end of cost control? The slippery slope is never far away no matter how many safeguards we propose.

The medical profession has historically opposed euthanasia. Respect for life has been central to its practice Does medicine have the 'competence to manage the meaning of life and death' or only some manifestations of the problems they bring, like suffering? Human death is not a right or a good, but something inevitable. It would be an illusion to believe that medicine can master any and all aspects of our human condition. Keeping that in mind, doctors have the duty to use all the means possible to help patients go through difficult times, but not to the extent of annihilation. As Daniel Callahan has written: 'It is a strange kind of community that would require consensual homicide to realize its members 'individual dignity'.[23]

Ms F. is reassured that every thing will be done to make her comfortable. The intravenous line and heparin are discontinued. She is put on continuous subcutaneous infusion of morphine for pain and midazolam for dyspnoea, with upwards titration to effect. She remains comfortable and dies peacefully 2 days later. During this difficult time she is accompanied by her loved ones. Everyone is at peace because they have the impression that they could express their feelings and discuss issues freely. The door is left open for communication and support. An autopsy is performed, revealing abdominal carcinomatosis and pulmonary metastases, primary tumour unknown.

Bibliography

Baudouin, J.L., and Blondeau, D. (1993) *Ethique de la mort et droir à la mort.* Paris: PUF.

Anonymous (1994) Futility in clinical practice: report on a Congress of Clinical Societies. *J Am Geriatr Soc,* **42**, 861–98.

Katz, J. (1984) *The Silent World of Doctor and Patient.* New York: Free Press.

Roy, D., William, J., and Dickens, B. (1994) *Bioethics Canada.* Scarborough, ON: Prentice-Hall.

Senate of Canada (1995) *On Life and Death. Report.* Ottawa: Minister of Supply and Services, Canada.

References

1. **Beauchamp, T.L., and Childress, J.F.** (2001) *Principles of Biomedical Ethics* (5th edn). New York: Oxford University Press.
2. **Latimer, E.J.** (1991) Caring for seriously ill and dying patients: the philosophy and ethics. *Can Med Assoc J,* **144**, 859–64.
3. **Latimer, E.J., and Dawson, M.R.** (1993) Palliative care: principles and practice. *Can Med Assoc J,* **148**, 933–4.
4. **May, W.F.** (1975) Code, covenant, contract or philanthropy. *Hastings Center Rep,* **5**, 29–38.

5. **Pellegrino, E., and Thomasma, D.** (1993) *The Virtues in Medical Practice.* New York: Oxford University Press.
6. **Latimer, E.J.** (1998) Ethical Care at the End of Life. *Can Med Assoc J,* **158(13)**, 1741–1747.
7. **Beauchamp, T.L., and Veatch, R.M.** (eds) (1996) *Ethical Issues in Death and Dying* (2nd edn). Englewood Cliffs, NJ: Prentice-Hall.
8. **Baylis, F., Downie, J., Freedman, B., Hoffmaster, B., and Sherwin, S.** (1995) *Health Care Ethics in Canada.* Toronto: Harcourt Brace Canada.
9. **Latimer, E.J.** (1995) Ethical decision-making in the care of seriously ill and dying patients. Theory and practice. In: Sharp, J, Mason, P, Blackett, T, Berek, J (eds) *Ovarian Cancer.* London: Chapman & Hall, 281–91.
10. **Latimer, E.J., and Lundy, M.** (1993) *Health And Cultures. Programs, Services and Care.* Vol 11 *The Care of the Dying: Multicultural Influences.* Oakville, ON: Mosaic Press.
11. **Kuhl, D.** (2003) *What Dying People Want. Practical Wisdom for the End of Life.* Doubleday Canada.
12. **Barnard, D., Towers, A., Boston, P., and Lambrinidou, Y.** (2000) *Crossing Over. Narratives of Palliative Care.* New York: Oxford University Press.
13. **Latimer, E.J., Crabb, M.R., Roberts, J.G., Ewen, M., and Roberts, J.** (1998) The patient care travelling record in palliative care: effectiveness and efficiency. *J Pain Symptom Manage* **15**, 1–11.
14. **Latimer, E.J.** (1991) Ethical decision-making in the care of the dying and its applications to clinical practice. *J Pain Symptom Manage,* **6**, 329–36.
15. **Devita, V.T., Hellman, S., and Rosenberg, S.A.** (2001) *Cancer. Principles and practice of oncology* (6th edn). Philadelphia, PA: J.B. Lippincott.
16. **Committee Report.** (1992) Medical futility. *NY State J Med,* **92**, 485.
17. **Kubler-Ross, E.** (1982) *On Death and Dying.* New York: Macmillan, 25–6.
18. **Lesage-Jarjoura, P., Lessard, J., and Philips-Nootens, S.** (2001) *Eléments de Responsibilité Civile Médicale. Le Droit dans le Quotidien de la Médecine* (2nd edn). Cowansville, QE: Yvon Blais, 141–6.
19. **Cherny, N., and Portenoy, R.K.** (1994) Sedation in the management of refractory symptoms: guidelines for evaluation and treatment. *J Palliat Care,* **10**, 31–2.
20. **Seale, C., and Addington-Hall, J.** (1994) Euthanasia: why people want to die earlier. *Soc Sci Med,* **39**, 647–54.
21. **van der, Mass, P.J., van der Wal, G., Averkate, I., *et al.*** (1996) Euthanasia, physician-assisted suicide, and other practices involving the end of life in The Netherlands 1990–1995. *N Engl J Med,* **335**, 1699–1705.
22. **Foley, K.** (1991) The relationship of pain and symptom management to patient requests for physician-assisted suicide. *J Pain Symptom Manage,* **6**, 289–90.
23. **Callahan, D.** (1993) *The Troubled Dream of Life. In Search of a Peaceful Death.* New York: Simon and Schuster, 115.

Chapter 22

Ethics in palliative care research

David J. Roy

Attitude

To enable each student to:

- Appreciate the purposes and the importance of clinical and social sciences research in palliative medicine and palliative care.
- Be attentive to the ethical questions raised by research with human beings, and particularly by research with persons who are at the end of life.
- Criticise stereotyping ideas about the dying and about research conducted with those who are approaching death.
- Develop a balanced understanding of the complex relationships that can arise between care of those who are at the end of life and the various kinds of research needed both to validate and to improve that care.

Skill

To enable each student to:

- Identify the varied needs for research with persons at the end of life, the good likely to result from that research, and the diverse ways in which the dying might be either helped or harmed by participation in research.
- Perform an ethical analysis of protocols for the conduct of research with those who are at the end of life.
- Master the conditions for the ethical conduct of research with the dying.
- Recognize the potential ethical pitfalls of research in palliative medicine and palliative care.

Knowledge

To enable each student to:

- Evaluate whether withholding standard treatments in a clinical trial is ethically justifiable.
- Master the conditions for, and the possible limitations on, informed, comprehending, and voluntary consent to participate in research.
- Ascertain whether and when the dying are experiencing certain kinds of vulnerability that would limit or annul their ability to consent to participation in research.

- Evaluate whether a research protocol presents a remote or very proximate chance of physical, psychological, or social harms that are proportionate or disproportionate to the knowledge sought in the search *and* to the requirements of optimal care of those at the end of life.

Research ethics: background

The following summary presentation of basic ideas about research ethics sets up a background for this chapter's more particular discussion of ethics in palliative care research.

First, it is a mistake to view research ethics as an external and authoritarian imposition of regulations or possibly arbitrary constraints on the conduct of clinical or social sciences research. Quite to the contrary research ethics is as integral a part of scientific and professional judgement as clinical ethics is of clinical judgement.

Secondly, research ethics and scientific research—be it clinical research, social sciences research, epidemiological research, or health services research—pursue a common cognitive goal: to distinguish mere appearance from reality. Scientific research, using measurement as a cardinal procedure, seeks to ascertain the actual relationships between phenomena. Uncritical reliance on initial observations, potentially distorted by numerous possible forms of bias, can lead to systematic divergence from the truth.[1] Rigorous research methods are devised precisely to counter the tendency to mistake mere semblances of correlation for judgements of causality or of fact.

Analogously, research ethics, a process of critical reflective and collaborative analysis carried out by people from diverse disciplines and walks of life, acts against the tendency to diverge systematically from what is right. As initial observations may fail to demonstrate true correlations or causal relationships, it may also happen that what appears to be good or right within a limited perspective may contradict a greater or more commanding value. The order between values at stake in a research project may not be immediately obvious. As a consequence, working out the ethics of research requires the exercise of critical intelligence and judgement by a community of persons engaged in attentive and mutually corrective discourse.[2]

Thirdly, the conduct of methodologically sound research is an ethical imperative. If we restrict attention here to clinical research, it is right to emphasize that a physician's ethical obligation to offer each patient the best available treatment cannot be separated from clinical and ethical obligations to base choices of treatment on the best available evidence. The tension between the interdependent responsibilities of giving care that is personal and compassionate, and treatment that is scientifically sound and validated, is intrinsic to the practice of medicine, nursing, and other health care professions.[3] This is a tension between two goods a physician owes each patient (compassionate care *and* validated treatments), not only or primarily a conflict between the good of an individual patient now and the good of other patients tomorrow.

Fourthly, the idea that methodologically sound clinical research constitutes an ethical imperative can only be maintained if, and to the extent that, it is possible to conduct this research in an ethically acceptable way.

If the practice of medicine is both morally mandatory and inherently experimental,[4] controlled clinical trials, and clinical research generally, cannot be inherently unethical. This research, whatever the tactics used to control for bias, will be unethical only to the extent that the research protocols and the actual conduct of research fail to meet a set of necessary and sufficient interrelated conditions. Research ethics is conditioned ethics, and the conditions for ethically justifiable research, worked out over many years and published in countless articles and books, centre around the following considerations.

- Is the research plan methodologically sound and likely to produce the knowledge that is sought?
- Is the knowledge sought critical, important, or trivial relative to the needs of care and treatment?
- Is the research project's plan for the recruitment of participants equitable or discriminatory?
- Are the participants recruited able to consent in an informed, comprehending, and voluntary fashion?
- Does the project's information plan adequately explain the purposes, methods, possible benefits or lack of benefits to participants, and the burdens or harms that participants may incur during or as a result of the research?
- Does the research project involve conflicts of interest, responsibilities, or loyalties that might provoke exercises of pressure that could reduce the voluntariness of a participant's consent?
- Does the research project subject participants to unacceptable probabilities and magnitudes of burden or harm to body, mind, life plans, reputation, or relationships?
- Does the research project respect the possible cultural diversities of potential participants?
- Is the research plan sensitive to and protective of the potential special vulnerabilities of certain populations of potential research participants?
- Does the research plan display awareness of and respect for four essential characteristics of an authentic human relationship (autonomy, lucidity, fidelity, humanity)?
- Is the research plan protective of privacy and confidentiality, not only with respect to the research participants themselves, but also with respect to their families?

These considerations are not exhaustive, but they do centre on a number of conditions, recently summarized in a set of seven requirements,[5] that have to be satisfied if clinical research, social sciences research, and other forms of research with human beings is to be ethically acceptable. Several of these conditions will be highlighted in the following discussion of research ethics in palliative medicine and palliative care, a discussion motivated by a case presentation. The case presented here as the focus for a discussion of research ethics in palliative care combines elements from a real-life case with elements from a published case presentation.[6]

Mr M.W.D. was diagnosed as having multiple myeloma early in the year 2000. He and his wife were of East European origin, had one adult son, lived alone, could communicate fairly well in everyday English, but had difficulty understanding English explanations of complex matters. M.W.D. had always been highly active, and continued to be so in his retirement. He was also a very independent and quite singularly uncommunicative man. His threshold for pain was high; his wife commented that he never complained.

When M.W.D.'s disease stopped responding to chemotherapy, his haematologist mentioned the possibilities of palliative care as well as the option of participating in a clinical trial of a vaccine therapy, a phase I trial designed to gauge safety. The haematologist explained that this vaccine might shrink M.W.D.'s tumour, but he also emphasized that there was currently no way of knowing if this beneficial effect on the tumour would ever occur. The haematologist also explained to M.W.D. and to M.W.D.'s wife that an essential condition of his being accepted into the vaccine trial was that M.W.D. would agree not

Continued

to take systemic steroids, such as megestrol and corticosteroids, or bisphophonates, such as pamidronate.

M.W.D.'s wife emphasized that her husband had benefited from biphosphonate treatment and she was adamantly opposed to his participation in the vaccine trial under the specified exclusion criteria. However, M.W.D. insisted that he could no longer bear his increasing incapacitation. Less than 3 years ago he was climbing a ladder while shouldering heavy roofing tiles to repair his house, and now here he was, hardly able to drag himself around the house. M.W.D. saw this vaccine trial as his chance, very likely his last chance, to stop or decelerate his deterioration, maybe even to regain lost ground. He decided to participate in the clinical trial.

At the end of the first part of this case history, several questions arise regarding the ethics of conducting research with persons who have entered the final stage of their disease and are at the end of their lives.

Question 1. Should persons requiring palliative care ever be invited to participate in research?

M.W.D.'s situation is a particular example of the more general question about the ethical acceptability of asking persons to participate in research, clinical research in this instance, when they are close to death or are in the final stages of an incurable disease.

Some have answered this question with a quite apodictive negative, essentially stating that attempting to conduct research with people close to death is a failure to respect the dignity of these people as well as their physical, emotional, and psychological fragility.[7] Over the last 10 years or so more differentiated answers have been given to this question.[8,9] These answers have emphasized at least the following considerations.

1. Terminally ill and dying people should not be stereotypically grouped into the class of the vulnerable.
2. These persons are very heterogeneous regarding their capacities to decide competently and to consent validly to participate in research.
3. Exclusions of these persons from participation in research when the exclusions are based upon their belonging to a class (of the dying), rather than upon careful assessment of each person's capacities, strengths, and weaknesses, are unjustly discriminatory and depersonalizing.
4. If research with persons close to death honours the essential characteristics of authentic human relationships, it is unjust and intellectually short-sighted to state that researchers are just using dying people as means to attain their own ends. Research is an opportunity to mobilize a community of people (researchers, physicians, nurses, very sick people, and their families) to achieve the knowledge to perfect care and treatment and to reject useless or harmful interventions. Everyone has a stake in these ends.

The realization has emerged over the last decade that it is wrong to exclude the dying in principle from participation in research, particularly research dealing with the multiple medical and psychological aspects of their condition. However, some may continue to wonder whether research with those at the end of life is so necessary as to justify intrusions into the lives of those who have so little time left to them. Moreover, even if research with those close to death is acceptable in principle, is it not ethically necessary to pay close attention to the multiple kinds of suffering that are particular to people in the final stages of their disease.

Question 2. Is research with dying people really necessary?

The leading principle to guide a response to this question is that physicians, nurses, psychologists, counsellors and other health care professionals are supposed to *know* what they are doing when they intervene in the bodies, psyches, and lives of very sick and dying people. Obtaining the knowledge required to bring about a desired and controlled change in an utterly undesirable or even intolerable condition—be it a disease progression, unrelenting pain, multiple debilitating symptoms, or collapses in the capacity to cope with loss—is the essential obligation of a health care professional.

If that is the leading principle, the corresponding fact is that many kinds of knowledge needed for effective palliative medicine and palliative care are not available. The catalogue of necessary research for the improvement of treatment and care of people close to death is long and includes at least:

- the development of staging systems and therapies for nausea, dyspnoea, cognitive failure, mood disorders, asthenia, anorexia, and other symptoms
- acquisition of the data required to master both the complex interactions between various kinds of pain, nutritional deficiencies, confusional states, and dyspnoea, as well as the possible interactions between treatments of these varied symptoms
- obtaining precise knowledge from those most affected by pain, symptoms, and losses—terminally ill people and their families—about how they are affected by these causes of suffering and the treatments and care they are receiving.[10]

Research in palliative medicine and care is not only necessary, but is also ethically imperative because it is ethically intolerable that treatment and care of people experiencing the highest peaks of human suffering should be guided by untested and unfounded ideas. At this point, we return to Question 1. Without the collaboration of dying people and their families, the development of the validated knowledge needed for safe and effective palliative medicine and care will remain a utopian dream.

Question 3. Should research ethics centre attention on the vulnerability of those close to death?

Those who would insouciantly downgrade the need to pay close attention in research to the particular frailties of terminally ill and dying people have either never studied, or have forgotten, the many kinds of careless and dangerous research that have been conducted on dying people under the assumption that the dying are invulnerable to harm. Reports about such research span the twentieth century.[11,12]

Vulnerability is a complex concept. It refers to deficiencies in power, resources, strength, intelligence, or emotional equilibrium resulting in greater or lesser inabilities:

- to protect one's person, life plans or interests
- to resist physical interventions
- to resist emotional, psychological, economic, or social inducements
- to take one's own decisions
- to choose freely without coercion and pressure.[13–15]

People at the end of life may very well be, and usually are, living under the pressure of multiple, often interacting, symptoms and treatments. Moreover, their levels of intellectual lucidity, emotional stability, or volitional strength may be intermittently, or continuously, more or less profoundly perturbed. While persons receiving palliative medicine and care may, as a group, be no more vulnerable than persons in emergency or intensive care or psychiatric units, it is ethically essential, in the research context as in the clinical care context, to pay careful and comprehensive attention to the particularities of each person under consideration for an invitation to participate in research.

Research ethics rightly emphasizes what those at the end of life need to know to consent meaningfully to participation in research. At least equal emphasis has to be placed on what researchers need to know about the symptoms, anxieties, weaknesses, fears, and desires of those whom they are inviting into their research projects. This is a knowledge, in sum, of a dying person's body, psyche, and biography sufficient to maximize the likelihood that the research relationship will exhibit the marks of an authentic human relationship (autonomy, lucidity, fidelity, humanity)[16] and avoid any exploitation of a research participant's vulnerabilities.

After M.W.D. received the first two administrations (2 weeks apart) of the vaccine without experiencing any appreciable side effects, he returned for his third vaccine dose at 4 weeks. However, he was now having increasing difficulty in getting out of bed, standing and attempting to shuffle around the room caused intense pain, and urine control was increasingly difficult. Imaging showed diffuse tumour invasion of the lumbosacral spine and cord compression at several sites.

At this point, M.W.D.'s haematologist recommended that he withdraw from the vaccine trial to receive corticosteroid treatment for the cord compression. M.W.D.'s wife and family physician were present during this discussion. His wife was extremely upset and insisted that her husband drop out of the trial immediately to start treatment for his symptoms. The family physician, who had known M.W.D. and his family for years, was of the same ethnic background, and spoke the same language as M.W.D. and his wife, accused the haematologist's invititation to M.W.D. into this research project as being unethical because

- M.W.D. was so obsessed with prolonging his life that he could not adequately appreciate that the project's exclusion criteria posed major risks of harm to his own quality of life;
- it is wrong to invite people to forego validated treatments of devastating symptoms when the possibility of the research drug having beneficial effects on the tumour progression were so utterly uncertain.

M.W.D.'s wife and family physician could not convince him that now was the time, if it was not already too late, to drop out of the vaccine trial. It was not only that M.W.D. held onto the straw of hope that the vaccine would shrink his tumour. There was more to it than that hope alone. M.W.D. had known all his life that he just was not the kind of man to quit something he had started. He always saw things through to the end.

Question 4. When does a person's decision and consent to participate in research become ethically questionable?

A person's decision and consent to participate in research become ethically questionable if they are based upon:

- incomplete information about the objectives, methods, potential benefits, possible restrictions (exclusion criteria), likely risks of harm and special burdens, and conflicts of interest, if any, of the research
- deficient understanding of the information given, even if that information is complete

- an enfeebled ability to appreciate or evaluate the implications and consequences of participation in the research, even if the information given is complete and the understanding of that information is conceptually correct
- pressures or inducements that diminish freedom and increase coercion of choice.

Decisions and choices to participate in research remain below the threshold of ethical questionability if they are informed, comprehending, discriminating, and voluntary.

Did M.W.D. and his wife receive adequate information about the vaccine trial? They probably did, even if the case description is too scanty to really know. However, a second question is equally important. Was that information adequately presented? There is a fine line between presenting information about a research project in a factually correct and objective fashion, and presenting the same information with sufficient emphasis on sensitive points, such as risks of harm, that those being invited to participate will have their attention alerted to, not diverted from, points that should call for careful deliberation on their part.

There is reason to wonder if M.W.D. really appreciated the dangers of this trial's exclusive criteria—the dangers of his not having access to corticosteroids and biphosphonates for as long as he remained in the study. M.W.D.'s wife quite clearly appreciated this danger, but there is little evidence that the haematologist pursued or tried to resolve this discrepancy of appreciation between M.W.D. and his wife. Could the lack of a really common language between the haematologist and M.W.D. and his wife have contributed to a diminished quality of the consent discussions? It is not only that M.W.D. and his wife had difficulty understanding English language explanations of complex medical matters. The English-speaking haematologist was utterly ignorant of the Eastern European language of M.W.D. and his wife. The haematologist could not follow the emotionally laden and heated discussions M.W.D. carried on with this wife in their own language. Moreover, M.W.D. and his wife were unable to convey to the haematologist in English the emotional overtones and undertones of their heated discussions, tones that could have alerted the haematologist to proceed with caution in inviting M.W.D. to participate in the research. One might also ask why M.W.D.'s family physician, who had known M.W.D. and his wife for years and spoke the same language as they did, was not invited to participate in the research discussions from the very beginning.

There is scant cause to suspect that M.W.D. was cognitively impaired or required formal assessment of his decision-making capacity. Many patients at the end of life do suffer some cognitive impairments and should be formally assessed, particularly if the research involves notable risks of harm and burden.[17] However, M.W.D. was singularly uncommunicative, particularly with strangers. Had the haematologist acquired a deeper knowledge of M.W.D., something he could have done with some pointed questions to M.W.D. and to his wife, he might have been more sensitively alerted than he apparently was to the limits on M.W.D.'s abilities to appreciate adequately the negative implications for his quality of life of his participation in the trial.

Question 5. Is it ethically acceptable to withhold validated treatments from patients in a clinical trial?

Validated treatments were withheld from patients in a recent clinical trial that compared *Hypericum* (St John's wort), sertraline (Zoloft), and placebo in the treatment of major depression.[18] There is currently considerable controversy about the use of placebos in controlled clinical trials and also about clinical equipoise as a prime ethical condition for randomizing patients to one or another of the treatment arms in a clinical trial.[19,20] Since even a summary of this controversy would far exceed the limits of the chapter, we return to the case presentation to discuss the ethical justifiability of excluding use of proven treatments as a condition for patients' participation in a clinical trial.

One of the ethical issues that is quite unique to research in palliative medicine and palliative care, it has been said, is the difficulty of assessing the balance between risks of harm and the potential benefits when the research participants are in the final stages of disease. Patients may shift emphasis from prolongation of life to control of symptoms and distress as they near death, and that shift will probably modify what those patients consider to be harms or benefits.[14]

M.W.D. insisted that the most important benefit he sought from participation in the vaccine trial was shrinkage of his tumour and prolongation of his life, however slim the chances of this occurring might be. M.W.D. seemed to have been unable to grasp the proper balance between that slim chance of benefit and the far more likely occurrence of serious harm to his quality of life that would result from his being barred from using corticosteroids and osteoclast inhibitors. In fact, M.W.D. paid a heavy price, increasing debilitation to the point of paraplegia, for his hope of achieving benefits that never occurred.

Those who designed the trial and who invited M.W.D. to participate also seemed to have underestimated the gravity of harm that could befall multiple myeloma patients who would be asked to forego use of validated treatments in advanced stages of their disease. It would not be excessive to say that this magnitude of harm definitely surpassed the limits of what should be ethically tolerable in a clinical trial.

This case presentation also contains two other lessons about the ethics of research in palliative medicine and palliative care. Informed consent, one should recall, is definitely a necessary, but is often not a sufficient, condition for the ethical acceptability of a clinical trial.[5]

Secondly, the exclusion criteria in this vaccine clinical trial not only increased the harm that multiple myeloma patient participants were likely to suffer, but also greatly reduced the generalizability of trial results to that restricted subset of multiple myeloma patients who would not be receiving steroids or osteoclast inhibitors.[21] If research ethics requires that a balance has to be obtained between harms participants may suffer and the value of the knowledge to be gained from the research, it would not be imprudent to say that this trial suffered from an imbalance sufficiently great to make the trial ethically questionable.

References

1. **Sackett, D.L.** (1979) Bias in analytical research. *J Chronic Dis*, **32**, 60.
2. **Roy, D.J., Black, P.M.cL., McPeek, B., and McKneally, M.F.** (1998) Ethical principles in research. In: Troidl H *et al.* (eds) *Surgical Research: Basic Principles and Clinical Practice* (3rd edn). New York: Springer Verlag, 581–604.
3. **Levine, R.J.** (1992) Clinical trials and physicians as double agents. *Yale J Biol Med*, **65**, 65–74.
4. **Bernard, C.** (1949) *An Introduction to the Study of Experimental Medicine.* New York: Henry Schuman, 101–261.
5. **Emanuel, E.J., Wendler, D., and Grady, C.** (2000) What makes clinical research ethical? *JAMA*, **283,** 2701–11.
6. **Casarett, D.J.** (1999) Case presentations: are dying patients too vulnerable to participate in research? *J Pain Symptom Manage,* **18,** 143.
7. **de Raeve, L.** (1994) Ethical issues in palliative care research. *Palliat Med*, **8**, 298–305.

8. **Casarett, D.J., Knebel, A.L., and Helmers, K.** (2003) Ethical issues of palliative care research. *J Pain Symptom Manage,* **25,** S3–5.
9. **MacDonald, N., and Weijer, C.** (2004) Ethical issues in palliative care research. In: Doyle D, Hanks G, Cherny N, Calman K (eds) *Oxford Textbook of Palliative Medicine* (3rd edn). Oxford: Oxford University Press, 76–83.
10. **Bruera, E.** (1998) Research into symptoms other than pain. In: Doyle D, Hanks GWC, MacDonald N (eds) *Oxford Textbook of Palliative Medicine* (2nd edn). Oxford: Oxford University Press, 179–85.
11. **Veressayev, V.** (1916) *The Memoirs of a Physician.* New York: Knopf.
12. **Annas, G.J.** (1996) Questing for grails: duplicity, betrayal and self-deception in post modern medical research. *J Contemp Health Law Policy,* **M12,** 297–324.
13. **Levine, R.J.** (1986) *Ethics and Regulation of Clinical Research* (2nd edn). Baltimore, MD: Urban and Schwartzenberg, 68ff.
14. **Casarett, D.J., and Karlawish, J.H.T.** (2000) Are special ethical guidelines needed for palliative care research? *J Pain Symptom Manage,* **20,** 130–9.
15. **Dickens, B.M.** (1999) Vulnerable persons in biomedical research: 50 years after the Nuremberg Code. *Int J Bioethics,* **10,** 13–23.
16. **Fried, C.** (1974) *Medical Experimentation: Personal Integrity and Social Policy.* New York: Elsevier, 101–4.
17. **Casarett, D.J.** (2003) Assessing decision-making capacity in the setting of palliative care research. *J Pain Symptom Manage,* **25,** S6–13.
18. Hypericum Depression Trial Study Group. (2002) Effect of *Hypericum perforatum* (St John's wort) in major depressive disorder: a randomized controlled trial. *JAMA,* **287,** 1807–14.
19. **Freedman, B.** (1987) Equipoise and the ethics of clinical research. *N Engl J Med,* **317,** 141–5.
20. **Miller, F.G., and Brody, H.** (2003) A critique of clinical equipoise: therapeutic misconception in the ethics of clinical trials. *Hastings Center Rep,* **33,** 19–28.
21. **Casarett, D.J.** (1999) Commentary. Looking beyond vulnerability: the ethics and science of research involving dying patients. *J Pain Symptom Manage,* **18,** 144–5.

Chapter 23

When palliative care involves children: Talking with the child as a family member, and as a patient, pain and symptoms highlights

Gerri Frager and Kim Blake

Introduction

Many of you will not encounter children as patients at their end-of-life. You will care for children like Nicholas who are impacted by the serious illnesses and death of a family member. The principles relating to talking with a child who is dying or a child whose family member is dying are much the same and are useful skills for any clinician.

The approach to paediatric palliative care is often broader than solely end-of-life. The principles of palliative care are often incorporated concurrently, while pursuing attempts at curative treatment. Jennifer's story demonstrates timely opportunities to talk with the paediatric patient and their family, and the possibilities for meaningful input and preparation.

This chapter highlights some of the important differences in palliative care involving children when caring for them as patients and/or as family members.

Talking with the child as a family member, and as a patient

Attitude

To enable each student to:

- Learn that death and dying are **not** beyond a young child's comprehension.
- Learn that difficult truths and hope can coexist.
- Learn that, with open communication, children can discuss and benefit from being involved in end-of-life events.

Skill

To enable each student to:

- Learn ways to be more competent and feel more confident when talking with children about serious illness and/or death.
- Learn practical ways to assist the family to support their children.

Knowledge

To enable each student to:

- Understand the basic developmental concepts and some moderating factors that determine how children understand serious illness and/or death.
- Learn how children are masters at playing through their grief.

A young brother's story: talking with the child as a family member

Nicholas was 5 years old when his baby sister Jenica was born. At 4 weeks of age, Jenica was diagnosed with a rare type of leukaemia (acute myeloblastic leukaemia) and received chemotherapy at a tertiary care centre (Fig. 23.1). During the several months that Jenica spent in hospital, Nicholas and other family members travelled for hours to visit Jenica and her mother.

Jenica's treatment involved a bone marrow transplant and Nicholas, being a perfect match, was her donor. This required travel to a distant hospital. After 5 long months, Nicholas was very happy to have his sister and mother back home with the family. Jenica did well for almost a year after her transplant (Fig. 23.2).

At 15 months of age, Jenica's leukaemia recurred. Sadly, there were no prospects for curative treatment. Jenica was again admitted to hospital and the family chose to continue end-of-life care there. It is during this hospitalization that we meet 6½-year-old Nicholas and his family.

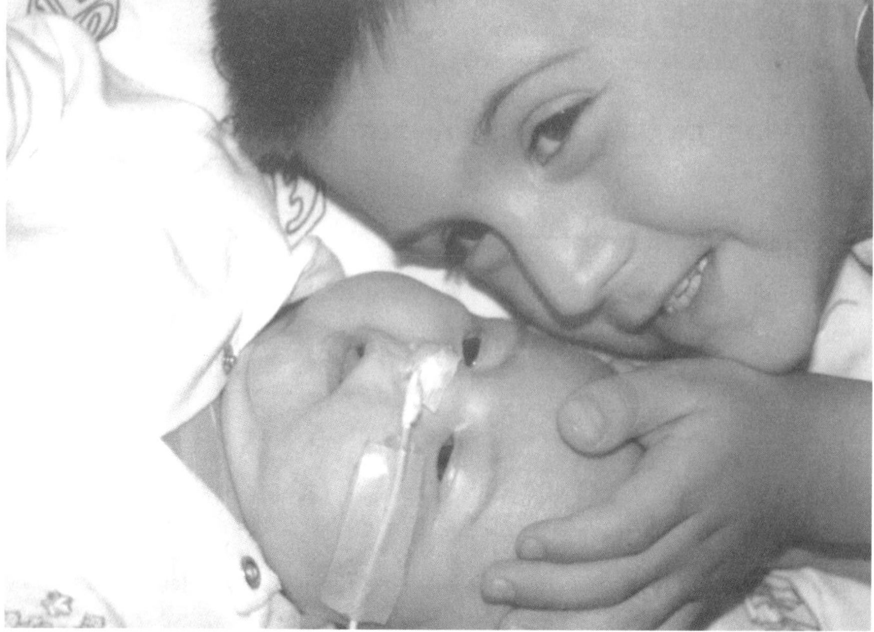

Fig. 23.1 Nicholas aged 5½ years and Jenica, aged 4 weeks.

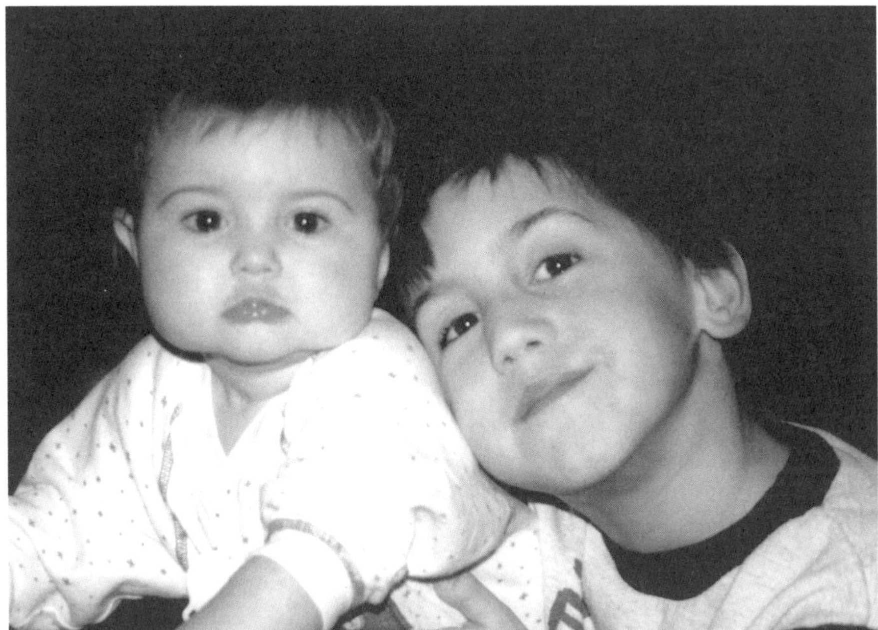

Fig. 23.2 Nicholas and Jenica, aged 12 months.

Question 1. Do you think that Nicholas should know how ill Jenica is now?

- Many adults have the perception that understanding death would be too hard on children, often based on their own level of distress, thinking: 'If it's hard for me as an adult, how could it be for a child?'
- Many adults erroneously assume that dying and death are beyond a young child's comprehension.

Question 2. What do we know about involving the child in discussions about significant illness and death?

- Children frequently possess, understand, and misunderstand more information than may be overtly shared with them.[1]
- We know that children benefit from honest communication and from being exposed to and included in the family's expression of sadness and grief.[2]

Question 3. What might a child understand about serious illness and death?

The child's age and their developmentally based concepts of death are linked (Table 23.1). However, they are elastic and may be superimposed and are not necessarily sequential. Many factors

Table 23.1 Children's concepts of death

Stage of development	Key concepts	Example	Practical implications
Infancy (0–2 years)	Experience the world through sensory information	Aware of tension, the unfamiliar, and separation	Comforted by sensory input (touch, rocking, sucking), familiar people, and transitional objects (favourite toys, tapes with a familiar song or voice, article of clothing from their familiar world)
Early verbal childhood (2–6 years)	See death as reversible Death is not personalized Magical thinking	May play with stuffed animal, alternately lying it down 'dead' and standing it up 'alive' May not believe that death can happen to them May equate death with sleep May believe that they can cause death by their thoughts, such as wishing someone would go away	Provide concrete information about the state of being dead, e.g., 'A dead person no longer breathes or eats.' Address the concept of feeling responsible and guilty because of their thoughts
Middle childhood (7–12 years)	Aware that death is final Death is personalized Earlier stage: understand causality by external causes Later stage: understand causality by internal causes	Aware that death can happen to them Believe that death is caused by event such as accident, may view death as a monster ('bogey-man') Understand that death can also be caused by an illness	Child may request graphic details about death, including burial and decomposition May benefit from specifics about an illness
Adolescence (>12 years)	Appreciate universality of death but may feel distanced from it	May engage in risky behaviour, with the view 'It can't happen to me' or 'Everyone dies anyway'	Ensure access to supportive peers and ensure their peers are supported. Adolescents who themselves are facing premature death may have a need to talk about unrealized plans such as schooling,relationships, and marriage

Modified with permission from G. Frager (1999) Pediatric palliative care. In: Joishy SK (ed) *Palliative Medicine Secrets*. Philadelphia, PA: Hanley & Belfus, 157–73.

influence the child's understanding of serious illness and death, including culture, the expression of grief from adults around them, and religious and spiritual beliefs. Previous and ongoing exposure to illness and/or death either though personal experience or through that of a family member impacts on a child's capacity for understanding beyond that attributable solely on the basis of developmental age.[1,3]

Question 4. What are the ingredients for sharing information about serious illness and death with a child?

1. First explore the family's mode of communication: how they share information and express emotions in front of one another. This may be assimilated from observation and from other members of the multidisciplinary team members. The family can be asked directly: 'If you have given your son/daughter some difficult news, how have you done this or how might you do this?'
2. Find out how the family would wish the information about serious illness and/or death to be shared. Some parents opt to talk with their children themselves. Others want or require someone there as a support.
3. Assist the family in talking with their children but do not do it for them. Long after you have left the room, it is the family unit which remains left to its own devices. Your most beneficial intervention for this family is to have them identify their strengths and build on them.
4. Use understandable, honest, and gentle language.
5. Let the child pace you with how much information you share, how much the child wants and can take in at intervals (see the detailed discussion following Question 8).
6. Rather than bringing your own belief system into the discussion, find out what the beliefs of the child and family are.
7. Reflect on some of the emotions that the child might be feeling, including sadness, confusion, and anger.
8. Clarify the child's understanding without subjecting him or her to what may feel like a test.

Question 5. How might you start the discussion with Nicholas about how ill his sister is?

A suggested approach to starting the discussion with Nicholas is as follows.

- Ask those who know him: 'Does Nicholas like a little or a lot of information?' 'Does Nicholas ask many questions and to whom does he turn?'
- Try to establish how much Nicholas understands: 'What has Nicholas been told about how ill Jenica is?' 'In what way does Nicholas show he understands?'
- Nicholas should be spoken with in a way that is clear and straightforward, as in: 'I wish that things were different for Jenica.' 'I am very sad that we have not been able to make her better.'
- Clarify that Nicholas has understood: 'We have talked about a lot of things. Can you tell me about the part you remember best?' or 'If a friend asked you what is happening to Jenica, what do you think you would tell them?'

Question 6. What might you say if an individual asks how they could talk about the serious illness and/or death of someone close to them without crying?

You can provide the information that children are comforted to see that the people whom they care about and whom they look to as role models are also upset by the illness/death. Parents and health professionals can be reassured that if they cry while talking about how ill the individual is or the anticipated death, it is absolutely acceptable. However, the expression of grief should not be so intense that the child is put in the position of having to comfort and support the parent or health professional.

As a health professional or a concerned individual who wants to help, providing concrete and practical approaches can both support those who are grieving and increase the comfort of those who are seeking to be supportive to the bereaved.[4] Providing some developmentally appropriate toys for the grieving/bereaved child to play with and/or spending some time playing with the child are helpful actions that serve as a bridge to others in a time of emotional turmoil. Talking about some of the child's favourite videos, cartoon characters, or songs can be a gentle introduction to help the child and those interacting with him or her to feel more at ease. Children may draw pictures or use their stuffed toys as puppets, as media to express their emotions and questions about what is happening around them.[3]

Question 7. What do we know is helpful in supporting the child though a serious illness or death?

Families can be helped to find the language that is congruent with their spiritual beliefs while providing comforting and developmentally appropriate concepts for the child about death and the afterlife (Table 23.2).

Misinformation can lead to unnecessary confusion and fear. Young children who have been misinformed by well-meaning adults may become fearful of going to sleep, angry at religious symbols, or frightened every time a family member leaves on a business trip. Honest information

Table 23.2 Tips and suggested language for talking with children about dying and death

What children may ask	What to say (whether or not asked)
Children need the facts about death 'Is he sleeping?'	'He may look like he's asleep. Being dead is very different from sleep'
They need to hear what being dead means 'What is dead?'	'Dead means that a person's heart is not beating anymore...that they don't need to eat anymore...that they are not hungry or thirsty...that they don't breathe anymore, etc.'
They need simple honest information to answer their questions 'What happened to my sister?'	Use honest language. Do **not** use clichés like: 'He's gone away', 'She's gone to sleep', 'God needed an angel'
The information children receive should inform and reassure them.	Use the words 'dead' and 'death' (if not precluded by cultural exceptions)
'Why did she die?'	'Your sister died because she was born with something very wrong with her lungs that just couldn't be fixed'

about what happened and what to expect carries more reassurance than leaving such concerns to a child's wonderful imagination.

Families should be encouraged to answer the child's questions about the end-of-life process thoughtfully and honestly. It is worth a reminder that saying 'I don't know' and 'I think I know who we can ask' is preferable to making something up.

There are many helpful resources, including video materials, websites, and books, that can be selected according to the level of understanding of the child. A list of several of these resources is given at the end of this chapter.

Children often demonstrate a remarkable capacity to combine grief and play. It is important that families and clinicians understand this as part of normal childhood development and not a reflection of the profound impact that the anticipated death is having on the child or a measure of the degree of grief they are experiencing.

Question 8. How do you imagine that Nicholas might be best supported through Jenica's end-of-life?

- Make sure that Nicholas has someone he trusts available **for him** and for **his** questions. It may be difficult to predict how his parents may be feeling and reacting, and how able they are to support Nicholas, particularly when Jenica is dying.
- Pace the information shared according to Nicholas's needs. Let him take the lead on how detailed and how quickly his questions are answered. For example, Nicholas should be prepared for how Janica's appearance is different, such as oxygen given through a plastic tube to her nose. He would then pace others for further information, such as by asking, 'Will Jenica always need the tube in her nose?' or 'Does that make her nose itchy?' Providing some information and waiting to see what questions are then generated is more helpful to Nicholas than trying to detail what one imagines his questions might be.
- Arrange the environment so that things are readily accessible for Nicholas, such as a stepstool so that he can readily interact and touch Jenica, who is cared for in a hospital crib.
- Have developmentally appropriate play materials and a support person available for Nicholas. This ensures that Nicholas is part of the family's activities while being able to move in and out of sadness, play, and grief.

> When Jenica's death appears imminent and many friends and family are arriving from her home community, Nicholas is told 'There will be many people coming to see Jenica, you, and your Mum and Dad. They will be very sad because of how sick Jenica is.'
>
> Nicholas: 'I'm sad too. If there will be more people that will give me more people to play with.'
>
> Nicholas is in Jenica's room when she dies.
>
> Mother to Nicholas: 'Jenica has died. Do you want to come over and see her?'
>
> Nicholas: (climbs up to her crib) 'How do you know Jenica is dead?'
>
> Mother: 'Do you remember what we had talked about before, about what being "dead" means?'
>
> Nicholas places his ear near his sister's chest to listen to her heartbeat and breathing. Not convinced, he asks for a stethoscope. Placing it on Jenica's chest, he listens for a long time and hands the stethoscope back to his mother.
>
> Mother: 'What did you hear?'
>
> Nicholas: 'It beat one last time' ... climbing down ... 'Can I go play?'

The aspect of combining play and grief is well demonstrated by these conversations.

Nicholas was well informed about what was happening to Jenica. He had a good understanding of what 'dead' meant, although he expressed a need to confirm her death for himself. Nicholas's family and the health professionals **allowed** him to state what he needed, **listened** to him, and supported him through this difficult time by following **his** lead.

Question 9. What do we know about supporting the child's involvement at the time of death?

- Children generally do better if involved in the care of their dying family member.[5,6] Some practical examples are letting the child bring the soap for a bath, drawing a picture for the ill family member, or singing them a song.
- For some children, it is helpful to have someone available to them who is not a friend or family member. This could be a child-life specialist, volunteer, or medical personnel. This enables the individual to give their full attention to the child, without being overwhelmed by their own grief. Some emotional relief is provided for the child in having an occasional 'break' from the focus on the dying individual.
- Children need to be prepared for what the room will look like and what their family member will look like ('There may be some machines around her bed. Some of them may be making beeping noises. She has a tube in her nose to help her breathe, or a tube in his arm to give him special medicines, etc.').
- Children also need information about what their family member looks like at the time of or after death as in: 'Her skin is not pinkish like ours, it looks a bit bluish. If you touch her, she'll probably feel a bit cool, like someone who has come in from a cold day outside.'
- Let them know they can talk to their family member and, if they wish, they can touch and kiss them.
- Ideas for ways for the child to say 'I love you, I remember', and 'Goodbye' can be facilitated through human resources, such as individuals with paediatric psychosocial expertise and/or the resources noted at the end of the chapter.

Every child will react differently to the death of their loved one and process their thoughts and emotions in their own ways. Provide opportunities for the child to express their needs. Listen. Provide support by following **the child's** lead.

Question 10. What about the child's guilt and imagination?

- A child's imagination is wonderful and can create images and fears worse than the graphic nature of reality. It is best to be honest even when challenged by the distressing reality.
- Children have a great capacity for what is referred to as magical thinking or make-believe.

This can lead to things like the child wanting to leave toys or food for the dead family member.

It can also be expressed by potentially destructive thoughts, such as thinking that they were responsible for the death of their family member because they wished they would go away because the ill person gets all the attention and toys.

This can result in the child harbouring tremendous guilt, so terrible to them that they may not volunteer their worry since they feel responsible. This is always a potential issue for all children, but particularly so if the family member has been involved as a tissue or organ donor.

Question 11. Are there concerns that need to be aired even if Nicholas does not raise them?

> Nicholas is given excellent pro-active preparation from his family assuring him that he is in no way responsible for what is happening to Jenica.
>
> Nicholas is given information that her condition is not contagious, as in: 'Jenica is sick and dying from a very different kind of sickness. It does not happen often at all. It is not something that you, your Mum, or Dad could catch.'

Question 12. Do you think that children should attend a funeral?

Children generally do better if included in the rituals that other family members and friends are participating in. This gives children an opportunity to see first-hand that people are sad and that showing this is permissible, that someone can be sad but still go to work, cook, and live despite the sadness. They are given the message directly that crying is all right, and this can help them to feel safe in expressing their own feelings.

- It is best to prepare the child for what he or she will encounter at the funeral. Saying things like, 'There will probably be a lot of people there who will be sad and showing they are sad by crying' 'There will be singing or a talk by the minister, etc.'
- Let him or her know details, such as 'Pictures of (the name of the family member) will be around the room as well as pictures of you, and Mum and Dad.'
- Provide details about whether or not there will be a coffin, and whether the body will be seen.
- Provide information in a simple manner, including whether there will be food and something to drink.
- Ensure that the child's questions are answered.
- Have someone the child trusts and likes accompany them, just for them, in case there are more questions, or he or she needs some comforting and wants to leave and come back.
- Provide the child with the choice to attend the funeral or not. Additional or alternative ways for the child to say how they are feeling and to say their goodbyes to their family member should be available.[4]

> Following Jenica's death, her family are packing and preparing to return home. During this time, Nicholas is busy drawing a picture. When the drawing is complete, Nicholas folds the paper many times and asks if he can place it in the memory box. The memory box contains a snip of Jenica's hair, footprints, and other mementos collected by her family. As Nicholas places his drawing into the memory box, he says aloud, 'I'll always remember my baby sister'.

Question 13. What can be done to support Nicholas as he grows?

Children like Nicholas, who experience the death of a brother, sister, parent, or other important person in their lives, will have new ways of feeling about the death as they grow. Reflections on what life might have been like if Jenica had continued to be his living sister may become a focus as Nicholas matures and has some of his own important lifetime milestones, such as graduating from high school.

Nicholas's comprehension of death will develop as he matures, and so he may need different and rather more sophisticated details to better match his continuing and enhanced capacity for understanding. He may have more elaborate questions about her illness which should be raised proactively, in pace with his increased understanding.

Nicholas may benefit from stories of his relationship with Jenica, including being shown pictures of them together and other ways that reinforce the message of their mutual affection and importance in one another's lives.

A young patient's story: talking with the child as patient

A frequent feature of paediatric palliative care is the need to integrate the principles of palliative care with measures that may be focused on curing or ameliorating the illness, so that both approaches can coexist in order to best support the child and family. Jennifer's story serves as an example reflecting such a concurrent approach to care.

> Jennifer is a 13-year-old with advanced cystic fibrosis, ineligible for a lung transplant at the time of her admission. She is admitted for a severe exacerbation managed with parenteral and aerosolized antibiotics, aggressive chest physiotherapy, and supplemental oxygen and nutrition. Breathlessness is her most prominent symptom. The paediatric palliative care service is asked to see Jennifer to discuss some anxieties that she has expressed about her illness. For the first part of the conversation, Jennifer (J) clarifies the source of the worry with the physician (P).
>
> J: I'm not worried… It's everybody else that's worried.
>
> P: What do you think everybody else might be worried about?
>
> J: They're all worried because they think I'm going to die.
>
> P: Oh! They all think that you're going to die. What do you think about that?
>
> J: I'm too young to die. I want to live long enough to do more stuff. I want to live long enough to become a marine biologist. I want to live long enough to have my own children. I want to live long enough to do some bad stuff. I'm only 13 and I haven't done any really bad stuff yet.

It should be noted that the recent decades have been positive for many patients with cystic fibrosis, who are living well into adulthood, with the expected survival based on the extent of their lung disease.

> P: I really hope that you get to live long enough to do all those things. I know that everyone here is working really hard on getting you better and getting you through this. I wonder, though, **just in case**, if it is not possible, if you have any worries about that.
>
> J: I'm not worried about dying. I know I won't have any pain, or anything.

The remainder of the conversation continues with Jennifer mentioning a wish for her short-term goal of holding and feeding an infant. This is arranged for the next day and Jennifer holds the baby while a staff member takes pictures for her family.

Over the next few days, Jennifer, her parents, and her sister share intimate thoughts and important moments together, led by the shared theme of 'getting better ... but **just in case**, I want you to know ...'). This occurs at a time when Jennifer is able to express her concerns and wishes relating to end-of-life while continuing to maintain hope. Jennifer and her parents, with the support of a spiritual care clinician, also discuss Jennifer's expressed concerns about whether she would see her parents in heaven.

Jennifer becomes unresponsive within several days and dies within a week of her initial conversation about possibly not being able to recover.

(Modified with permission from Y. McConnell and G. Frager G. Decision-making in paediatric palliative care module. The Ian Anderson Continuing Education Program in End-of-Life Care. A Joint Project of Continuing Education and the Joint Centre for Bioethics, University of Toronto and The Temmy Latner Centre for Palliative Care, Mount Sinai Hospital, www.cme.utoronto.ca/endoflife)

Question 14. How might you address Jennifer's worries without causing her additional distress? Do you believe that discussing the possibility of not getting better can steal away hope from the hopeful?

Reflective Question. Have you been part of a similar conversation about 'hoping for the best but preparing for the worst'? Of what potential benefit is it to address such concerns?

Patients who have been living with a chronic illness for some time, as well as their families, have thought about these issues and may have talked about them amongst themselves. In such instances, early mention of palliative care treatment options can reduce the fear associated with such discussions, allow plenty of time for thought, plant the seeds for later discussions and decisions without eroding hope, and enable decisions to be made over time.[7–9] The myth that the introduction of such topics can remove a patient's or family's hope for cure or improvement is unfounded. Discussing probable death with parents who have not yet recognized that there is no realistic chance for cure does not usually reduce the parents' capacity for hope.

Earlier recognition by physicians and parents of the probability of a child's death has been associated with earlier integration of palliative care interventions and improved quality of life for children during the palliative phase.[9] Such discussions provide opportunities to reassure the child about their concerns, that they will not be abandoned, and that they will be remembered, a concern expressed by critically ill children. Difficult discussions early on, by building on trust and rapport, can facilitate subsequent discussions and decisions at a time when the accompanying distress may preclude thoughtful planning.[10,11] The talking may help the greatest worries to become smaller by discussing them. A large Swedish study examined the subsequent impact on bereaved parents who had discussions about death with their children. No parent regretted having had these discussions. Only those parents who had not discussed death with their children expressed regret. This was noted at a greater frequency when parents sensed that their child had awareness of the extent of their illness.[12]

Knowing the child's and family's expressed wishes, enables the team to provide care congruent with their wishes.[7] The creation of memories and mementos, which will be important later in the lives of the survivors, can be supported throughout this time.

Pain and symptoms highlights

Attitude

To enable each student to:

- Learn that a child's pain or other symptoms can be measured.
- Learn how to include risk–benefit considerations in your overall approach to care.

Skill

To enable each student to:

- Learn how to help to reassure the child and family about a difficult symptom, such as breathlessness.

Knowledge

To enable each student to:

- Understand the common and unique aspects of pain and symptom management in the palliative care of children compared with adults.
- Learn that resources exist for this aspect of care and how to access them.
- Learn that non-pharmacological measures are available to help relieve breathlessness.

Pain and symptom assessment and management common to both children and adults

The intensity of the pain or symptom is best rated by self-report. Self-report scales, such as the basic numerical 0–10 scale used in adults, can be used in children who have the developmental capacity of 7–8-year-olds. Modified pain rating scales, using photographs or pictorial representations of children in varying degrees of apparent distress, have been well validated for younger children, such as in 3–4-year-olds or those not able to rate the intensity of their pain with the 0–10 numerical scale. An example of such a scale is the Faces Pain Scale–Revised (FPS–R).[13] (Fig. 23.3)

In introducing the scale, the clinician should use the same words as used by the child for pain, such as 'owie', 'hurt', or 'pain', and say 'These faces show how much something can hurt.

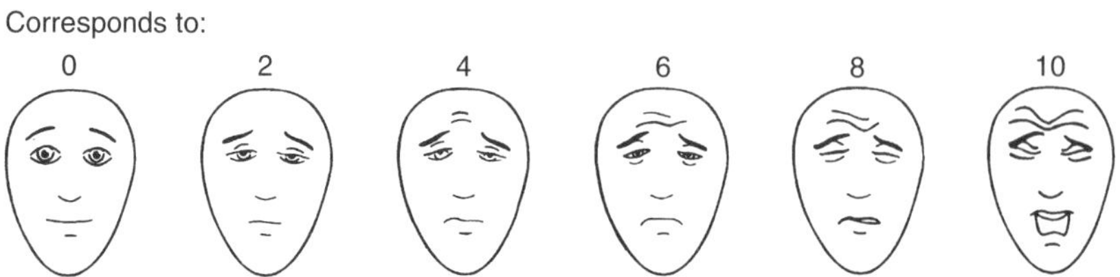

Fig. 23.3 Faces Pain Scale–Revised (FPS–R) (for administration instructions and details consult http://www.painsourcebook.ca). Reproduced with permission from C.L. Hicks *et al.* (2001) *Pain*, **93**, 173–83.

This face (point to furthest left face) shows **no pain**. The faces show more and more pain (point from left to right) up to this one (point to furthest right face)—it shows **very much pain**. Point to the face that shows me how much you hurt (right now).' Score the chosen face 0, 2, 4, 6, 8, or 10. Do not use words that reflect affect, like 'happy' or 'sad', as the scale reflects how children feel, not how their face may appear. It can be helpful to add, 'You don't have to look like any of the faces to feel the hurt or pain'.

The child may be more or less able to use the scales appropriate for their developmental level, as some children regress with illness whereas others appear more advanced.

When self-report cannot be determined, use behavioural observations. Impressions of the child's behaviour and apparent comfort/discomfort are ideally made by someone who knows the child. This should include the parent/family members and health professionals, such as nurses, who spend time with the child and are attuned for such observations.

Principles of management

The principles of management parallel those for adults. They include the following.

- Anticipate and prevent pain.
- Provide regular 'around-the-clock' medication.
- Use the oral route, if possible.
- Use an immediate release preparation for breakthrough pain.
- Titrate to pain relief.
- Anticipate and prevent adverse effects.
- Have an alternative analgesic plan if there are adverse effects.
- Add adjuvants to act as co-analgesics. (Adjuvants are medications with inherent analgesic effects generally used for a primary indication other than pain.)
- Begin a bowel regimen when starting opioids:
  - never limit opioids because of concern of constipation.
  - use a stool softener combined with a cathartic (i.e. docusate and senna extract).
  - re-assess regularly as constipation does not lessen over time and its absence ensures greater comfort.

Unique aspects of pain and symptom assessment and management in children

- Do not ignore, underestimate, or undertreat pain in children, as is the tendency.
- Children in pain may present with non-specific symptoms (e.g. be irritable, withdraw, be less communicative).
- Tailor pain measurements according to the according to the child's development.
- The child's medical condition can affect pain assessment.[14] For example, a non-verbal child with severe cerebral palsy may at times have facial grimacing and increased tone unrelated to discomfort/pain.
- Compared with adults:

  children are less likely to express specifics about their discomfort, including pain, nausea, itching, and bowel/bladder dysfunction among other sources of distress the intravenous route is used more commonly than the subcutaneous route, as there is often established central/peripheral venous access.

opioid rotation is used more commonly:

children with significant pain problems are often on many concurrent medications, and the side effects may be managed by changing opioid rather than adding an adjuvant to counteract them.

- A child may lack the understanding of the cause–effect relationship; for example, a child with opioid-related pruritus will be less likely than an adult to continue with the analgesic even when experiencing pain relief.

Pharmacokinetics/pharmacodynamics

- Start with milligram per kilogram dosing.
- When treating non-ventilated infants, the initial dose is generally reduced to approximately one-third of the 'usual' milligram per kilogram starting dose in infants and then titrated to effect. (Infants may be at increased risk toropioid toxicity because of the factors of increased surface area, fat-to-muscle ratio, decreased glycoproteins, and renal/hepatic clearance capacities.[15])
- Many medications have not been formally studied in paediatric populations, and hence children could be considered pharmacological orphans. Thus many medications are being used according to rough extrapolations from adult studies.

Fears and facts

- Since someone other than the child provides access to medication, it is critical to address misperceptions that might limit the child's access to pain relief. Ensure that misperceptions and worries are addressed.
- Compared with adults:

  children are **not** at increased risk for adverse effects (e.g. respiratory depression) (refer to pharmacokinetics/pharmacodynamics text above with respect to infants)

  children are **not** at increased risk for addiction.
- Pain medications (even large doses) **will not** generally impair the child's ability to interact, play, and be themselves—**uncontrolled pain will.**

Mitchell: a story of ensuring comfort

Figure 23.4 shows 11-year-old Mitchell with his father on a motorcycle. Mitchell had a malignant brain tumour, an astrocytoma. His symptoms were seizures, intermittent and severe nausea, vomiting, and headache.

Question 1. How common is pain in children with cancer compared with adults?

Pain is common in children with advanced cancer. Procedures and treatment-related interventions are the greatest contribution to cancer pain in children rather than the predominance of disease-related pain, typically seen in adults. This pattern, documented over a decade ago, persists despite interim improvements in procedural and treatment-related pain management.[16,17]

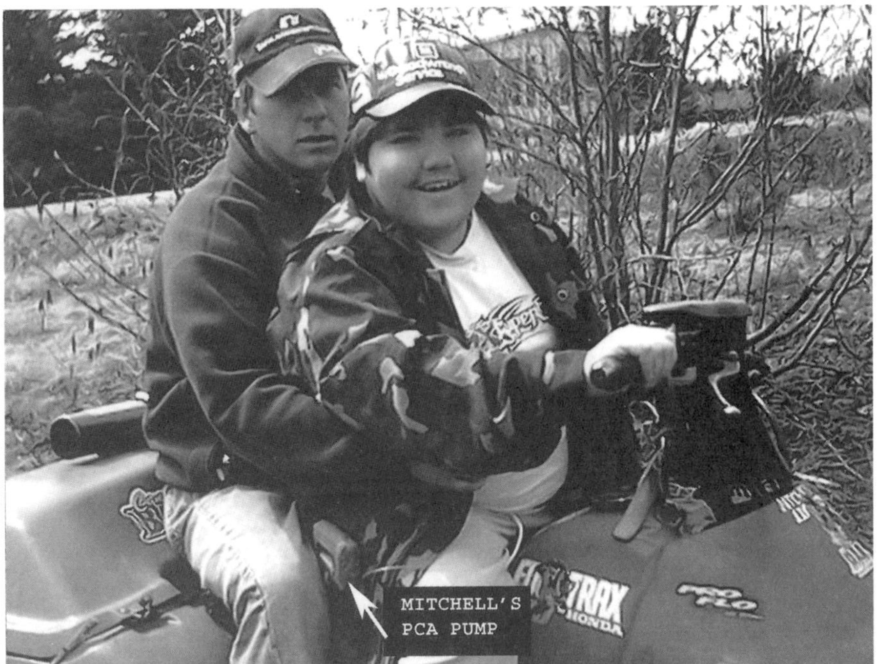

Fig. 23.4 Mitchell and his father.

Mitchell's symptoms were managed with a parenteral infusion of morphine and dexamethasone (6.6 times the potency of prednisone/prednisolone), antiemetics, and anticonvulsants. Mitchell was able to self-administer additional doses for breakthrough pain in addition to a continuous background opioid infusion delivered via a patient-controlled analgesia (PCA) pump.

Mitchell lived for 10 days after this picture was taken, having continued with his analgesic, antiemetic, and anticonvulsant regimen along with the addition of a benzodiazepine.

Question 2. Is Mitchell's activity and function what you might expect for a child at their end-of-life? Is it common for pain in children living with and dying from advanced cancer to be relieved with 'standard' or 'conservative' opioid therapy?

Most children want to continue with their activities at the end-of-life as they have through their life. Pharmacological and non-pharmacological therapies assist in this goal.

Despite the prevalence of pain and the concern engendered by the possibility of pain in children with advanced cancer, much as in the adult population, the profoundly important goal of pain relief is attainable. In fact, patients and families can be reassured that pain relief with preservation and enhancement of the child's quality of life is a reasonable expectation for the vast majority of children with advanced cancer, even at the end-of-life. It is the exception to require what would be considered 'extraordinary' opioid doses or to give opioids in unusual ways, such as via the subarachnoid route or to provide sedation for comfort.[18]

Occasionally, titration to 'extraordinarily' high doses or unusual routes of opioid adminstration may be required. There is 'no maximum' opioid dose for the agents used for moderate to severe pain, such as morphine, hydromorphone, or fentanyl. Even children requiring gradual titration to several grams of parenteral morphine equivalents per kilogram can have preservation of cognitive and haemodynamic function. Infrequently, sedation with the attendant compromise of cognition may be required to ensure comfort.

PCA can be used by developmentally appropriate 6 year-olds. Even younger children can use such a device, provided that they understand the cause and effect concept of relieving their intermittent pain by pushing the 'button'.

A checklist for analgesic therapy in children

- Aim for pain relief with the lowest effective dose
- Anticipate, prevent, and actively treat side effects
- Use around-the-clock (ATC) dosing
- Use non-noxious routes for analgesic administration:
  - Use oral administration, if possible
  - Check the equianalgesic when changing routes; the oral route is less bio-available and will always be a higher dose (Table 23.3)
  - Ensure that the preparation is acceptable to the child (palatability, dosing frequency, etc.)
  - **No** intramuscular injections
  - Avoid rectal administration
  - **Do not** use transdermal fentanyl in the opioid-naive child or in unstable pain
  - If the child already has a central line, use it rather than subcutaneous administration
  - If using subcutaneous access, use a small gauge needle (25G–27G)
  - Use topical anesthetics before inserting a subcutaneous or Port-a-Cath needle
- Use an analgesic that matches the pain intensity
  - Acetaminophen for mild pain (thrombocytopenia precludes the use of non-steroidal anti-inflammatory drugs)

Table 23.3 Opioid table

Drug	IV/SC starting dose		Ratio of IV/SC to oral dose	Oral starting dose	
	<50 kg	>50 kg		<50 kg (mg/kg)	>50 kg (mg)
Morphine	0.05–0.1 mg/kg every 4 h	2.5–5 mg every 4 h	1:3	0.15–0.3 mg/kg every 4 h	5–10 mg every 4 h
Codeine	0.5 mg/kg SC every 4 h ***Do not give IV***	15–60 mg SC every 4 h	1:1.5	0.5–1 mg/kg every 4 h	30–60 mg every 4 h
Hydromorphone	0.015 mg/kg every 4 h	1–2 mg every 4 h	1:3–1:5	0.06 mg/kg every 4 h	1–2 mg every 4 h
Oxycodone	SC/IV preparation not available			0.2 mg/kg every 4 h	5–10 mg every 4 h

Meperidine is ***not recommended*** for chronic or increasing pain.

  - Codeine for mild-to-moderate pain
  - Morphine/hydromorphone/diamorphine for moderate to severe pain
  - **Do not** use meperidine for pain that lasts more than a couple of days (meperidine has a toxic metabolite that causes significant adverse effects)
  - **Do not** use mixed agonist–antagonists preparations for moderate to severe pain and increasing opioid requirement
- Check if known differences in pharmacokinetics compared with adults
  - For children <50 kg: use a dose based on a milligram per kilogram calculation (Table 23.3)
  - For children >50 kg: start with the 'usual' adult starting dose (Table 23.3)
  - For infants <6 months: use a third to a quarter of the usual starting dose and titrate to relief
  - There is no 'maximum' for the opioids used for moderate to severe pain
- Start with an immediate release preparation to determine opioid requirements
- Change to a sustained release preparation once opioid requirements are determined
- Always provide a breakthrough opioid dose
  - Use their ATC opioid in the immediate release form
  - At a usual dose equal to 10% of their daily opioid requirement
  - Provide at a frequency related to peak onset of action (every 30 min–1 h)
  - If more than four breakthrough doses in 24 h—increase ATC dose
- Always start a bowel regimen (softener and cathartic) when starting opioids
  - Re-assess, adjust, and continue bowel regimen with opioid use
- Use adjuvants as co-analgesics
  - Pharmacological, e.g. gabapentin, steroids, amitriptyline, low-dose ketamine (refer to the detailed resources listed at the end of the chapter)
  - None contraindicated but exercise caution with neuroleptics (possible dystonia)
  - Physical: massage, transcutaneous electrical nerve stimulation (TENS)
  - Cognitive: distraction, hypnotherapy, guided imagery
- Reassure the child and family about options; try alternative opioid if there are adverse effects
- Proactively and repeatedly address misperceptions and concerns; the child is reliant on another's confidence and comfort for their medications.

Breathlessness: a difficult and distressing symptom

Breathlessness is a significantly distressing and frequent symptom in the oncological population. Breathlessness assumes greater prominence than pain in children living with and dying from a myriad of illnesses including multiple neurodegenerative illnesses, cystic fibrosis, muscular dystrophy, spinal muscular atrophy, cerebral palsy and intercurrent infections, complex congenital heart disease, and the metabolic storage diseases such as the mucopolysaccharidoses. Children with such diverse and unusual illnesses represent the demographics of serious illness and death in childhood.

Jennifer is the 13 year old with advanced cystic fibrosis we met earlier in this chapter. While hoping for improvement and directing treatments to resolve Jennifer's current exacerbation, her accompanying breathlessness and anxiety are concurrently addressed.

Question 1. How do you measure the intensity of breathlessness?

Breathlessness or dyspnoea is a subjective phenomenon. Like pain, its intensity is based on how it is reported by the person who is experiencing it.

Intensity is measured by self-report, if possible, with a lack of reliance on physical parameters. The tool used should be appropriate for the child's developmental level. Tools used in the adult population are frequently in language that is not applicable to a younger child's activities or level of understanding.[19]

The child could be asked:

- 'Are you a little or a lot breathless?' as with a categorical scale
- 'Can you show me how breathless you feel?' (with the aid of a visual analogue scale)
- 'What can you do or not do because your breathing is bothering you?'
- To use a newly tested visual analogue scale for dyspnoea in children.[20]

Jennifer rates her breathlessness as 6/10. She is working harder at breathing and appears anxious, both these observations are worse with minimal exertion. Although the best measure of someone's breathlessness is to hear it from them, when this is not possible, behavioural observations, as for pain, are the default assessment.

Question 2. Is there anything that you would like to check in the way of investigations?

Ensure that Jennifer is provided with measures directed to symptomatic relief whether or not you pursue investigations.

It is important to pursue diagnostic tests or interventions always considering the relative burden and benefit in the context of goals of care. You may feel a complete blood count, chest radiograph and/or other investigation is warranted.[7,21] In addition to directing your interventions to relieving a child's breathlessness, sometimes having additional information may be useful for symptomatic relief by treating the cause of the breathlessness. For example, a chest radiograph may guide you in treating pneumonia or a pleural effusion, and a complete blood count may indicate significant anaemia for which you may consider a transfusion

Some investigations may not be warranted or appropriate. An example in the majority of situations of breathlessness at end-of-life would be a nasopharyngeal aspirate to test for respiratory syncitial virus. This is a distressing test and is not linked with any therapeutic intervention for the majority of children with this context of breathlessness.

Question 3. If the chest radiograph had shown a pneumothorax, what would you suggest doing about it?

It is reasonable to consider a chest tube, taking into account the likelihood and degree of relief, how distressing it may be for Jennifer, whether there are any significant risks, and what might be a rough estimate of her expected survival.

Question 4. What do you recommend for monitoring Jennifer's oxygen saturation or blood gases?

Monitoring should be based on goals of care. During end-of-life care, monitoring may contribute to the anxiety of the patient and family. When, the usual interventions in response to the 'numbers' and clinical state are not being pursued (e.g. the child will not be ventilated in the setting of progressive respiratory compromise), monitoring is not indicated and may actually be a burden to the child and family. It may also depend on the orientation of the child and family to such monitoring; they may view this as part of 'care' and 'caring'. This is often seen in the patient population living and dying with cystic fibrosis, where the monitoring of oxygen saturation and other parameters is viewed as continuity of care.[22] Anything else may be perceived as abandonment.

It also depends on how distressing or invasive the monitoring may be to the child and family. Blood gas monitoring involves some physical discomfort, whereas oxygen saturation monitoring does not. The approach needs to be considered in light of the goals of care and the wishes of the child and family.[7,21]

Question 5. What is your recommendation about providing supplemental oxygen in end-of-life care?

Supplemental oxygen should be administered according to the comfort of the child and not based on or influenced by the degree of oxygen saturation. The options for supplemental oxygen administration are none, a facemask, nasal prongs, or blow-by, where supplemental oxygen is directed towards but not over the child's face, all according to the child's expressed preferences or apparent comfort when a verbal response is not possible.

Question 6. Describe other non-pharmacological measures to help decrease the sensation of breathlessness.

Non-pharmacological interventions can include physical measures, such as a cold facecloth, air to face by fan, a favourite scent in the room or positioning.

Children will assume a position of comfort if they are able to move into such a position. There are times when it will not be feasible for the child to find his or her own position of comfort because of developmental limitations, such as an infant who is unable to sit up or a child with a neuromuscular condition (e.g. spinal muscular atrophy) who cannot shift position or clear their secretions. In these instances, it is helpful to change the child's position and observe apparent changes in comfort.

Question 7. Describe some pharmacological measures to help decrease the sensation of breathlessness.

Pharmacological measures to reduce the sensation of breathlessness include systemic opioid therapy[23] and a benzodiazepine as an anxiolytic (breathlessness is very anxiety provoking).[24] Occasionally, sedation may be required for symptom relief, even if this further compromises the child's respiratory or cognitive function.[25]

Details relating to opioid dosing, routes, titration, and other aspects of pain and symptom management in the context of paediatric palliative care can be found in the publications cited in the bibliography at the end of the chapter.

Other medications may be given concurrently with those directed to symptomatic relief. These medications are directed to the cause of the breathlessness, such as diuretics in the setting of congestive heart failure, antibiotics for pneumonia, and steroids for disseminated pulmonary leukaemic infiltrates.

The family, friends, and staff attending the child should be informed that the pharmacological measures may not change the pattern of the child's breathing. The child may continue to have nasal flaring, tracheal tug, or noisy inspiration/expiration, but the medications help the child to not mind the sensation of breathlessness.

When the child is unresponsive, the noisy breathing associated with increased secretions can be distressing to those attending him or her. First, acknowledge that the sound is distressing to hear but reassure them, often repeatedly, that this is in no way bothersome to the child. The addition of an anticholinergic agent, such as glycopyrrolate, hyoscine, or scopolamine can help reduce the accumulation of secretions and therefore the sound. These medications should be initiated at the first sign indicating retained secretions, as they do virtually nothing to clear the large airway secretions that are already present. Staff can model continuing to talk to the unresponsive child, allowing opportunities for friends and family to say what they want to say, and continue to support the child and themselves through talking and touching.

Despite the immense tragedy of a child's death, clinicians can improve the way that the child and family feel throughout this time. Ensuring comfort at the end-of-life also provides the possibility of a durable comfort for the family, friends, and staff who carry these memories throughout their lives.

Acknowledgements

Grateful thanks are given to the families of Nicholas and Jenica Saulnier, and to Jennifer Rozee and Mitchell Fraser who so generously allowed the pictures and stories of their children to be shared.

Resources

Websites

www.virtualhospice.ca

Canadian Virtual Hospice. An interactive network for people dealing with life-threatening illness and loss.

www.nap.edu/catalog/10390.html When Children Die: Improving Palliative and End-of-Life Care for Children and their Families Washington, DC: National Academies Press, 2003.

www.act.org.uk and www.CNPCC.ca

Policies, resources, links to other sites, and a place to connect with other health professionals for this specialized area of care.

www.dougy.org

The Dougy Center: a resource accessible by web, mail, telephone for materials relating to grief and bereavement in childhood. Tel: +1 503 775 5683; Fax: +1 503 777 3097.

www.growthhouse.org

Growth House: a clearing house for reviewed and rated resources relating to life-threatening illness, end-of-life care, and grief and bereavement.

www.ich.ucl.ac.uk

A joint initiative by Great Ormond Street Children's Hospital and the Institute of Child Health providing resources for children, families, and health professionals.

www.winstonswish.org.uk

Provides on-line and other practical resources including memory boxes and printed material for supporting bereaved children and youth.

Sources/suppliers of books

Meditec, Jackson's Yard, Brewery Hill, Grantham, Lincs NG31 6DW Tel: +44 (0)476) 590505.

Book list and mail order resource relating to parental and child grief.

www.centering.org

The Centering Corporation: suppliers of a wide variety of books for the bereaved including children.

Videos

A Death in the Lives of Children National Child's Bureau. Huntington, UK: Childhood Bereavement Network, 2002.

What Do I Tell My Children? Aquarius Productions, 31 Martin Road, Wellesley, MA. Tel: +1 02181 617 237 0608.

Bibliography

For all ages—parent and child

Hanson, W. (1997) *The Next Place.* Minneapolis, MN: Waldman House Press.

For children aged 2–6 years (preschool)

Buscaglia, L. (1982) *The Fall of Freddie the Leaf.* Thorofare, NJ: Slack.

Dodge, N. (1984) *Thumpy's Story: A Story of Love and Grief Shared by Thumpy the Bunny.* St Charles, MO: Share Pregnancy and Infant Loss Support.

Mellonie, B., and Ingpen, R., (1993) *Lifetimes.* Limpsfield, UK: Paper Tiger/New York: Bantam Books.

For children aged 6–12 years (school-age)

Crossley, D. (2000) *Muddles, Puddles, and Sunshines.* Stroud, UK: Hawthorn Press (an activity book)

Krasny Brown, L., and Brown, M. (1996) *When Dinosaurs Die: A Guide to Understanding Death.* New York: Little, Brown.

Wolfelt, A.D. (2001) *Healing Your Grieving Heart for Kids.* Fort Collins, CO: Companion Press.

For adolescents

Byers Crawford, B., and Lazar, L. (1999) *In My World.* Omaha, NE: Centering Corporation (a workbook for an adolescent facing their own premature death).

Traisman, E.S. (1992) *Fire in my Heart, Ice in my Veins.* Omaha, NE: Centering Corporation (a workbook for adolescents experiencing a loss through another's death).

Wolfelt, A.D. (2001) *Healing Your Grieving Heart for Teens.* Fort Collins, CO: Companion Press.

For school

Bennett Blackburn, L. (1991) *The Class in Room 44: When a Classmate Dies.* Omaha, NE: Centering Corporation.

Smith, S.C., and Pennells, M. (1995) *Interventions with Bereaved Children.* London: Jessica Kingsley.

Sutherland Fox, S. (1988) *Good Grief: Helping Groups of Children When a Friend Dies.* Boston, MA: New England Association for the Education of Young Children.

For parents and health professionals (to help bereaved children and youth)

Hamilton, J. (2001) *When a Parent is Sick—Helping Parents Explain Serious Illness to Children.* Lawrencetown Beach, Nova Scotia: Pottersfield Press.

Nussbaum, K. (1998) *Preparing the Children: Information and Ideas for Families Facing Terminal Illness and Death.* Kochick, AK: Gifts of Hope.

Wolfelt, A.D. (2001) *Healing a Child's Grieving Heart. Healing a Teen's Grieving Heart.* Fort Collins, CO: Companion Press.

For health professionals

Adams, D., and Deveau, E. (eds) (1995) *Beyond the Innocence of Childhood.* Amityville, NY: Baywood.

Davies, B. (1999) *Shadows in the Sun: Experiences of Sibling Bereavement in Childhood.* Philadelphia, PA: Brunner–Mazel.

Sourkes, B.M. (1995) *Armfuls of Time: The Psychological Experience of the Child with a Life-Threatening Illness.* Pittsburgh, PA: University of Pittsburgh Press.

Stevens, M. (2004) Psychological adaptation of the dying child. In: Doyle D, Hanks GWC, Cherny N, Calman KC (eds) *Oxford Textbook of Palliative Medicine* (3rd edn). Oxford: Oxford University Press, 798–806.

General paediatric palliative care

Armstrong-Dailey, A., and Zarbock Goltzer, S. (1993) *Hospice Care for Children.* New York: Oxford University Press

Doyle, D., Hanks, G.W.C., Cherny, N., and Calman, K.C. (eds) (2004) *Oxford Textbook of Palliative Medicine* (4th edn). Oxford: Oxford University Press. (Several chapters are devoted to paediatric palliative care.)

Galloway, K.S., and Yaster, M. (2000) Pain and symptom control in terminally ill children. *Pediatr Clin North Am,* **47**, 711–46.

Goldman, A. (1999) *Care for the Dying Child.* New York: Oxford University Press.

Hilden, J., and Tobin, D. (2003) *Shelter from the Storm, Caring for a Child with a Life-Threatening Condition.* Cambridge, MA: Perseus.

Liben, S. (1998) Home care for children with life-threatening illness. *J Palliat Care,* **14**, 33–8.

Wolfe, J., and Grier, H.E. (2002) Care of the dying child. In: Pizzo P, Poplack D (eds) *Principles and Practice of Pediatric Oncology* (4th edn). Baltimore, MD: Lippincott–Williams and Wilkins, 1447–93.

World Health Organization (1998) *Cancer Pain Relief and Palliative Care in Children.* Geneva: World Health Organization. (Although cancer is the focus, principles are applicable to children with other conditions; available in several languages.)

References

1. **Bluebond-Langner, M.** (1978) *The Private Worlds of Dying Children.* Princeton, NJ: Princeton University Press.
2. **Pettle, S., and Lansdown, R.** (1988) The psychological care of children with malignant disease. *J Child Psychol Psychiatry,* **29**, 556–67.
3. **Sourkes, B.M.** (1995) *Armfuls of Time: The Psychological Experience of the Child with a Life-Threatening Illness.* Pittsburgh, PA: University of Pittsburgh Press.
4. **Widger, K.A., MacDonald, V.E., and Frager, G.** (2004) Death of a child. In: Jones R, Britten N, Culpepper L, ***et al*** (eds) *Oxford Textbook of Primary Medical Care,* Vol. 2. Oxford: Oxford University Press, in press.
5. **Davies, B.** (1987) Family responses to the death of a child: The meaning of memories. *J Palliat Care* **3**, 9–15.
6. **Lauer, M.E., Mulhern, R.K., Bohne, J.B., and Camitta, B.M.** (1985) Children's perceptions of their siblings' death at home or hospital. The precursors of differential adjustment. *Cancer Nurs,* **6**, 21–7.
7. **McConnell, Y., and Frager, G.** *Decision-Making in Pediatric Palliative Care Module.* The Ian Anderson Continuing Education Program in End-of-Life Care. A Joint Project of Continuing Education and the Joint Centre for Bioethics, University of Toronto and The Temmy Latner Centre for Palliative Care, Mount Sinai Hospital, www.cme.utoronto.ca/endoflife.
8. **James, L., and Johnson, B.** (1997) The needs of parents of pediatric oncology patients during the palliative care phase. *J Pediatr Oncol* **14**, 83–95.
9. **Wolfe, J., Klar, N., and Grier, H.E., *et al.*** (2000) Understanding of prognosis among parents of children who died of cancer: impact on treatment goals and integration of palliative care. *JAMA,* **284**, 2469–75.
10. **Bartel, D.A., Engler, A.J., Natale, J.E., Misra, V., Lewin, A.B., and Joseph, J.G.** (2000) Working with families of suddenly and critically ill children: physician experiences. *Arch Pediatr Adolesc Med,* **154**, 1127–33.
11. **Hinds, P.S., Oakes, L., and Furman, W.** (2001) End-of-life decision making in pediatric oncology. In: Ferrell BR, Coyle N (eds) *Textbook of Palliative Nursing.* Oxford: Oxford University Press, 450–60.
12. **Kreicbergs, U., Valdimarsdottir, U., Onelov, E., Henter, J.I, and Steineck, G.** (2004) Talking about death with children who have severe malignant disease. *N Engl J Med,* **351**, 1175–86.
13. **Hicks, C.L., von Baeyer, C.L., Spafford, P., van Korlaar, I., and Goodenough, B.**(2001) The Faces Pain Scale—Revised: toward a common metric in pediatric pain measurement. *Pain,* **93**,173–83.
14. **Hunt, A.M., and Burne, R.** (1995) Medical and nursing problems of children with neurodegenerative disease. *Palliat Med,* **9**, 19–26.
15. **Yaster, M.** (2003) Clinical Pharmacology. In: Schechter NL, Berde CB, Yaster M (eds) *Pain in Infants, Children, and Adolescents.* Philadelphia, PA: Lippincott Williams & Wilkins, 71–84.
16. **McGrath, P.J., Hsu, E., Capelli, M., Luke, B., Goodman, J.T., and Dunn-Geir, J.** (1990) Pain from paediatric cancer: A survey of an outpatient oncology clinic. *J Psychosoc Oncol,* **8**, 109–24.
17. **Ljungman, G., Gordh, T., Sorensen, S., and Kreuger, A.** (2000) Pain variations during cancer treatment in children: a descriptive survey. *Pediatr Hematol Oncol,* **17**, 211–21.
18. **Collins, J., Grier, H., Kinney, H., and Berde, C.B.** (1995) Control of severe pain in children with terminal malignancy. *J Pediatr,* **126**, 653–7.
19. **Franck, L.S., Greenberg, C.S., and Stevens, B.** (2000) Pain assessment in infants and children. *Pediatr Clin North Am,* **47**, 487–512.
20. **Pianosi, P., Smith, C.P., and McGrath, P.** (1998) Pictorial scales for the measurement of dyspnea in children. *Am J Respir Crit Care Med,* **157**(Suppl), A782.
21. **Frager, G.** (1999) Pediatric palliative care. In: Joishy SK (ed) *Palliative Medicine Secrets.* Philadelphia, PA: Hanley and Belfus, 157–73.

22. **Robinson, W.M., Ravilly, S., Berde, C., and Wohl, M.E.** (1997) End-of-life care in cystic fibrosis. *Pediatrics,* **100**, 205–9.
23. **Jennings, A.L., Davies, A.N., Higgins, J.P., Gibbs, J.S., and Broadley, K.E.** (2002) A systematic review of the use of opioids in the management of dyspnoea. *Thorax,* **57**, 939–44.
24. **Zeppetella, G.** (1998) The palliation of dyspnea in terminal disease. *Am J Hosp Palliat Care,* **15**, 322–30.
25. **Kenny, N.P., and Frager, G.** (1996) Refractory symptoms and terminal sedation of children: ethical issues and practical management. *J Palliat Care,* **12**, 40–5.

Chapter 24

Cognitive impairment

Peter G. Lawlor, Bruno Gagnon, and Wilma Falconer

Attitude

To enable the student to:

- Recognize that cognitive impairment is a component of both delirium and dementia.
- Appreciate the potential distress of delirium and its accompanying behavioural manifestations for the patient, family, and health care personnel.
- Be aware that cognitive impairment is frequently missed or misdiagnosed, and therefore appreciate the importance of objectively assessing cognition.
- Appreciate the educational and supportive needs of a delirious patient's family.
- Recognize that cognitive impairment is reversible in many episodes of delirium and therefore avoid an unduly nihilistic approach to investigation and management.
- Appreciate that cognitive impairment, as part of delirium, is a normal accompaniment of the last hours or days of life for most patients receiving palliative care.
- Appreciate the challenges in assessing other symptoms in the context of cognitive impairment.
- Recognize the importance of regular assessment and early diagnosis in situations where delirium is commonly encountered.

Skill

To enable the student to:

- Differentiate delirium from dementia and depression.
- Determine the reversibility of cognitive impairment based on the assessment and recognition of precipitants that are superimposed on pre-delirious vulnerability or risk profile.
- Recognize issues relating to the perception and response of family members to a patient with delirium.
- Develop skills in adopting an ethical perspective on the level of assessment and intervention, and therefore formulate a management approach that recognizes the goals of care.

Knowledge

To enable the student to:

- Be aware of the core diagnostic criteria and the other clinical features of delirium.
- Outline the epidemiology of cognitive impairment in end of life care.

- Recognize the multifactorial aetiology of delirium.
- Understand the pathophysiology and pathogenesis of delirium, and therefore know the rationale for pharmacological agents used in treatment.
- Appreciate the potential ethical dilemmas associated with total sedation.

You are called to the emergency room to assess Mr B.K., a 75-year-old man with a 5-year history of prostate cancer. He is known to have extensive metastatic bone disease, which is hormone refractory. He received palliative radiation therapy to painful lumbar metastases three months previously. At that time a chest radiograph showed three metastatic nodules in his right lung, and a CT scan showed a single metastatic deposit in his right hepatic lobe and extensive intrabdominal nodal disease. He was mobile with the aid of a walking frame at the time of completing his radiation therapy. Two weeks ago his family physician diagnosed a herpes zoster infection in the right T4 dermatomal distribution. He was initially treated with famciclovir for one week. In the last week he was started on amitriptyline for a burning pain in the same distribution. He has also been receiving escalating doses of oral morphine for relief of this pain. He complains of nausea and has vomited once or twice daily for the past 2 days. His last bowel movement was 1 week ago.

His wife has been giving him night sedation with lorazepam for the past week. However, he continues to have poor sleep. He gets some sleep during the day but he is restless at night, disoriented, calling out, trying to get out of bed, and having occasional episodes of urinary incontinence. He has been suspicious of his wife, thinking that she was trying to poison him when she was giving him his medication. His wife and family are fearful that he is either 'losing his mind or going senile', or that he is 'deeply depressed'. They are worried that he is very close to death. His youngest son has just made a 7-h flight to be with him. He is angry about the level of care as he perceives the major problem to be one of poor pain control.

Question 1. How common is cognitive impairment in patients like Mr B.K. with advanced cancer?

Cognitive impairment can present as part of either a delirium or dementia, or as part of a delirium superimposed on dementia. Occasionally, mild cognitive dysfunction can occur as part of a depression (depressive pseudodementia). Other psychotic disorders might also be considered but they are commonly associated with a prior history of similar episodes. The diagnosis of delirium superimposed on dementia is often only made when some of the features of delirium subside with treatment of underlying precipitating causes, revealing an underlying dementia. This chapter will focus predominantly on cognitive impairment as part of a delirium.

Cognitive impairment has been documented in 42–44 per cent of patients on admission to palliative care units.[1,2] The presence of cognitive impairment, as part of a delirium, has been detected in 40 per cent of advanced cancer patients on admission to a palliative care unit.[3] Cognitive impairment has been identified in hours to days before death in the vast majority of patients with advanced cancer.[4,5]

Question 2. What are the core criteria for a diagnosis of delirium? What are the additional associated clinical features?

The major DSM-IV criteria to make a diagnosis of delirium due to a general medical condition are summarized in Table 24.1.[6] In the case of delirium due to an exogenous substance

Table 24.1 DSM-IV diagnostic criteria for delirium due to a medical condition

A: Disturbance of consciousness (i.e. reduced clarity of awareness of the environment) with reduced ability to focus, sustain, or shift attention
B: A change in cognition (such as memory deficit, disorientation, language disturbance) or the development of a perceptual disturbance that is not better accounted for by a pre-existing, established, or evolving dementia
C: The disturbance develops over a short period of time (usually hours to days) and tends to fluctuate during the day
D: There is evidence from the history, physical examination, or laboratory findings that the disturbance is caused by the direct physiological consequences of a general medical condition

Reprinted with permission from the *Diagnostic and Statistical Manual of Mental Disorders* (4th edn). Arlington, VA: American Psychiatric Association.

(e.g. a psychoactive drug such as a tricyclic antidepressant), substance withdrawal (e.g. alcohol withdrawal), unknown or multiple aetiologies, the criteria A, B, and C are similar to the corresponding criteria for a general medical condition.

Other associated clinical features include disturbance of the sleep–wake cycle, delusional thinking, emotional lability, and altered psychomotor activity. Subtypes of delirium are classified according to the type of alteration in psychomotor activity, namely hyperactive, hypoactive, or a mixed form with both hyper- and hypoactive features. Although the clinical features of common underlying causes should be sought and identified, the presence of delirium may sometimes be the sole clinical manifestation of a major life-threatening problem such as sepsis.

A prodromal period, often with single symptoms of mild intensity such as temporal disorientation, may sometimes precede the onset of a full-blown delirium by a few days.[6]

Question 3. Why might delirium be either missed or misdiagnosed? What are the consequences of missing the diagnosis or misdiagnosing the syndrome in the case of Mr B.K.?

Failure to recognize delirium or misdiagnosis occurs commonly.[7–9] Ambiguous terms used to describe symptoms of delirium, such as pseudosenility, confusional state, or terminal restlessness, can contribute to some physician 'confusion' and possibly discourage further investigation. Other reasons cited for its under-recognition include failure to conduct an objective test of cognition, fluctuation in the intensity of delirious symptoms (e.g. the occurrence of a lucid interval), and the presence of the hypoactive subtype. The hypoactive delirious patient is often quiet and withdrawn, and therefore behaves as a 'good' patient, in contrast with the agitated hyperactive patient, whose behaviour is more likely to attract attention and possibly thereby prompt recognition of delirium. Delirium superimposed on dementia is arguably more difficult to diagnose.

Delirium most commonly tends to be misdiagnosed as depression or dementia. Cognitive impairment, perceptual disturbances, and psychomotor abnormalities occur in both dementia and delirium. In the case of the hypoactive or emotionally labile patient, depression is often erroneously diagnosed.

Missing the diagnosis in Mr B.K.'s case could result in his death, especially if potentially reversible underlying causes of delirium were not sought and identified. Dementia is rarely reversible, whereas delirium has been reported as being reversible in approximately 50 per cent of episodes in patients with advanced cancer.[3] Misdiagnosing Mr B.K.'s delirium as depression and commencing an antidepressant could have led to worsening of his delirium.

Question 4. How might your history-taking and physical assessment help to clarify the diagnosis?

A collateral history from Mr B.K.'s wife would be essential to establish the fluctuating nature of Mr B.K.'s mental status and the temporal onset of his cognitive decline. Dementia is characterized by an insidious onset over months to years, whereas delirium has an onset over hours to days. Fluctuation in the clinical presentation of symptoms, especially awareness, is much more likely to occur in delirium than dementia. Your interaction with Mr B.K. and a formal cognitive assessment should identify the attentional deficit, which is typically characteristic of delirium as opposed to dementia. Delusions in patients with delirium tend to be loosely held (i.e. not always present), whereas psychoses such as schizophrenia are characterized by more firmly held delusions. One might ask about the presence of opioid-induced neurotoxicity features such as 'jerky movements' or myoclonus, tactile hallucinations, hyperalgesia, or allodynia (pain associated with touch).[10]

Physical examination should be comprehensive in an effort to identify underlying causes of delirium, such as dehydration and infection, and neurological signs such as cranial nerve deficits associated with leptomeningeal disease. Unlike leptomeningeal metastases, metastatic disease of the brain parenchyma very rarely occurs in prostate cancer. Abnormal movements such as asterixis (e.g. with hepatic encephalopathy) and myoclonus should be identified. Commonly, signs of bifrontal dysfunction such as the palmo-mental, snout, and grasp reflexes can be detected in diffuse encephalopathies.

Question 5. What tools are most appropriate to use in your initial and ongoing assessment of Mr B.K.?

A large number of instruments have been developed to assess delirium, each with varying strengths and weaknesses for use within the palliative setting.[11] Some of these instruments involve a large component of active patient participation and therefore are unduly burdensome in patients such as Mr B.K. The Mini-Mental State Examination (MMSE) and the Confusion Assessment Method (CAM) are two well-validated yet suitably brief instruments that have been widely used in the screening and diagnosis of delirium.[12,13] The MMSE is used to detect the cognitive impairment component of delirium, and norms are established for age and educational level.[14] The CAM is rated on the basis of physician or nurse interaction with the patient, and assesses the presence or absence of four criteria:

- acute onset and fluctuating course
- inattention
- disorganized thinking
- altered level of consciousness.

The CAM algorithm for diagnosis of delirium requires the presence of both the first and the second criteria and either the third or the fourth criterion. Tools such as the Confusion Rating Scale (entirely observational and nurse rated) or the Memorial Delirium Assessment Scale (partly observational and physician rated) capture the behavioural changes of delirium and could be used to monitor the severity of delirium. The MMSE does not capture behavioural disturbance, and this renders it less useful in monitoring the severity of delirium.

A collateral history from Mr B.K.'s wife suggests that the cognitive deficit and behavioural disturbance began a week ago. It has fluctuated over the course of the day with some periods of relative lucidity on some mornings. He has no past history of any psychiatric disorder. Mr B.K. was able to give a history of tactile and visual hallucinations. Mr B.K.'s MMSE score was 16/30 (the expected low norm for age and grade 8 educational level is 23). His CAM assessment was positive for the first three criteria, and therefore you make a diagnosis of delirium. The relevant positive findings on physical examination are signs of dehydration, moderate cachexia, multifocal myoclonus, and mild pedal oedema. Mr B.K. is mildly agitated and intermittently tearful.

Question 6. What impact does the diagnosis of delirium have for Mr B.K., his family, and you or other health care professionals?

The wide spectrum of thought and behavioural disturbance involving hallucinations and delusions with a background of disorientation means that this is a highly distressing experience for Mr B.K. His intermittent urinary incontinence is also related to his delirium. Despite many attempts at climbing out of bed, he has not sustained any falls or injuries. The presence of delirium has rendered Mr B.K. mentally incompetent in relation to conducting his financial affairs and participating in the therapeutic decision-making process. For both Mr B.K. and his family, delirium impedes meaningful communication at a very critical time. This is particularly distressing for his son, who has made a long journey to be with his father and finds that he now cannot discuss many issues with him like he used to. The perception of his father in unrelieved pain and the son's consequent anger could potentially complicate bereavement. Furthermore, the memory of this image could have a negative impact if he or another family member were to encounter a terminal illness at a later date.

For the nursing staff and the other members of the health care team, the presence of delirium creates great difficulty in assessing pain and other symptoms. Delirious patients have been noted to receive a higher number of breakthrough doses of opioid analgesics in the evening and night, whereas non-delirious patients use more doses in the daytime.[15] This suggests that either restlessness associated with 'sundowning' could give rise to more movement-associated pain or the agitation could be misinterpreted as pain related. Conflict commonly arises in this situation among the patient, family, and staff concerning the level of analgesia and the need for opioid dose escalation. A common scenario that can emerge is when the patient's distress causes marked emotional distress in relatives, who advocate for an increase in opioid dose to reduce the patient's distress (and indirectly their own distress).[16] This could further fuel the problem if the opioid is already contributing to the delirium. It is possible that Mr B.K.'s son may vent some anger towards the health care team.

Question 7. What are the major aetiological factors associated with delirium in the palliative care setting? What are the risk factors and possible precipitants in Mr B.K.'s case?

The aetiology of delirium is generally multifactorial, invariably involving organic factors; environmental factors such as movement out of a familiar home setting can also potentially contribute to the process. The organic factors have been classified as primary cerebral disease, systemic disease affecting the brain secondarily, exogenous toxic agents such as medications or drugs of abuse, and withdrawal from certain psychoactive substances such as alcohol or benzodiazepines.[17] These organic factors are outlined in Table 24.2. The underlying vulnerability to

Table 24.2 Aetiological factors associated with delirium in advanced cancer

Causal category	Cause
Intracranial disease	Primary and metastatic brain neoplasms; leptomeningeal metastatic disease; post-ictal
Medication	
Psychoactive	Opioids; benzodiazepines; tricyclics; anticholinergics; selective serotonin-reuptake inhibitors; neuroleptics; antihistamines
Others	Steroids; H2 blockers; ciprofloxacin
Systemic disease	
Organ failure	Cardiac; hepatic; renal; respiratory
Infection	Any site but especially pulmonary and urinary
Haematological	Anaemia; disseminated intravascular coagulation
Metabolic	Dehydration; hypercalcaemia; hyponatraemia; hypomagnesaemia; hypoglycaemia
Withdrawal reaction	Alcohol, psychoactive medications such as benzodiazepines

Adapted and reproduced with permission from *Home Health Care Consultant* **8**, 10–16, 2001.

the development of delirium in patients with advanced cancer is high owing to underlying factors such as:

- cachexia
- hypoalbuminaemia
- advanced age or pre-existing dementia.

Various precipitants such as medications or infection, are superimposed on this high level of underlying vulnerability, culminating in an episode of delirium.

In the case of Mr B.K., potential risk factors to consider include his age, nutritional status, hepatic impairment (unlikely with a single liver metastasis unless there is underlying pre-existing liver disease), possible anaemia, and possible renal insufficiency associated with obstructive uropathy (a common scenario in retroperitoneal tumour from prostate as well as other malignancies). In addition, precipitants such as infection, amitriptyline, famciclovir, morphine, lorazepam, electrolyte disturbance, hypoxia, and dehydration need to be considered.

Question 8. What is the pathogenesis of delirium?

Delirium is considered to be a global disorder of brain dysfunction reflecting reduced cerebral oxidative metabolism and an imbalance in neurotransmission. At the cerebral neurotransmission level the most widely accepted explanation is a reduction in cholinergic transmission or at least an altered balance with a relative reduction of cholinergic in comparison with dopaminergic transmission.[18] Alterations in other neurotransmitters have been implicated in the pathogenesis of delirium, but their roles remain unclear. Cytokine production in the setting of Mr B.K.'s advanced disease is also considered to have a role in this complex process.

Many medications, for example tricyclic antidepressants such as amytriptiline, have an anticholinergic potential.

Morphine is metabolized mainly to morphine-6-glucuronide (M-6-G) and morphine-3-glucuronide (M-3-G). The M-6-G metabolite is active at the μ opioid receptor and contributes to analgesia. However, the M-3-G metabolite does not bind to opioid receptors.

It has been shown to be neuroexcitatory in animal studies, and it is postulated that it may contribute to the neurotoxicity (myoclonus, delirium, allodynia) associated with morphine. Hydromorphone-3-glucuronide, a metabolite of hydromorphone, has also shown to be neuroexcitatory in animal studies. However, the precise mechanisms subserving this opioid-induced neurotoxicity have yet to be elucidated. Some of the most florid examples of opioid-induced neurotoxicity have been reported in patients with renal impairment and consequent opioid and opioid metabolite accumulation.[19,20]

> In his advanced directive, Mr B.K. has named his only daughter, Fiona, as a proxy decision-maker. His son is feeling guilty about being so far away from home. In addition, he indicates that he is exhausted after his long journey, despondent at the level of his father's deterioration since he last saw him 6 months ago, and angry about what he perceives as his father's uncontrolled pain. He proceeds to advocate strongly for his father, and he expresses his concerns in an abusive way towards the nursing staff.

Question 9. What is your initial approach to management of a potentially reversible delirium?

An algorithm for a general approach to management of delirium might involve the following steps:

- Identify the underlying causes and assess its impact on the patient's quality of life.
- Rank the distress of delirium in the context of the patient's overall symptom burden.
- Assess the potential burden associated with correcting the underlying causes of delirium and the consequent impact on quality of life (e.g. establishing an intravenous line for bisphosphonate administration)
- Consider the pros and cons of correcting underlying causes and providing symptomatic treatment versus intervention directed exclusively at symptomatic control.
- Meet with the patient (who may be capable of some input in the case of mild cognitive impairment) and his or her family to facilitate informed decision-making and a consensus on the appropriate level of intervention.

Question 10. How do you apply this management strategy in Mr B.K.'s case? In particular, how do you approach Mr B.K.'s verbally abusive son?

Following your initial history and physical examination, you meet with Mr B.K.'s family to discuss your preliminary findings and the goals of care. You explain the nature of delirium, particularly the seriousness of this diagnosis but also the potential for reversal in some episodes depending on the cause. You explain that while pain should be treated, the presence of emotional lability and agitation are also probably associated with the delirium. Mr B.K.'s son is able to express his feelings in this meeting, including his guilt. Further meetings are arranged for him to have some counselling from the team social worker. Mr B.K.'s son now appears to have acquired a better understanding of his father's presentation and is grateful for your informative efforts. He personally acknowledges that some of his anger was projected onto the nursing staff, and is extremely apologetic.

The consensus reached at the family meeting was that reversible precipitants of Mr B.K.'s delirium should be sought and treated, and that the goal of treatment was to optimize his quality of life and comfort. The family were assured that they would be regularly kept appraised of Mr B.K.'s status. Team communication on the medical unit was emphasized so that Mr B.K. and his family received consistent and non-conflicting responses to their questions from staff members. Mr B.K.'s advanced directive refers to his wishes not to have aggressive resuscitation measures such as cardiopulmonary resuscitation, intubation, and defibrillation. This was clearly documented on his hospital chart.

The reversibility of delirium in this situation is likely to depend on the identification of reversible precipitants such as psychoactive medications, intravascular volume depletion, dehydration, hypercalcaemia, anaemia, obstructive uropathy, and infection. Underlying factors associated with progressive disease such as cachexia, hepatic impairment, and hypoalbuminaemia are less amenable to treatment. The association of cachexia and hypoalbuminaemia with delirium may relate to aberrant cytokine activity. The approach to opioid toxicity is either to reduce the dose or switch to a different opioid, and hydrate the patient (usually using a subcutaneous infusion known as hypodermoclysis, as it can be easier to start and maintain than an intravenous line), in addition to symptomatic management (see Question 12 below).

Question 11. What laboratory and radiological investigations might you perform in the case of Mr B.K.?

Preliminary laboratory tests aimed at identifying some reversible causes might include a complete blood count, electrolytes, urea, creatinine, calcium, albumin, magnesium, bilirubin, liver enzymes, urinalysis, and urine culture. Radiological investigation might include a chest radiograph and a plain abdominal film to assess constipation. Moderate elevation of Mr B.K.'s urea and creatinine levels might prompt an abdominal ultrasound scan to assess for obstructive uropathy.

Question 12. Apart from treating underlying causes, what other options do you have for symptomatic management?

Haloperidol is the drug of choice for the symptomatic treatment of hyperactive and mixed delirium.[21] It is a potent neuroleptic with dopamine-blocking properties. Therefore it may serve to redress the balance between dopaminergic and cholinergic neurotransmission (see Question 8). It can be administered orally, intramuscularly, intravenously, or subcutaneously. It can be associated with extrapyramidal side effects, such as dystonia and akathisia, although this is uncommon in the palliative setting. However, newer agents such as olanzapine, respiridone, and quetiapine have an even lower risk of extrapyramidal toxicity and are now being used more frequently. Methotrimeprazine can be used in preference to haloperidol if a greater level of sedation is required. Benzodiazepines such as lorazepam are considered as drugs of choice specifically for delirium related to alcohol withdrawal, but are generally avoided in other causes of delirium in cancer patients.[21]

Efforts aimed at environmental modification may help. These include reorientation efforts such as encouraging the family to engage in conversation with the patient, strategic placement of a calendar or clock, optimal lighting, noise reduction, and limiting staff changes or allocation of a specific nurse. Palliative care institutions will try to avoid physical restraints.

Constipation frequently accompanies delirium. It is unclear whether constipation is a contributory cause of delirium or perhaps more likely occurs in association with delirium and its underlying causes such as opioid treatment, dehydration and hypercalcaemia. Decreased mobility associated with delirium is also likely to contribute to constipation. The symptom distress associated with constipation and its frequent occurrence in association with delirium warrant adequate prevention and treatment (see Chapter 18).

Mr B.K. was found to have hypercalcaemia, opioid toxicity, and dehydration. Amitriptyline and lorazepam were discontinued. He received hydration with normal saline via hypodermoclysis. He had an infusion of intravenous pamidronate (a bisphosphonate) and his opioid was switched to a lower equianalgesic dose of hydromorphone with the addition of breakthrough doses. He was also administered haloperidol 1 mg subcutaneously every 8 h, and every hour if needed for agitation. A chest radiograph revealed progression of metastatic lung nodules and two small pleural effusions. However, oxygen saturation remained at 94 per cent on room air. His constipation was managed with enemas and an increase in his regular laxatives. An abdominal ultrasound scan showed only mild ureteric dilatation and mild ascites.

Within 48 h his agitation and perceptual disturbance subsided and he became more oriented. An MMSE performed on the third day of admission was scored at 22/30, virtually normal for his age and educational level. His family were most appreciative of the supportive care that they and Mr B.K. received. He was discharged home after a week. His expressed wish was to remain at home with his wife for as long as possible. You contacted the patient's community nurse and family physician to discuss discharge plans, and in particular the need to monitor calcium levels regularly and treat as necessary at home with a subcutaneous infusion of clodronate (a bisphosphonate).

In your discharge letter you surmise that Mr B.K. became drowsy as a result of hypercalcaemia, amitriptyline, and lorazepam, nauseated as a result of constipation and hypercalcaemia, consequently drank less fluid, became dehydrated, and then developed signs of opioid toxicity. This episode of delirium has highlighted for you the reversibility and multifactorial aetiology of delirium, in addition to the importance of addressing family concerns.

***

At this point Mr B.K. has been back in his home for 3 months. He truly enjoyed his first 6 weeks at home. He was initially mobile with the help of a walker and enjoyed sitting in his garden, which was his pride and joy. He spent some precious time with his son, who spent an additional 2 weeks with his parents before flying back to Europe. Mr B.K.'s daughter was granted compassionate leave from work and moved back home to assist her mother in caring for her father. The community care nurse and family physician visited regularly. Mr B.K. required clodronate infusions for hypercalcaemia on two occasions with good results.

His pain had been well controlled for the first couple of months at home but he then began to experience increasing bone pain in his shoulders and lower back, complete loss of appetite, progression of his cachexia, increasing abdominal girth, and uncomfortable scrotal and leg oedema. He began to spend more and more time in bed, and by the third month after his hospital discharge he was completely bedbound.

He developed episodes of both urinary and fecal incontinence. On a home visit 3 days ago, his family physician described the patient to be mildly jaundiced and dyspnoeic at rest despite home oxygen. The patient was prescribed haloperidol 1 mg subcutaneously at bedtime and hourly as needed for intermittent agitation and visual hallucinations, especially at night-time. A serum calcium level was reported in the normal range, when corrected for a very low albumin level of 18 g/l (**normal 36–47g/L**).

Continued

A further home visit was made by his family physician this morning. He was told by Mr B.K.'s daughter that he had been agitated most of the previous night despite four additional doses of haloperidol. At one stage he appeared to be talking to his dead mother and at another he was convinced that the house was invaded by soldiers. Both the patient's daughter and wife are completely exhausted. His daughter spoke earlier to her brother in Europe, who planned to get a flight as early as possible in order to see his father. Collectively, the family feels that he has 'gone through enough' and request that no further blood tests be done. Concerned regarding suboptimal symptom control and the family's exhaustion, the family physician raises the possibility of admission to hospice. He reassures them regarding the excellent care that has already been provided and, in accordance with their wishes, he plans to discuss further management and care with one of the palliative care consultants at the nearest hospice.

You are the palliative care consultant on call and receive a telephone call from Mr B.K.'s family physician. He outlines the history and physical findings for you Neurological examination is difficult and he cannot rule out the possibility of spinal cord compression. He is requesting hospice admission, and informs you that Mr B.K.'s proxy decision-maker is requesting no bloodwork. He also seeks advice in the interim regarding what can be done for agitation, and whether a diuretic would help with Mr B.K.'s discomfort from his leg and scrotal oedema.

Question 13. How do you respond to the family physician regarding Mr B.K.'s status? How would your response be different if there was no advanced directive in place? What do you suggest regarding the agitation and the value of giving a diuretic?

At this point it is clear that Mr B.K. is in another delirium. Primarily, it is necessary to respect the expressed wish of the patient (through his daughter as proxy) not to have any further bloodwork done. You agree to accept Mr B.K. for admission to hospice.

Even if Mr B.K. had no advanced directive, given the major progression in his disease, the associated dramatic decrease in his functional status, and the likelihood of delirium being less reversible on second or later episodes,[3] following the algorithm outlined in Question 9, it seems very reasonable to conclude that the management of his delirium and the goals of care should largely be restricted to symptomatic treatment. Searching for underlying precipitants would be inappropriate in the context of his pre-terminal status. However, such decisions are often difficult to make, and need to be individualized for each patient and each episode of delirium. Recall that Mr B.K. had a previous reversed episode of delirium, and it is wise not to prematurely adopt a nihilistic approach to therapeutic interventions.

You suggest a more sedating neuroleptic and suggest that the community nurse give methotrimeprazine 6.25 mg subcutaneously prior to moving him to hospice. Regarding the diuretic, it is likely that Mr B.K. has intravascular fluid loss to third-space sites (ascites and pleural effusions). His leg and scrotal oedema is probably arising from adenopathy-related lymphatic obstruction and possibly venous compression, and further aggravated by hypoalbuminaemia. Therefore you suggest that a diuretic will not improve his symptoms; indeed, it could actually worsen his intravascular volume depletion and consequently worsen his delirium.[22]

Mr B.K. is admitted to hospice. Your findings are consistent with those already described by his family physician. There was some mild myoclonus, which could reflect some mild opioid toxicity, renal impairment, or both. You continue hydration at 60 ml/h via hypodermoclysis. Following two doses of methotrimeprazine his agitation subsides to some extent. You meet with the Mr B.K.'s wife and daughter, who are relieved to see some reduction in his agitation. You decide to increase his methotrimeprazine to 12.5 mg subcutaneously every 8 h round the clock and hourly if needed for control of agitation. Overnight his methotrimeprazine was further increased to 25 mg using the same dosing schedule as previously prescribed.

On the following morning, Mr B.K. is again intermittently agitated, and as a result his family, who maintained an overnight vigil by his bedside, are very distraught. Because his agitation is refractory to standard measures, you propose inducing a deeper level of sedation with a continuous infusion of midazolam. You outline the benefits and risks to Mr B.K.'s family, including the son who has now arrived. After some discussion, they indicate their agreement with deep sedation. They appreciate that his prognosis is short (hours to days), irrespective of whether or not he receives midazolam. They also understand that he will be maintained in a state of deep sleep, and therefore will not be able to communicate. A medical student is spending the morning in the hospice and has accompanied you during your assessment of Mr B.K. and the subsequent family meeting.

Question 14. The medical student asks you what total sedation is and whether it is the same as euthanasia. How do you respond?

Voluntary euthanasia refers to the process of deliberately intending to end a patient's life at the request of the patient. Total sedation (sometimes called palliative sedation) refers to the deliberate intent to induce and maintain a deep level of sedation (deep sleep) pharmacologically, but not to cause death intentionally, in a dying patient with otherwise medically refractory symptoms and a high level of distress.[23] In clinical practice there is considerable variation in what physicians view as refractory symptoms, and consequently the rates of total sedation vary considerably, ranging from 10 to 52 per cent in published studies.[24] The ethical framework most commonly used in making a decision on total sedation is the doctrine of double effect. The primary intent of achieving relief from refractory symptom distress (positive outcome) outweighs the foreseen potential of actually but not intentionally hastening death (negative outcome).[25]

Delirium is one of the most common reasons for initiating total sedation. The most commonly used agent is midazolam. Alternatives include higher doses of more sedating neuroleptics such as methotrimeprazine or chlorpromazine, or use of other agents such as phenobarbital or intravenous propofol.

Question 15. In general, what safeguards should be implemented prior to initiating sedation with a continuous infusion of midazolam?

- Establish the diagnosis of delirium.
- Pursue appropriate efforts within the context of the goals of care to assess the reversibility of delirium.
- Clarify the intent of sedation.

- Discuss with family members and health care staff regarding the level of patient distress, the benefit versus burden of assessing reversibility in the context of the goals of care, and the intent of sedation.
- Consider temporary use of this type of sedation. This could arise in the event of refractory symptom distress associated with a potentially reversible delirium, and while awaiting the outcome of therapeutic interventions aimed at reversal.

Question 16. What safeguards should be in place once the infusion of midazolam has commenced?

- Frequent monitoring of level of sedation and respiratory status.
- Careful documentation of the infusion rate changes and the level of sedation.
- In the case of a potentially reversible delirium, the level of infusion can be reduced cautiously to assess the response to therapeutic interventions aimed at treating the underlying precipitants of delirium.

Mr B.K. is commenced on a midazolam infusion. The dose is titrated up to 6 mg/h and this helps to maintain him in a deep sleep. Mr B.K. dies peacefully about 36 h later with his family at his bedside.

Future trends and research objectives

The projected change in society with a great increase in the elderly population warrants a greater awareness and understanding of the spectrum of cognitive dysfunction in palliative care. Therefore further educational efforts are necessary to improve the recognition of these disorders and their consequences. For delirium, future research should focus on:

- phenomenological studies to characterize the syndrome better
- the development of low-burden assessment instruments
- the critical evaluation of communication strategies and the psychosocial impact of delirium on the family
- predictive models of delirium reversibility
- evidence-based guidelines on the use of sedation in symptomatic management.

References

1. **Pereira, J., Hanson, J., and Bruera, E.** (1997) The frequency and clinical course of cognitive impairment in patients with terminal cancer. *Cancer,* **79**, 835–42.
2. **Minagawa, H., Uchitomi, Y., Yamawaki, S., and Ishitani, K.** (1996) Psychiatric morbidity in terminally ill cancer patients. A prospective study. *Cancer,* **78**, 1131–1137.
3. **Lawlor, P.G., Gagnon, B., Mancini, I.L.,** ***et al.*** (2000) Occurrence, causes, and outcome of delirium in patients with advanced cancer: a prospective study. *Arch Intern Med,* **160**, 786–94.
4. **Massie, M.J., Holland, J., and Glass, E.** (1983) Delirium in terminally ill cancer patients. *Am J Psychiatry,* **140**, 1048–50.
5. **Bruera, E., Miller, L., McCallion, J., Macmillan, K., Krefting, L., and Hanson, J.** (1992) Cognitive failure in patients with terminal cancer: a prospective study. *J Pain Symptom Manage,* **7**, 192–5.

6. **American Psychiatric Association** (1994) Delirium, dementia and amnestic and other cognitive disorders. In: *Diagnostic and Statistical Manual of Mental Disorders* (4th edn) (DSM-IV) Washington, DC: American Psychiatric Association, 123–33.
7. **Breitbart, W., and Cochinor, H.M.** (2004) Psychiatric symptoms in palliative medicine. In: Doyle D, Hanks GWC, Cherny N, Calman K (eds) *Oxford Textbook of Palliative Medicine* (3rd edn). Oxford: Oxford University Press, 746–71.
8. **Inouye, S.K.** (1994) The dilemma of delirium: clinical and research controversies regarding diagnosis and evaluation of delirium in hospitalized elderly medical patients. *Am J Med,* **97**, 278–88.
9. **Meagher, D.J.** (2001) Delirium: optimising management. *BMJ,* **322**, 144–9.
10. **Lawlor, P.G.** (2002) The panorama of opioid-related cognitive dysfunction in patients with cancer: a critical literature appraisal. *Cancer,* **94**, 1836–53.
11. **Smith, M.J., Breitbart, W.S., and Platt, M.M.** (1995) A critique of instruments and methods to detect, diagnose, and rate delirium. *J Pain Symptom Manage,* **10**, 35–77.
12. **Folstein, M.F., Folstein, S., and McHugh, P.R.** 1975) 'Mini-Mental State': a practical method for grading the cognitive state of patients for the clinician. *J Psychiatric Res,* **12**, 189–98.
13. **Inouye, S.K., van Dyck, C.H., Alessi, C.A., Balkin, S., Siegal, A.P., and Horwitz, R.I.** (1990) Clarifying confusion: the confusion assessment method. A new method for detection of delirium. *Ann Intern Med,* **113**, 941–8.
14. **Crum, R., Anthony, J.C., Bassett, S.S., and Folstein, M.F.** (1993) Population-based norms for the Mini-Mental State Examination by age and educational level. *JAMA,* **269**, 2386–91.
15. **Gagnon, B., Lawlor, P.G., Mancini, I.L., Pereira, J.L., Hanson, J., and Bruera, E.D.** (2001) The impact of delirium on the circadian distribution of breakthrough analgesia in advanced cancer patients. *J Pain Symptom Manage,* **22**, 826–33.
16. **Fainsinger, R.L., Tapper, M., and Bruera, E.** (1993) A perspective on the management of delirium in terminally ill patients on a palliative care unit. *J Palliat Care,* **9**, 4–8.
17. **Lipowski, Z.J.** (1990) Etiology. In: Lipowski ZJ (ed) *Delirium: Acute Confusional States.* New York: Oxford University Press, 109–40.
18. **Trzepacz, P.T.** (2000) Is there a final common neural pathway in delirium? Focus on acetylcholine and dopamine. *Semin Clin Neuropsychiatry,* **5**, 132–48.
19. **Sjogren, P., Dragsted, L., and Christensen, C.B.** (1993) Myoclonic spasms during treatment with high doses of intravenous morphine in renal failure. *Acta Anaesthes Scand,* **37**, 780–2.
20. **Hagen, N., and Swanson, R.** (1997) Strychnine-like multifocal myoclonus and seizures in extremely high-dose opioid administration: treatment strategies. *J Pain Symptom Manage,* **14**, 51–8.
21. **American Psychiatric Association** (1999) Practice guideline for the treatment of patients with delirium. *Am J Psychiatry,* **156** (Suppl), 1–20.
22. **Lawlor, P.G.** (2002) Delirium and dehydration: some fluid for thought? *Support Care Cancer,* **10**, 445–54.
23. **Chater, S., Viola, R., Paterson, J., and Jarvis, V.** (1998) Sedation for intractable distress in the dying—a survey of experts. *Palliat Med,* **12**, 255–69.
24. **Fainsinger, R.L.** (2000) Treatment of delirium at the end of life: medical and ethical issues. In: Portenoy RK, Bruera E (eds) *Topics in Palliative Care.* Oxford: Oxford University Press, 261–77.
25. **Cherny, N.I., and Portenoy, R.K.** (1994) Sedation in the management of refractory symptoms: guidelines for evaluation and treatment. *J Palliat Care,* **10**, 31–8.

Chapter 25

Dehydration

Robin Fainsinger

Attitude

To enable each student to:

- Recognize that dehydration is a potential cause of symptom distress in patients with advanced disease.
- Recognize that overhydration of chronically ill patients can cause symptom distress.
- Recognize that not all chronically ill patients require the institution of parenteral hydration, and that some patients receiving parenteral hydration should have this therapy discontinued.
- Recognize the need for regular assessment of the hydration status and needs in chronically ill patients.

Skill

To enable each student to:

- Use appropriate history and physical and investigational methods to assess the patient's hydration status.
- Demonstrate clinical judgement in management decisions over the need to use parenteral hydration, stop parenteral hydration, or decide against treating a dehydrated patient.
- Use appropriate rehydration techniques when parenteral hydration is deemed necessary.
- Demonstrate the ability to involve other team members, including the patient and/or family, in decisions regarding parenteral hydration.

Knowledge

To enable each student to:

- Recognize that the management of dehydration in patients with advanced disease is a controversial issue, best managed by taking an individual approach to each patient.
- State the arguments for and against use of hydration in patients with advanced disease.
- Describe an approach to an individual assessment and management plan for the treatment of a dehydrated patient.
- Identify hypodermoclysis as an alternative to intravenous parenteral hydration, and know how this technique can be utilized.
- Describe the difficulties of parenteral hydration at home compared with in hospital, and how these problems can be managed.

Mr N.D. is a 65-year-old man who presented with a 2-month history of vague upper-abdominal discomfort. Over the 2-month period he was treated and investigated for peptic ulcer disease with no benefit. He has no history of significant medical problems. His only medication was an antacid, which had not relieved the abdominal discomfort. An abdominal ultrasound revealed a mass in the head of the pancreas with two lesions, compatible with metastatic deposits, noted in the liver. A liver biopsy revealed adenocarcinoma that was probably secondary to primary pancreatic cancer. He was evaluated at the cancer clinic. Treatment options were discussed with him and his family by the oncologist. He decided to receive 'palliative' measures only.

The pros and cons of a coeliac plexus block for pain management were discussed with Mr N.D. However, he felt that he would prefer the less invasive option of oral medication.[1] The oncologist started the patient on morphine for the moderately severe epigastric pain, together with laxatives.

Four days later you make a house call at the request of the patient's wife. The history is of persistent nausea and vomiting since starting morphine. The patient's wife indicates that her husband is unable to keep any fluids down. The patient weighed 91 kg when his symptoms first began 2 months previously, and now weighs 88.6 kg. On examination he shows signs of dehydration. Blood tests show an elevated sodium of 150 mmol/l (normal 135–145 mmol/l), urea of 14 mmol/l (normal 2.4–8 mmol/l) and creatinine of 160 mmol/l (normal 50–110 mmol/l).

Question 1. In making an assessment of hydration status, what information would you look for from the history and the physical or laboratory tests? Having diagnosed dehydration in this patient, explain your approach to managing the dehydration and nausea, including where and how you will treat Mr N.D. (home versus hospital)

The following factors would assist with a hydration assessment.[2,3]

- History: estimated oral intake and presence of nausea or vomiting and diarrhoea.
- Physical findings: pulse, blood pressure (supine and erect), oral secretions, sweating, tissue turgor, exclude urinary retention, measurements of input and output.
- Laboratory tests: haematocrit, sodium, urea, creatinine. However, under some circumstances laboratory tests might be considered excessive or unnecessary.

This patient is clearly at a relatively early stage in his trajectory of illness. The evidence strongly suggests that his vomiting is opioid induced, resulting in dehydration. This deterioration is readily reversible.

In a region with sufficient home care support, parenteral rehydration by hypodermoclysis or the intravenous route could be managed in the patient's home. If there is inadequate palliative home care support for the patient, family and attending physician, a short admission to an acute care hospital can be justified (perhaps admission to a daycare centre would suffice).

The regular opioid could be continued with the addition of oral metoclopramide 10 mg four times daily. If the patient continues to vomit, replacing metoclopramide with prochlorperazine suppositories (domperidone suppositories are available in the UK) would be an option. Obviously it would have been preferable to have prevented the opioid-induced nausea by prescribing a regular or as-needed antiemetic at the initiation of opioid therapy.[4] Other options to consider are parenteral or rectal opioid administration until the nausea settles, or a switch to an alternative opioid such as hydromorphone using recognized guidelines of opioid equivalents.[5,6]

Mr N.D. recovered during the first few days of your treatment. He was able to resume some activities, such as walking and gardening. Over the next few weeks he had progressively increasing abdominal pain and required an increase of his morphine to 25 mg orally every 4 h. Other medications include oral metoclopramide 10 mg four times daily, two tablets of senna twice daily, and docusate 200 mg twice daily. Six weeks after your initial home visit Mr N.D. has lost 13.6 kg, his poor appetite has resulted in poor fluid intake, and his wife has noted that he is confused.

On visiting Mr N.D. at home you again note that he is dehydrated and confused. You find that his son and daughter have returned home for a brief visit. His 35-year-old son is an intensive care physician in another city, and is very concerned that his father is dehydrated and wants him admitted to the hospital for intravenous fluids. Mr N.D.'s 32-year-old daughter is a nurse working for a hospice programme near Chicago. She is clearly angry with her brother's opinion, feeling that her father should stay at home with hydration only offered orally. Mr N.D.'s wife is undecided, but wants 'the best' for her husband.

Question 2. How would you summarize the 'dehydration controversy' for this family to allow them to see the alternative viewpoints? Explain how and where *you* would prefer to manage this patient's problems at this stage of the disease.

Controversies surrounding the rehydration of chronically ill patients can be summarized as follows.[7–9]

- Arguments against:
  - Obtunded or comatose patients do not experience pain, thirst, etc.
  - Fluid may prolong the dying process.
  - Less urine output means less need for bedpan, urinal, commode, or catheter.
  - Less gastrointestinal fluid and less vomiting occur.
  - Less pulmonary secretion, along with less cough, choking, and congestion.
  - Decreased fluids and electrolyte imbalance may act as a natural anaesthetic for the central nervous system, with decreased level of consciousness and decreased suffering.
  - Parenteral hydration is uncomfortable and limits patient mobility.
  - Thirst is readily controlled with minimal oral fluids and good mouth care.
- Arguments for:
  - Dehydration is recognized as a cause of confusion and agitation.
  - Dehydration is a cause of renal failure which may result in accumulation of medications such as opioids or opioid metabolites, with the potential development of myoclonus, seizures, and agitated confusion.
  - Dehydration is suggested as an increased risk factor for bed sores.
  - Constipation is reported to be more problematic in dehydrated patients.
  - Dying patients may be more comfortable if they receive adequate hydration.
  - There is no evidence that fluids alone prolong life to any meaningful degree.
  - Water is administered to dying people who complain of thirst, so why not give parenteral hydration.
  - Arguments regarding poor quality of life detract from efforts to find ways to improve comfort and life quality.

- Parenteral hydration is a minimum standard of care, and discontinuing this treatment is to break a bond with the patient.
- Withholding fluid to dying patients is the 'thin edge of the wedge' of withholding therapies to other compromised patient groups.

This is arguably the controversial midpoint of this patient's illness. Arguments can be found for an approach to reverse the confusion, and a case can be made that the patient has deteriorated to the point that he could be considered to be actively dying.

Perhaps the dehydration has resulted in opioid metabolite accumulation and caused the confusional syndrome. Rehydration could reverse pre-renal failure and allow the opioid metabolites to clear more rapidly, and improve Mr N.D.'s cognition. The opioid should be decreased in view of probable drug accumulation, or an alternative opioid such as hydromorphone could be prescribed.[1] The presence of renal failure and the concept of incomplete cross-tolerance between opioids suggests that reduced starting doses of hydromorphone should be used.[6,9,10]

If the arguments for not hydrating the patient prevail, it would be important to recognize the need to decrease or switch opioids, and to avoid increased toxicity due to opioid accumulation. The most important component of any answer is a clear rationale for the treatment approach proposed.

Question 3. Explain how you would work with this family with conflicting viewpoints to achieve a compromise treatment approach with which they could all agree

Family conference

A major conflict is developing within this family. The physician needs to recognize this potentially devastating complication, and explain how a family conference could help to resolve the crisis to everyone's mutual satisfaction. Other members of an interdisciplinary palliative care team (e.g. social worker, nurse, psychologist) may need to be included in the team conference.

The conference should have a number of goals.

- Clarify that all family members are aware of the patient's diagnosis and understand the management approach to this point.
- Allow family members the opportunity to express their viewpoint or ask questions regarding Mr N.D.'s treatment.
- Discuss the problems that now confront the patient and the alternative approaches to management of his dehydration and confusion.
- The crucial point is a family understanding and compromise on what is perceived to be in Mr N.D.'s best interest. The family might find this easier to answer if they are aware of what Mr N.D.'s previous expressed wishes were, and whether they see an advantage to attempting to reverse his confusion and prolonging his life for a further period of time.

The answers and management approach can be expected to vary with different patients and families. The crucial point is to discover what is right for this patient and this family, and to make the decision with them.[11–13]

It is worth remembering that patient and family decisions regarding hydration (as in other medical decisions) are clearly influenced by the manner in which health care professionals present information to them. In addition, while advanced directives may provide a useful guideline, they may not provide answers for potentially reversible conditions or cover the complexity of some complications. Thus obtaining clear patient-directed guidelines for every situation is often impossible.

Question 4. Hypodermoclysis is mentioned in the course of the discussion. The family requests further information. What will you say?

Hypodermoclysis

Hypodermoclysis[14–16] is a method of providing parenteral fluids by the subcutaneous route. It has many advantages over the intravenous route.

- It is easy for a health care professional, or even a family member, to learn to insert a subcutaneous needle.
- Infusion can be stopped and started without concern that the needle will clot.
- Hospitalization can be avoided or shortened.
- Subcutaneous sites often last for several days.

Hyaluronidase is an enzyme that breaks down hyaluronic acid and aids the rapid diffusion and absorption of injected fluids by temporarily lysing the normal interstitial barrier. The amount of hyaluronidase recommended varies from 0 to 300 U/l. Many patients will be able to tolerate hypodermoclysis without the addition of hyaluronidase. This is fortunate, as the major supplier of hyaluronidase to the North American market has recently ceased production. Most authors recommend the use of solutions with electrolytes, such as normal saline or 2:1 dextrose 5%–normal saline, since non-electrolyte solutions draw fluid into the interstitial space. Rates of infusion in the range 20–120 ml/h have been suggested; however, there are reports of success using bolus infusions of 500 ml over 1 h two or three times daily.

During the family conference, Mr N.D.'s wife indicated that her husband had expressed the wish to live as comfortably as possible, without having to endure 'useless medical intervention'. The family agreed that he was enjoying his quality of life prior to the development of confusion. Thus a more active management approach including rehydration was not a contradiction of his viewpoint, and was acceptable to all the family members.

With the help of the home care nurse, the patient was given parenteral hydration by hypodermoclysis at home for a period of 1 week. In addition, the morphine was discontinued and replaced with oral hydromorphone 3 mg every 4 h. He was stable over the next few weeks with improvement in his cognition . However, he continues to lose weight and is increasingly weak, and 10 weeks after your visit is now on hydromorphone 6 mg subcutaneously every 4 h. His daughter has moved home temporarily to nurse her father, and asks you to visit, as over the previous days she has noted progressive myoclonus and agitated confusion. She feels that her father might be having more pain, causing agitation, and suggests an increase in the opioids and possibly a benzodiazepine for sedation. She notes that he has been drinking nothing in recent days, and is occasionally incontinent of small amounts of urine. Your examination reveals a severely cachectic, confused, and dehydrated man with myoclonus of the arms and legs every 1–2 min, constant purposeless arm and leg movements, and indecipherable moaning and muttering. His daughter is determined to help her father die at home. His wife is ambivalent, and tells you that her son telephones twice a day, and during the last call stated that his father should be admitted to hospital, or at the very least be given parenteral fluid at home.

Question 5. State the main problems that you now have to manage. Explain how and where *you* would prefer to manage the problems you now identify. Explain how you will work with the family to find agreement on a management approach that is in the best interest of an increasingly symptomatic patient and an increasingly tired and distressed family

The main presenting problems at this time are dehydration, agitated delirium, myoclonus, pain assessment in a confused and agitated patient, a tired and exhausted family, and potential family conflict over appropriate treatment.

Once again there are a number of treatment options in managing this patient at home with appropriate support or opting for a hospital admission. The most important aspect of the answer is the rationale that is used to deal with all the presenting problems. The following points need to be recognized.

- This dehydrated patient, with no oral intake and minimal urine output, has pre-renal failure. The opioid dose of 36 mg of parenteral hydromorphone daily is causing side effects of metabolite accumulation with myoclonus and agitated delirium.
- The family is making the common error of seeing the agitation as a manifestation of pain.[17] Agreeing to the request to increase the opioid can worsen the delirium and myoclonus, cause seizures, and lead to further opioid increases to treat the perceived pain. Inevitably other medications will be added to treat the myoclonus, delirium, and seizures.
- The management approach must include the decision whether or not to hydrate the patient. It can be argued that hydration will assist in the excretion of offending opioid metabolites. In any event, the opioid needs to be switched and/or the dose decreased. The need to decrease the opioid is even more imperative if the decision is made not to hydrate the patient.
- The delirium[9,18,19] needs to be treated aggressively, as this has been shown to be a major cause of distress to the family and dissatisfaction with care. Management might include sedating treatments on a temporary or permanent basis.[19] (Management of delirium is covered in Chapter 24.)
- Care can be continued at home with sufficient explanation and education of the family, as well as intensive ongoing nursing and physician support to monitor the patient's progress and change treatment if symptoms are not improving. If insufficient support is available, or the family are no longer able to cope physically or psychologically, admission to an acute care hospital or palliative care unit is appropriate.

A family conference will probably be required to understand the family's stress and treatment preferences. The family is confronting the death of a close relative who is deteriorating with a number of distressing symptoms. They will probably be experiencing grief, fear, and anger, all compounded by the physical and psychological exhaustion of caring for a relative through a prolonged illness. Adequate use of community options such as palliative home care, other family members or friends, or hospital admission needs to be evaluated and discussed appropriately. The family needs to understand the care proposed, and come to an agreement with the caregivers on where and how Mr N.D. will be managed.

Commentary: trends and research

Despite starting from different perspectives, there is consensus from a number of palliative care groups[8] that available data are inadequate for final conclusions, individual assessment of dehydration relevance in each clinical situation is required, and further research would be helpful.

Research in this area has tended to focus on three areas:[20]

- the association between biochemical findings and hydration status
- biochemical findings and clinical symptoms
- hydration status and clinical symptoms.

However, there are significant challenges to research in this area. A systematic review attempted to clarify the physical diagnosis of hypovolaemia in adults, and concluded that few findings, with the exception of serum electrolytes, urea, and creatinine levels, have proven value in patients with vomiting, diarrhoea, or decreased oral intake.[21] We need more rigorous designs to test hypotheses regarding the effects of fluid deficiency and fluid therapy on mental status, thirst, and dry mouth.[22] In addition, the subpopulation of chronically ill to whom the parenteral hydration controversy applies is not that clear. We need to agree on a common set of outcome and measurement tools for use in palliative care research in order to allow comparison and synthesis of data across a variety of studies.[9,22] Consideration of how a randomized double-blind controlled study could be applied to aspects of the parenteral hydration debate further highlights the difficulty of definitive research designs.[23]

References

1. **Cherny, N., Ripamonti, C., Pereira, J., *et al.*** (2001) Strategies to manage the adverse effects of oral morphine: an evidence-based report. *J Clin Oncol,* **19**, 2542–54.
2. **Sarhill, N., Walsh, D., Nelson, K., *et al.*** (2001) Evaluation and treatment of cancer-related fluid deficits: volume depletion and dehydration. *Support Care Cancer,* **9**, 408–19.
3. **Jackson, K.C.** (2000) Nutrition and hydration problems in palliative care patients. *J Pharm Care Pain Symptom Control,* **8**, 183–97.
4. **Ripamonti, C., and Bruera, E.** (2002) Chronic nausea and vomiting. In: Ripamonti, C., and Bruera, E. (eds) *Gastrointestinal Symptoms in Advanced Cancer Patients.* Oxford: Oxford University Press, 169–206.
5. **Fainsinger, R.L.** (2002) Pain. In: Rakel RE, Bope ET (eds) *Conn's Current Therapy.* Philadelphia, PA: W.B. Saunders, 1–5.
6. **Pereira, J., Lawlor, P., Vigano, A., *et al.*** (2001) Equianalgesic dose ratios for opioids: a critical review and proposals for long-term dosing. *J Pain Symptom Manage,* **22**, 672–87.
7. **Fainsinger, R.L., and Bruera, E.** (1997) When to treat dehydration in a terminally ill patient? *Support Care Cancer,* **5**, 205–11.
8. **Fainsinger, R.L.** (2002) Hydration. In: Ripamonti C, Bruera E. (eds) *Gastrointestinal Symptoms in Advanced Cancer Patients.* Oxford: Oxford University Press, 395–410.
9. **Lawlor, P.G.** (2002) Delirium and dehydration: some fluid for thought? *Support Care Cancer,* **10**, 445–54.
10. **Kappel, J., and Calissi, P.** (2002) Nephrology: safe drug prescribing for patients with renal insufficiency. *Can Med Assoc J,* **166**, 473–7.
11. **Latimer, E.J.** (2002) 'Matters of the Heart …' Feeding and hydration in palliative care. *Can J Continuing Med Educ,* **3**, 97–106.
12. **Parkash, R., and Burge, F.** (1997) The family's perspective on issues of hydration in terminal care. *J Palliat Care,* **13**, 23–7.

13. **Morita, T., Tsunoda, J., Inoue, S., *et al.*** (1999) Perceptions and decision-making on rehydration of terminally ill cancer patients and family members. *Am J Hospice Palliat Care,* **16**, 509–16.
14. **Fainsinger, R.L., MacEachern, T., Miller, M.J., *et al.*** (1994) The use of hypodermoclysis (HDC) for rehydration in terminally ill cancer patients. *J Pain Symptom Manage,* **9**, 298–302.
15. **Steiner, N., and Bruera, E.** (1998) Methods of hydration in palliative care patients. *J Palliat Care,* **14**, 6–13.
16. **Centeno, C., and Bruera, E.** (1999) Subcutaneous hydration with no hyaluronidase in patients with advanced cancer. *J Pain Symptom Manage,* **17**, 305–6.
17. **Bruera, E., Fainsinger, R., Miller, M.J., *et al.*** (1992) The assessment of pain intensity in patients with cognitive failure: a preliminary report. *J Pain Symptom Manage,* **7**, 267–70.
18. **Fainsinger, R.L., Tapper, M., and Bruera, E.** (1993) A perspective on the management of delirium in the terminally ill. *J Palliat Care,* **9**, 4–8.
19. **Fainsinger, R.L.** (2000) Treatment of delirium at the end of life: medical and ethical issues. In: Portenoy RK, Bruera E (eds) *Topics in Palliative,* Vol 4. Oxford: Oxford University Press, 261–77.
20. **Morita, T., Ichika, T., Tsunoda, J., *et al.*** (1999) Three dimensions of the rehydration—dehydration problem in a palliative care setting. *J Palliat Care,* **15**, 60–1.
21. **McGee, S., Abernethy, W.B., and Simeld, L.** (1999) Is this patient hypovolemic? *JAMA,* **21**, 1022–9.
22. **Viola, R.A., Wells, G.A., and Peterson, J.** (1997) The effects of fluid status and fluid therapy on the dying: a systematic review. *J Palliat Care,* **13**, 41–52.
23. **Bruera, E., Sala, R., Rico, M.A., *et al.*** (2005) Effects of parenteral hydration in terminally ill cancer patients: a preliminary study. *J Clin Oncol,* **23**, 2366–71.

Chapter 26

Mouth care

Dominique Dion and Bernard Lapointe

Attitude

To enable each student to:

- Appreciate the importance of early recognition of mouth problems in persons living with cancer or HIV/AIDS.
- Practise regular examination of the patient's mouth (at least twice weekly).

Skill

To enable each student to:

- Demonstrate skills in recognizing the common oral pathologies.
- Demonstrate skills in preventing and treating the most common conditions such as: candidiasis, xerostomia, and mucositis.

Knowledge

To enable each student to:

- Recognize that a dry mouth is a common feature of patients with advanced illness and state the principal reasons why this occurs.
- State the differential diagnosis of stomatitis, with or without ulcerations.
- Describe the syndrome of candidiasis, and state the common presenting features of *Candida* infection.

Mrs H., a 46-year-old woman, is referred for radiotherapy. She has been diagnosed with a neglected and now ulcerated left breast carcinoma that has metastasized to the left axilla and lower cervical spine. Mrs H. is of low socioeconomic status, has a history of chronic alcoholism, and continues to drink a half-bottle of wine and five or six bottles of beer daily.

She was started on amitryptiline 25 mg at bedtime 1 week ago by her oncologist for two reasons: depression and mild neuropathic pain radiating from her left shoulder down to the left elbow, presumed secondary to either her cervical spinal metastases or axillary invasion. Her main complaints today are dryness of the mouth with decreased and distorted taste and mild ill-described left arm pain with fleeting dysaesthetic discomfort around the elbow. She has not made up her mind yet about a proposed course of 'heavy' chemotherapy.

Continued

On examination, she appears well nourished, but her facies and attitude betray depression and her general appearance is somewhat neglected. Abnormal physical findings are limited to the mouth and the left breast and adjacent axillary area.

Question 1. Identify five areas of the mouth that you would examine in this patient.

The health care professional needs to examine the oral cavity systematically and discern normal from abnormal. The oral cavity is composed of hard and soft tissues. We should systematically review the following.

1. **Teeth**. The adult can have a maximum of 28 teeth. They may appear to have varying colours from white to yellow. This colour differential is affected by the amount of remaining enamel, the quantity and nature of the plaque, and the influence of medications. Note should be made of severely carious teeth as potential foci of infection.
2. **Lips.** Lips should not normally be cracked, and should be soft and pink. As the lips are retracted Fordyce granules can be seen; these are minor salivary glands.
3. **Gingiva and oral mucosa.** The gingiva and oral mucosa should appear to be pink, moist, and glistening from the presence of saliva. The gingiva around the teeth should be strippled and firm.
4. **Tongue.** The tongue should have a regular texture, but with age it can appear fissured. It should not be either bald or hairy in appearance. The tongue increases in size with the loss of teeth.
5. **Presence and quality of saliva.** Saliva is produced by three paired major salivary glands: the submandibular, sublingual, and parotid glands. In addition to these glands, minor salivary glands are present in the lips, oral mucosa, and palate. The volume of saliva secreted daily is between 500 and 1500 ml. It was once speculated that salivation decreased with age; however, recent evidence indicates that salivation rate is affected by medications and systemic disease, and that age does not affect significantly salivary flow in healthy individuals.[1,2]

Saliva's function is often viewed to be primarily that of digestion via salivary amylase, lipase, and proteases. However, saliva's principal role in the oral cavity is protection. The oral cavity is a major route for bacterial invasion, and saliva is the body's first line of defence. Saliva is a complex solution containing inhibitory factors such as lysozyme, peroxidase, and immunoglobins G, M, and A (IgG, IgM, and IgA) as well as normal bacterial flora competing with pathogens for growth.[3] It also contains buffers which aid in the establishment of a relatively neutral pH[2,4] in the mouth, as well as ions such as calcium which aid in the remineralization of the teeth. Saliva also dissolves chemical mediators which are important in taste perception.[5]

The examination of Mrs H.'s mouth reveals the following.

- Halitosis is readily perceived.
- The lips and corners of the mouth are normal.
- Several lower teeth are in obviously poor condition, and she wears a well-fitted upper denture.
- There is no evidence of gingivitis or pyorrhoea.
- The tongue looks dry but otherwise normal.
- No candidiasis is seen or suspected, but the oral cavity, including the pharynx, is dry and slightly hyperaemic, with some thick saliva.

Question 2. How common and how important are oral problems in palliative care patients?

We do not fully appreciate the oral cavity's contribution to our quality of life until such time as its functioning is impaired or lost. The mouth is vital in communication and expression (speaking, singing, kissing, laughing, crying) and in the appreciation of food and drinks (chewing, swallowing). Also, it is the easiest route for administering medications.

Oral complications can contribute to the development of pain, infection(s), malnutrition, speech difficulties, and taste alterations. These problems, in turn, may contribute to a patient's decreased self-esteem. Thus it is important for the professional to detect and treat abnormalities before the patient's quality of life is affected.

The oral cavity is often one of the first sites of pain and loss of function. The prevalence of oral symptoms is shown in Table 26.1. As the health of the oral mucosa mirrors the status of the patient's immune system, we have witnessed a significant decrease in the prevalence of mucosal complications in patients living with HIV who are receiving antiretroviral therapy (ART). However, the prevalence of oral symptoms in HIV/AIDS patients not receiving ART remains very high.[8]

The palliative care team should strive to maintain or improve the patient's level of oral hygiene to prevent complications such as dental decay, periodontal disease, and stomatitis. However, as complications arise, it is important to treat reversible conditions rapidly or institute symptom control. These measures would probably decrease the incidence of loss of function and improve the patient's quality of life.

Table 26.1 Prevalence of oral symptoms among palliative care patients

	Prevalence (%)	
Symptoms	**Jobbins *et al.*[6]**	**Aldred *et al.*[7]**
Taste disturbance	37	26
Dysphagia	35	37
Oral soreness	33	42
Xerostomia	77	58
Candidiasis	85	70
Denture problems[a]	45	71

[a]Among those patients wearing dentures

Question 3. What types of oral problem do you identify in this patient?

This patient's oral problems include basic oral hygiene and denture care, halitosis, and xerostomia.

Question 4. How would you advise Mrs H. on her basic oral hygiene?

Basic oral hygiene: tips and traps

Oral hygiene measures can be divided into two classes of treatment modalities.

Mechanical plaque control

The most effective mechanical means to improve oral hygiene in palliative care patients is the prudent use of a toothbrush with soft rounded bristles. Anti-tartar toothpaste may cause discomfort in some sensitive mouths; in this case, substitute a children's fluoridated or low-abrasive toothpaste. The toothbrush should be replaced every 3 months. As the patient's ability to combat infection decreases with time, it must be remembered that the toothbrush can actually be a reservoir for many organisms.[9] The toothbrush can be soaked in either a commercial mouthwash or 0.12 per cent chlorhexidine to decrease the levels of pathogenic and opportunistic organisms. As the dexterity and mobility of the palliative patient may become compromised, an electric toothbrush may be advantageous for both patient and caregiver. Modification of the toothbrush can enhance the patient's ability to maintain oral hygiene and thus improve their self-worth.

Toothettes or foam toothbrushes are often perceived as a more gentle technique for cleaning the teeth and gums. However, toothettes do not clean as effectively as a regular toothbrush.[10] Nevertheless, the toothette is a useful adjunct in the application of chemotherapeutic agents to the oral cavity. This will be discussed in the next section.

Chemical plaque control

Patients with decreased salivary flow rate and halitosis may seek salvation in mouthwashes. Many mouthwashes contain alcohol which has been demonstrated to be a potent drying agent and thus can increase xerostomia.[11] Alcohol-free mouthwashes are commercially available. An inexpensive alternative mouthwash consists of a baking soda and/or saline solution (1 teaspoon baking soda and/or 1 teaspoon salt in 500 ml water) followed by a plain water rinse. Although many commercial mouthwashes can help reduce the dental plaque, most of them will not have a significant impact on the occurrence of gingivitis or caries if used alone.

Chlorhexidine Chlorhexidine, used at 0.12 per cent dilution, is an effective chemotherapeutic agent against bacteria and fungi in the oral flora.[12,13] It has been shown to be an antiplaque agent that can help reduce gingivitis and caries.[14] It can be administered as an oral rinse (15 ml rinsed for 30 s, then spit out) twice daily after breakfast and at bedtime or by an oral applicator. A 4 × 4 gauze (wrapped around a tongue depressor) soaked in chlorhexidine can be used to remove dried mucus and debris in the mouth.

The prophylactic use of chlorhexidine in cancer patients or its prolonged use remains controversial.[14,15] Chlorhexidine mouthwash should be withheld during head and neck radiation therapy or in the presence of severe mucositis as one study showed that it was no better than placebo in such patients, and that it might have increased the severity of their mucositis.[16] Chlorhexidine can cause slight staining of teeth, which can be easily corrected by a simple dental cleaning. Chlorhexidine can cause taste alterations; therefore it should be taken after meals.

Hydrogen peroxide Hydrogen peroxide at a 0.5 per cent concentration is sometimes used to remove hardened debris and to clean a coated tongue. However, it should be used prudently because it can lead to the destruction of healthy granulating tissues, and may increase and prolong the severity of mucositis.[15,17] Following the use of hydrogen peroxide, patients should be advised to rinse their mouth with plain water.

Similarly, in many centres, chewing canned pineapple is recommended to remove debris in the oral cavity and to clean the tongue.

Glycerin–lemon swabs Glycerin–lemon swabs are not recommended as they have been found to be inadequate for the cleaning of the oral cavity, and in addition glycerin can increase oral drying.[18]

Question 5. What advice will you provide Mrs H. on denture care?

Denture care

Palliative care patients should never wear dentures for 24 hours a day. Dentures should be kept scrupulously clean as they have been found to be prominent reservoirs of *Candida* species. Commercial toothpastes can be too abrasive for the denture acrylic and teeth. Dentures are best cleansed with the use of non-abrasive paste or a mild soap and a denture brush. Dentures should not be boiled, as boiling will lead to the distortion of the denture base. Soaking the denture in bleach and water (15 ml:250 ml) for 30 min will help rid the denture of odours. Partial dentures should not be soaked in bleach solution as it will lead to metal fatigue; plain water suffices. Dentures should be stored in well-identified vessels containing warm water, denture-cleaning solution, or, if fungus is suspected, 0.12 per cent chlorhexidine or 100 000 IU nystatin suspension and water. Patients should be advised always rinse to their dentures under warm running water before putting them back in their mouth or before soaking.

The chronically ill often complain to dentists that their dentures are too loose because they have lost weight. Although physically the patient may appear emaciated, the hard tissues of the mouth do not decrease with weight loss. Loss of facial muscle tone and xerostomia can compromise the adherence and function of a denture, and the problem can be corrected by a denture reline at the bedside.

Question 6. Why does Mrs H. have halitosis?

Halitosis

Halitosis is an offensive odour of the breath. In over 90 per cent of cases, the cause of bad breath is to be found in the oral cavity.[19] Common oral causes include:

- poor oral hygiene
- xerostomia
- coated tongue—a common reservoir of bacteria
- infection (periodontitis, gingivitis, etc.)
- malignancy.

Common non-oral causes of halitosis are throat and sinus infections, lung abscess, and gastric stasis.

In Mrs H's case, halitosis may stem from poor oral hygiene with xerostomia and possibly low-grade unrecognized infection. Addressing the underlying intra-oral conditions would be expected to improve the halitosis.

Question 7. Why does Mrs H. have a dry mouth?

Xerostomia or dry mouth is a common complaint amongst palliative care patients. It is most commonly seen as a consequence of medication, head and neck radiotherapy, or progressive debilitation resulting in mouth breathing.

Several types of medications often used in palliative medicine can cause xerostomia:[2,20,21]

- tricyclic antidepressants
- neuroleptics (phenothiazines)

- antihistamines
- anticholinergics (atropine, scopolamine, etc.)
- opioids.

Diuretics, by contributing to dehydration, can be responsible for the feeling of oral dryness. Diabetes may be a further underlying cause of xerostomia.

Question 8. What measures can relieve xerostomia?

One of the first steps should be to review medications.[4] The patient and caregivers can also be educated about simple strategies that can bring appreciable relief.[2,22–24] Mrs H. should be advised to:

- Implement regular oral hygiene.
- Keep her mouth moist by sucking on ice cubes, ice lollies (popsicles), or semi-frozen/frozen fruit juice or tonic water.
- Take small sips of liquid (e.g. water, juices, or soft drinks). Keep fluids at bedside (within easy reach).
- Use a water spray. This is particularly useful in the gravely ill.
- Try saliva substitutes. Most preparations contain either mucin or methylcellulose (CMC).[2,4] These can be used as often as necessary, but their effect is of limited duration and some patients do not like the sensation or taste.
- Stimulate the production of saliva, using sugarless gum and sugar-free sweets (candy) or sialagogues, such as pilocarpine drops or tablets (administered 30 minutes before meal), if other measures do not prove sufficient.

Alternative therapies such as acupuncture merit further attention as some studies have shown that it could be an interesting option.[2,25,26]

Other measures that may be taken to relieve xerostomia include:

- Maintain room humidity.
- Take advantage of dietary tips such as softening food with milk, broth, gravy, melted margarine, or butter. Olive oil swabbed onto the mucosa can act as a lubricant.[2]
- Puree foods.
- Avoid foods such as dry crackers or cereal.
- Avoid tobacco and alcohol.

You explain to Mrs H. that although amitryptiline was a good suggestion, it is advisable to switch to another medication given her complaint of xerostomia. Any of the newer selective serotonin-reuptake inhibitors (SSRIs) would be less likely to contribute to mouth dryness, but the literature on their efficacy in neuropathic pain is scarce and they are generally not recommended (see Chapter 3). The use of desipramine or nortryptiline, tricyclics with less anticholinergic properties, would also be reasonable alternatives from the same medication class. Several other analgesic medications can be helpful in relieving neuropathic pain. You agree to re-assess the situation at your next encounter.

***

One week ago, Mrs H. commenced radiotherapy to her lower cervical spine and left breast and axilla areas. She now presents with a painful burning mouth and throat, which is worse with swallowing. On examination, you note that her dental caries has not yet been treated. Her lips appear normal, but the left corner of her mouth is slightly inflamed. The gingiva show no evident inflammation, but the entire oral mucosa is reddened and bears several white curdy patches which bleed slightly when scraped gently with a tongue depressor. Her tongue is also dry and reddened and also has similar white patches. The saliva is sparse and thick. You conclude that Mrs H. has acute stomatitis with signs of oral candidosis.

Question 9. How would you characterize stomatitis?

The terms mucositis and stomatitis are often used interchangeably to describe a state of mucosal irritation.[27] However, the term mucositis is usually reserved to describe the cytotoxic reaction due to chemotherapy or radiotherapy. Stomatitis can have multiple causes including infections.[11]

Question 10. What are the predisposing factors for candidiasis? Which of these does Mrs H. have?

Candidiasis (candidosis)[4,28–30]

Fungal infections are common in patients with cancer or HIV/AIDS. *Candida albicans* is the pathogen most frequently isolated. However, other *Candida* species can also be found. Although less frequently involved, *Aspergillus* species can also be responsible for oral fungal infections.

The major risk factors for candidiasis are:

- poor oral hygiene
- xerostomia
- immunosuppression
- corticosteroids
- broad-spectrum antibiotics
- poor nutritional status
- diabetes (and other systemic diseases)
- denture wear

Mrs H. has four of these predisposing factors.

Question 11. How would you diagnose oral candidiasis?

Clinical manifestations

Oral candidiasis has several different clinical manifestations

Pseudomembranous form (thrush).

Thrush is characterized by white or yellowish plaques (pseudomembranes) that can be wiped off, revealing an underlying erythematous mucosa. It can be found on any oral surfaces but the palate, buccal mucosa, and dorsal surface of the tongue are the most common sites.

Acute erythematous form (acute atrophic candidiasis).

Patients with this form demonstrate painful erythematous and atrophic areas which are most often found on the palate or dorsal surface of the tongue.

Chronic atrophic (erythematous) candidiasis

This form, also called 'denture stomatitis', is manifested by chronic erythema, oedema, and small erosions or plaques with a velvety texture. It is found characteristically on the hard palate where the upper denture fits but it can also affect other mucosal surfaces.

Chronic hyperplastic candidiasis

This variant may resemble leucoplakia, with white or discoloured plaques that cannot be wiped off. Common sites are the buccal mucosal near the commissures or the laterodorsal surface of the tongue. It is often associated with a painful burning sensation.

Angular cheilitis

In patients with this form of candidiasis, erythematous fissures are seen at the corners of the mouth. *Staphylococcus aureus* can also be a contributing pathogen.

Diagnosis

Clinical evaluation of the oral mucosa is often sufficient in the diagnosis of candidiasis. If laboratory proof is required, stained smears from the lesions may demonstrate characteristic hyphae. However, colonization shown in culture (hyphae) does not unequivocally confirm infection because *C. albicans* can be a normal inhabitant of oral flora. Nevertheless cultures can be important to confirm diagnosis of an acute erythematous form of candidal infection.

Question 12. Explain the treatment for candidiasis and what you would recommend for Mrs H.

Pseudomembranous and erythematous forms can be treated both topically and systematically. Hyperplastic candidiasis necessitates systemic agents. Angular cheilitis is best treated with antifungal ointments, sometimes used alternately with antibiotic ointment. The patient should be encouraged to maintain good oral hygiene. A variety of topical agents may be helpful in treating the infection.

Nystatin is used as a swish–swallow suspension; 200 000—500 000 IU may be given three to five times daily. To be effective, prolonged contact with the mucosa is needed. Nystatin ice cubes can be made up by adding water to the nystatin suspension and freezing it. However, the high sugar content of this preparation can lead to dental caries from prolonged use. An alternative is the oral use of nystatin lozenges (200 000 IU) or nystatin vaginal tablets (100 000 IU). Dissolve tablets in the mouth three to five times daily.

Clotrimazole lozenges can be administered topically three to five times daily. If lozenges are not available, the vaginal tablet form can be used. Dissolve the tablet in the mouth three to five times daily.

> You prescribe nystatin oral suspension 500 000 IU four times daily, to be 'swished and swallowed'. It should be swished for several minutes and then swallowed to prevent oesophageal spread. Mrs H. is to telephone you in 5 days (sooner if need be) if her infection has not improved.

The majority of oral candidal infections will resolve within 7–14 days with nystatin oral suspension. More severe cases, which are seen in more immunosuppressed patients (post-chemotherapy, post-radiotherapy, or with AIDS), will require more expensive and potentially more toxic systemic agents:

- fluconazole 100–200 mg on the first day followed by 50–100 mg daily by mouth for 7–14 days
- itraconazole 100–200 mg daily by mouth for 7–14 days (solution can be swished in the mouth before swallowing)
- ketoconazole 200–400 mg daily by mouth for 7–14 days.

Azole compounds are CYP-450 inhibitors and may cause drug–drug interactions such as accumulation of methadone, which can be life threatening.

Although further studies are warranted, a fluconazole rinse (suspension of 2 mg/ml of fluconazole in distilled water) may become a useful option to consider. In one study, fluconazole 2 mg/ml (in distilled water) used three times a day (as a rinse and spit solution) for 1 week provided complete symptomatic and clinical relief in a majority of patients.[31]

Recurrent candidiasis, particularly in the immunocompromised patient, could be managed with a prophylactic administration of oral fluconazole 50 mg/day.[32]

> A few months later, Mrs H. reconsidered her choices and opted for chemotherapy. A dental evaluation led to the extraction of two lower teeth followed by a broad-spectrum antibiotic for 2 weeks. She received chemotherapy and you are asked to see her again in hospital to offer suggestions to relieve the distress caused by the development of severe mucositis. Her blood counts have returned to just above 50 per cent of normal and she has a fever. When you see her, you find that her pain is so severe that she can barely speak. It is almost impossible for her to swallow her saliva, and total parenteral nutrition has been started. The oral examination is difficult to perform because of her severe distress. Although she can barely open her mouth, you are able to identify swollen inflamed gingiva with pyorrhoea and several ulcers on both buccal walls and the sides of her tongue.

Question 13. What is the cause of Mrs H.'s pain?

Pain[11,22,33–37]

Some forms of chemotherapy result in severe mucositis by a direct cytotoxic effect on oral mucosa because of cessation of epithelial replication. In addition, myelosuppression increases the patient's susceptibility to infections (bacterial, fungal, or viral). The oral cavity is a documented common source of septicaemia in neutropenic patients.

The common causes of oral pain are:

- xerostomia
- radiotherapy-induced mucositis
- chemotherapy-induced mucositis
- chemotherapy-induced neurotoxicity
- infections
- mechanical (ill-fitting dentures)
- idiopathic (aphthous ulcers).

Question 14. What would you recommend to manage Mrs H.'s severe pain?

This is a pain emergency! Mrs H. has severe stomatitis secondary to the cytotoxic effect of the chemotherapy and a superimposed mixed infection. This condition can cause severe pain and compromise nutrition and communication, increasing the patient's distress. Several approaches to the prevention and treatment of this condition (colony-stimulating factors, cytokine therapy) are currently being investigated but, at present, palliation remains the cornerstone of the approach.[37] A comprehensive approach should include:

- identification of all possible causes of oral pain
- reduction of factors that could contribute to further irritation
- modification of basic oral hygiene measures as tolerated
- active treatment of infections (fungal, viral, bacterial) if present or suspected (obtain cultures)
- analgesics, both topical and systemic.

Topical analgesics can be used alone or in combination with coating agents mixed in a 1:1 ratio. Most institutions have their own favourite mixture (Table 26.2). The relative efficacy of these preparations has not been solidly established. Because topical local anaesthetics may interfere with swallowing and epiglottic reflexes, food should not be taken for 60 min after application. An oral rinse with a morphine solution (15 ml of 2% morphine solution used six times a day) can also be tried.[38,39] Patients are instructed to hold the mouthwash for 2 min and then spit it out. Additional studies are currently underway to determine the optimal treatment regimen.

With severe mucositis, topical agents alone may not relieve the pain adequately. In these cases, a systemic opioid should be used in combination with local approaches.

Because Mrs H. has such difficulty in swallowing, opioid should be administered parenterally, either subcutaneously or intravenously; intermittent administration or continuous infusion are both reasonable options. At the same time, the dietician should meet with the patient to advise a soft and liquid diet best suited to her taste and ability to swallow. Once the acute phase resolves, a switch to oral opioids, non-steroidal anti-inflammatory drugs, or transdermal opioids and gradual tapering of local anaesthetics can be considered.

Other common oral problems in cancer or AIDS patients

Bacterial infections[37,40,41]

Bacterial infections in the mouth usually present as odontogenic, gingival, or mucosal infections. In patients receiving chemotherapy, they usually occur when myelosuppression is maximal (7–14 days after the initiation of chemotherapy). The usual signs of infection can be absent in granulocytopenic patients. The presence of pain, lesions, and fever should make one suspect an oral infection. Mixed infections can be present, justifying the use of broad spectrum antibiotics.

Necrotizing ulcerative periodontitis[42,43]

This bacterial infection, mainly seen in persons with HIV infection and AIDS, is characterized by a rapid localized destruction of alveolar bone and periodontal tissue. It is frequently associated with severe immune suppression. It presents with deep-seated pain, spontaneous gingival bleeding, and halitosis. Recommended treatment is scaling of affected areas (if possible), institution

Table 26.2 Oral care agents and mixtures

Topical anaesthetic or anti-inflammatory agents

- Methylcellulose-related mixtures
- Lidocaine viscous 2 per cent% 15 ml given every q 3–4 h up to a maximum 120 ml/day
- Lidocaine spray 10 per cent%
- Dyclonine oral lozenges or oral solutions 0,5% or 1%; not to be swallowed
- Benzydamide
- Diphenhydramine (The injectable or paediatric preparations do not contain alcohol)

Caution: Topical anaesthetic agents can cause irritation and suppress the gag reflex

Coating agents

- Antacid supension
- Sucralfate suspension or chewable tablets
- Attapulgite (Kaopectate)

Milk of magnesia should not be used as a vehicle as it can further increase mucosal dessication.

Miscellaneous mixtures

- Diphenhydramine–lidocaine (described below)
- Magic mouthwash (described below)
- Alcohol-free mouthwash–diphenhydramine (1:1 mixture)
- Diphenhydramine–magnesium hydroxide or aluminium hydroxide (1:1 mixture)

Diphenhydramine–lidocaine solution[22]

1.5 ml diphenhydramine injectable 50 mg/ml + 45 ml xylocaine viscous 2% + 45 ml magnesium aluminium hydroxide. Swish and hold 15 ml in mouth for 30 s

Magic mouthwash

153 ml diphenhydramine HCL 12.5 mg/5ml (382 mg) +
1.25 ml hydrocortisone sodium succinate 50 mg/ml (62.5 mg) + 38.75 ml nystatin oral suspension 100,000 units/cc (3,875,000 units)
Add sterile water to make a total of 500 ml.
Swish and hold 15 ml in mouth for 30 s

of systemic antibiotics (metronidazole 500 mg at once, followed by 250 mg four times daily), and the use of topical chlorhexidine.

Linear gingival erythema[42,43]

Another common gingival problem in immunocompromised people living with HIV/AIDS presents as a localized erythematous area(s) on the marginal gingiva associated with spontaneous bleeding. This bacterial infection, formerly referred to as HIV-associated gingivitis, can best be controlled with an antibacterial mouth rinse and scaling of affected areas.

Viral infections[30,37,40–43]

Herpes simplex infection (HSV-1)

Herpes simplex is a common oral viral infection in patients receiving chemotherapy or head and neck radiation. Reactivation of latent virus in a patient who has been previously exposed is the usual situation. It is commonly seen in severely immunocompromised patients (e.g. with leukaemia, AIDS, or following bone marrow transplantation).

Herpetic lesions usually appear late (18 days) following the start of chemotherapy. This timing can help distinguish this infection from direct chemostomatoxicity (5–7 days) and bacterial oral infection (7–14 days). Clinically, the lesions (small tense vesicles rapidly followed by ulcerations) are usually found on the fixed mucosa (hard palate, gingiva). They often look bland and lack specific identifiying characteristics. They can coalesce, form large ulcerations, appear haemorrhagic, and be covered by pseudomembranes. Extra-oral lesions may not be present. In the immunocompromised patient, severe herpetic ulcerations can be found on any or all mucosal surfaces and can become secondarily infected. The diagnosis of herpetic stomatitis is made from the clinical findings and laboratory tests, including viral culture, smears (to detect nuclear viral inclusions), and immunological tests.

Systemic antiviral agents are recommended for the treatment of severe oral HSV-1 infection in immunocompromised individuals as follows:

- oral acyclovir 200–400 mg five times daily for 7–10 days or more
- intravenous acyclovir 5.0 mg/kg every 8 h for 7 days
- oral famciclovir 500 mg twice daily for 7 days (approved for AIDS patients)
- foscarnet in cases of aciclovir-resistant strains (we recommend consultation with an infectious disease specialist).

Cytomegalovirus infection (HHV-5)

HIV patients with CD4+ counts <50–100/ml are at risk of reactivation of latent cytomegalovirus. This acute oral infection manifests itself as gingivitis and large erythematous ulcers.

Epstein–Barr virus (EBV) infection [oral hairy leucoplakia (OHL)]

This infection is characterized by the development of asymptomatic vertically corrugated white hyperkeratotic lesions usually found on the lateral border of the tongue. OHL can be confused with candidiasis (thrush), but typically the lesions in OHL cannot be wiped off and they have a characteristic vertical pattern. Although asymptomatic, these lesions can cause a cosmetic problem. Tretinoin gel (0.025–0.05 per cent) can be used twice daily and will cause exfoliation of the lesions.

Bleeding mouth[11,15,37,44]

Bleeding gums are a frequent problem in advanced leukaemia, and are psychologically (often more than physically) very distressing to some patients and families. Spontaneous bleeding rarely occurs if platelet counts are >20 000 cells/mm^3.

Regular basic oral hygiene can be continued if platelet counts are >50 000 cells/mm^3 and white blood cell counts are >1000 cells/mm^3. If counts are lower, patients can be advised to use a moist 2 × 2 gauze or a foam stick moistened in water instead of a toothbrush.

Localized therapies include the use of haemostatic dressings or products:

- absorbable gelatin (Gelfoam™), available in powder or compressed pack form
- thrombin (Thrombostat^{MD}) in powdered form can be sprinkled over the bleeding sites or a gauze impregnated by a thrombin solution (100 U/ml) can be applied with pressure to the bleeding site
- collagen clot-forming agents
- tranexamic acid (50 mg/ml) as a mouthwash.

The systemic administration of an inhibitor of fibrinolysis such as aminocaproic acid or tranexamic acid might be useful. The small (<0.5%) risk of thrombotic events (renal, cerebral, etc.) can be justified in view of the discomfort caused by the bleeding.

In certain circumstances, when oral bleeding is causing a great deal of distress or is complicated by epistaxis, platelet transfusion might be helpful. Because of the limited lifespan of the transfused platelets, transfusions might be needed every few days. It is also important to take into account that platelet transfusions often cause unpleasant febrile reactions.

AIDS-related malignancy

Kaposi's sarcoma[45,46]

This form of angiosarcoma, which is characterized by red, bluish, or purplish macular nodular lesions, is found very frequently in AIDS patients. Studies in oral medicine have reported oral mucosal manifestations in >50 per cent of patients with a diagnosis of Kaposi's sarcoma.

It is usually asymptomatic, but some lesions may be associated with ulceration and spontaneous bleeding. They can cause pain if located on the hard palate or gingiva, and occasionally can interfere with deglutition. In these cases, laser therapy or radiation therapy can be very helpful. Other treatment modalities include intralesional injection of chemotherapeutic agents or interferon-α.

Acknowledgements

We are indebted to Dr Michael Wiseman and Dr Marcel Boisvert for their participation as authors of the chapter on mouth care in the first edition. Their contributions are reflected in both the style and content of this chapter in the second edition

Bibliography

Sonis, S.T., and Fey, E.G. (2002) Oral complications of cancer therapy. *Oncology,* **16**, 680–6.

Ventafridda, V., Ripamonti, C., Sbanotto, A., and De Conno, F. (2004) Mouth care. In: Doyle, D., Hanks, G., and MacDonald, N. (eds) *Oxford Textbook of Palliative Medicine* (4th edn). Oxford: Oxford University Press, 673–87.

References

1. **Baum, B.J.** (1981) Evaluation of stimulated parotid saliva flow rate in different age groups. *J Dent Res,* **60**, 1292–6.
2. **Diaz-Arnold, A.M., and Marek, C.A.** (2002) The impact of saliva on patient care: a literature review. *J Prosthet Dent,* **8**, 337–432.
3. **Mandel, I.D.** (1987) Functions of saliva. *J Dent Res,* **66S**, 623–7.
4. **Sweeney, M.P., and Bagg, J.** (2000) The mouth and palliative care. *Am J Hosp Palliat Care,* **17**, 118–24.
5. **Spielman, A.I.** (1990) Interaction of saliva and taste. *J Dent Res,* **69**, 838–43.
6. **Jobbins, J., Bagg, J., Finlay, I.G., Addy, M., and Newcombe, R.G.** (1992) Oral and dental disease in terminally ill cancer patients. *BMJ,* **304**, 1612.
7. **Aldred, M.J., Addy, M., Bagg, J., and Finlay, I.** (1991) Oral health in the terminally ill: a cross-sectional pilot survey. *Spec Care Dentist,* **11**, 59–62.
8. **Greenwood, I., Zakrzewska, J.M., and Robinson, P.G.** (2002) Changes in the prevalence of HIV-associated mucosal disease at a dedicated clinic over 7 years. *Oral Dis,* **8**, 90–4.
9. **Glass, R.T., and Lare, M.M.** (1986) Toothbrush contamination: a potential health risk. *Quintessence Int,* **17**, 39–42.
10. **Krishnasamy, M.** (1995). The nurse's role in oral care. *Eur J Palliat Care,* **2**, 8–9.

11. **Chambers, M.S., Toth, B.B., Martin, J.W., Fleming, T.J., and Lemon, J.C.** (1995) Oral and dental management of the cancer patient: prevention and treatment of complications. *Support Care Cancer,* **3**, 168–75.
12. **Emilson, C.G.** (1977) Susceptibility of carious micro-organisms to chlorhexidine. *Scand J Dent Res,* **85**, 255–65.
13. **Ferretti, G.A., Brown, A.T., Raybould, T.P., and Lillich, T.T.** (1990) Oral antimicrobial agents—chlorhexidine. *NCI Monogr,* **9**, 51–5.
14. **FDI Commission** (2002) Mouthrinses and periodontal disease. *Int Dent J,* **52**, 346–52.
15. **Majorana, A., Schubert, M.M., Porta, F., Ugazio, A.G., and Sapelli, P.L.** (2000) Oral complications of pediatric hematopoietic cell transplantation: diagnosis and management. *Support Care Cancer,* **8**, 353–65.
16. **Foote, R.L., Loprinzi, C.L., Frank, A.R., *et al.*** (1994) Randomised trial of a chlorhexidine mouthwash for alleviation of radiation-induced mucositis. *J Clin Oncol,* **12**, 2630–3.
17. **American Medical Association** (1975) *AMA Drug Evaluation* (2nd edn). Acton, MA: Publishing Sciences Group.
18. **Van Drimmelen, J., and Rollins, H.F.** (1969) Evaluation of a commonly used oral hygiene agent. *Nurs Res,* **18**, 327–32.
19. **Leung, A.K.C., Robson, W.L., Gung, G.W.T., and Barsky, R.L.** (1995) Halitosis. *Ann R Coll Physicians Surg Can,* **28**, 213–16.
20. **Atkinson, J.C., and Fox, P.C.** (1992) Salivary gland dysfunction. *Clin Geriatr Med,* **8**, 499–511.
21. **Vissink, A., Johannes's-Gravenmade, E., Panders, A.K., and Vermey, A.** (1988) The causes and consequences of hyposalivation. *Ear Nose Throat J,* **67**, 179–85.
22. **Barker, G., Barker, B., and Gier, R.** (1992) *Oral Management of the Cancer Patient—A Guide for the Health Care Professional* (4th edn). Kansas City, KS: Biomedical Communications.
23. **Pray, W.S.** (1994) Dry mouth syndrome: causes and treatment. *US Pharm,* **19**, 16–24.
24. **Greenspan, D.** (1990) Management of salivary dysfunction. *NCI Monogr,* **9**, 159–61.
25. **Johnstone, P.A., Niemtzow, R.C., and Riffenburgh, R.H.** (2002) Acupuncture for xerostomia: clinical update. *Cancer,* **94**,1151–6.
26. **Rydholm, M., and Strang, P.** (1999) Acupuncture for patients in hospital-based home care suffering from xerostomia. *J Palliat Care,* **15**, 20–3.
27. **Specht, L.** (2002) Oral complications in the head and neck radiation patient. Introduction and scope of the problem. *Support Care Cancer,* **10,** 36–9.
28. **Garber, G.E.** (1994) Treatment of oral candida mucositis infections. *Drugs,* **47**, 734–40.
29. **Lynch, D.P.** (1994) Oral candidiasis. History, classification, and clinical presentation. *Oral Surg Oral Med Oral Pathol,* **78**, 189–93.
30. **Pallasch, T.J.** (2000) Antifungal and antiviral chemotherapy. *Periodontology,* **28**, 240–55.
31. **Epstein, J.B., Gorsky, M., and Caldwell, J.** (2002) Fluconazole mouthrinses for oral candidiasis in postirradiation, transplant, and other patients. *Oral Surg Oral Med Oral Pathol Oral Radiol. Endod,* **93**, 671–5.
32. **Regnard, C., Allport, S., and Stephenson, L.** (1997) ABC of palliative care. Mouth care, skin care, and lymphoedema. *BMJ,* **315**, 1002–5.
33. **McCarthy, G.M., and Skillings, J.R.** (1992) Orofacial complications of chemotherapy for breast cancer. *Oral Surg Oral Med Oral Pathol,* **74**, 172–8.
34. **Loprinzi, C.L., Foote, R.L., and Michalak, J.** (1995) Alleviation of cytotoxic therapy-induced normal tissue damage. *Semin Oncol,* **22** (Suppl 3), 95–7.
35. **Bavier, A.R.** (1990) Nursing management of acute oral complications of cancer. *NCI Monogr,* **9**, 123–8.

36. **Miaskowski, C.** (1990) Oral complications of cancer therapies. Management of mucositis during therapy. *NCI Monogr*, **9**, 95–8.
37. **Sonis, S.T., and Fey, E.G.** (2002) Oral complications of cancer therapy. *Oncology*, **16**, 680–6.
38. **Cerchietti, L.C., Navigante, A.H., Bonomi, M.R.,** ***et al.*** (2002) Effect of topical morphine for mucositis-associated pain following concomitant chemoradiotherapy for head and neck carcinoma. *Cancer*, **95**, 2230–6.
39. **Cerchietti, L.C., Navigante, A.H., Korte, M.W.,** ***et al.*** (2003) Potential utility of the peripheral analgesic properties of morphine in stomatitis-related pain: a pilot study. *Pain*, **105**, 265–73.
40. **Sonis, S.T.** (1993) Oral complications. In: Holland JF *et al.* (eds) *Cancer Medicine*, Vol 2. Philadelpha, PA: American cancer society, 2381–8.
41. **Sonis, S., Fazio, R., and Fang, L.** (1995) Oral complications of cancer chemotherapy. In: Sonis, S., Fazio R, and F and L. (eds) *Principles and Practice of Oral Medicine* (2nd edn). Philadelphia, PA: W.B. Saunders, 426–54.
42. **Narani, N., and Epstein, J.B.** (2001) Classifications of oral lesions in HIV infection. *J Clin Periodontol*, **28**, 137–45.
43. **Glick, M.** (ed) (1993) *Clinician's Guide to Treatment of HIV-Infected Patients*. Seattle,WA: American Academy of Oral Medicine.
44. **Perreira, J., Mancini, I., and Bruera, E.** (2000) The management of bleeding in advanced cancer patients. In: Portenoy RK, Bruera E (eds) *Topics in Palliative Care*, Vol 4. Oxford: Oxford University Press, 163–83.
45. **Robertson, P.B., and Greenspan, D.** (eds) (1988) *Perspective on Oral Manifestations of AIDS: Diagnosis and Management of HIV-Associated Infections*. Littleton, MA: PSG Publishing, 86–7.
46. **Convissar, R.A.** (2002) Laser palliation of oral manifestations of human immunodeficiency virus infection. *J Am Dent Assoc*, **133**, 591–8.

Chapter 27

Malignant wounds and pressure ulcers

Valerie Nocent Schulz

Attitude

To enable each student to:

- Recognize the physical, emotional, and functional concerns associated with malignant wounds and pressure ulcers in palliative patients.

Skill

To enable each student to:

- Learn to complete a comprehensive assessment of patients with malignant wounds and pressure ulcers that encompasses the physical, emotional, and functional perspectives of care provision.
- Learn management strategies based on assessment of patients with malignant wounds.
- Learn to adopt the practice of reducing the risk of pressure ulcer formation.
- Learn to assess the common sites of pressure ulcer formation on a regular basis.

Knowledge

To enable students to:

- Describe the classification of malignant wounds.
- Describe concerns common in patients with malignant wounds.
- Assess and manage patients with malignant wounds.
- Describe the pathophysiology of pressure ulcers.
- Understand risk, staging, assessment, and management of pressure ulcers.

Mrs J.L. is a 78-year-old women diagnosed with squamous cell carcinoma of the oral cavity. She underwent a radical neck dissection and adjuvant radiation therapy for positive resection margins 6 months ago. She had no signs of recurrent disease until recently, when she first noted a wound on the right side of her mandible, along the surgical scar. It grew rapidly and began to break down in the centre. Her family physician referred her back to the cancer clinic for an assessment; a biopsy was positive for recurrent squamous cell carcinoma. In addition to her other oncology consultations, she was seen by the palliative care team.

Question 1. What is the definition of a malignant wound? How does it occur? What are the common tumour types that cause malignant wounds?

A malignant wound has been defined as the invasion by cancer into the skin.[1,2] Spread of cancer to the skin is believed to occur along paths of least resistance, including the lymphatic system and blood vessels, along tissue planes, and by implantation (seeding) of malignant cells during procedures or surgery.[3] Malignant wounds most commonly develop in the following tumours:[4]

- primary skin tumours, i.e. basal cell, squamous cell, and malignant melanoma
- breast
- oral cavity
- lung
- ovary
- large intestine
- larynx
- kidney.

Question 2. What is the classification of Mrs J.L.'s malignant wound?

Malignant wounds can be classified according to their appearance (Table 27.1). This classification aids in communication with other health care providers and in predicting the course of disease progression. This classification system[1] was based on case-based literature reports[5] and on clinical experience. The tumour may be nodular, infiltrating subcutaneously, ulcerating, or fungating within the skin or on the surface of a large tumour mass.

Question 3. Mrs J.L. has an ulcerating malignant wound from squamous cell carcinoma of the oral cavity. What are the clinical problems common to patients with malignant wounds?

Patients with malignant wounds are a unique patient population as these wounds behave significantly different from non-malignant wounds. The wound bed is infiltrated with cancer or it is the surface of internal malignancy. Oncologists' attempts to 'cure' or 'control' tumour burden must be complimented by excellence in symptom management for patients with malignant wounds. The most common clinical concerns of these patients are pain, odour, exudate, bleeding, oedema, complications related to the location of the tumour, emotional distress, and social concerns.[1–3,5,8–15] Individual patients generally experience some but not all of these symptoms.

It is essential that patients with malignant wounds have an opportunity for the highest quality of life as the average life expectancy ranges from 1 to 3 months for gastric, gallbladder, and bile duct cancers, 18 months for colon and rectum carcinomas, and 31 months for breast cancer, the most common tumour site metastasizing to skin.[16] Therefore patients will potentially require wound care for extended periods of time.

Table 27.1 Classification of malignant wounds based on wound appearance

Malignant wound classification	Wound types within the classification
Nodules and induration	Subcutaneous nodules
Subcutaneous spread: four phases[5] of progressive increase in contiguous spread of malignancy within the skin	1. Carcinoma erysipeloides: biopsy reveals carcinoma in the dermis or lymphatics plus inflammation;[5] the tumour appears as cellulitis, but the inflammation and erythema is not cellulitis 2. Carcinoma *en cuirasse*: a phase of induration as the skin and subcutaneous tissue harden, appearing as dry flat indurated skin; the tumour often grows to involve large body surface areas, spreading extensively 3. Elephantiasic skin changes: dermal stasis, hyperkeratosis, and papillomatosis[5] appearing as thick raised indurated skin 4. Schirrhous dermal reaction: similar to morphea,[5] appearing as localized scleroderma
Fungating and ulcerating wounds	1. Fungating wounds have characteristics of both proliferation and ulceration. Inadequate blood supply to support the entire fungating mass results in infarcts, necrosis, and sloughing of the tumour, creating ulcers within the fungating mass. It occurs most commonly in breast cancer, but also in lung, stomach, head and neck, uterus, kidney, ovary, colon, bladder, melanoma, and lymphoma[5] 2. Ulcerating malignant wounds without features of a fungating mass occur in head and neck tumours, bowel, lymphoma,[4,6] squamous cell, and basal cell carcinoma,[6] amongst others. The ulcerating process can be so aggressive that fistulae develop from the wound into the underlying visceral cavity (e.g. oral cavity, pharynx, or bowel)
Other	1. Zosteriform lesions, which have a similar appearance to herpes zoster, result from perineural lymphatic spread of malignancy[7] 2. Wounds with mixed appearances

Question 4. How will you assess Mrs J.L.'s malignant wound?

A thorough patient assessment is the cornerstone of investigation and management of patients with malignant wounds. A patient assessment based on common concerns is beneficial[1,3,9,10,13,17] and will help in guiding management. The Malignant Wound Assessment Tool[1,2] was designed to be a comprehensive assessment for patients with malignant wounds. The first iteration of that tool is the Schulz Malignant Wound Assessment Tool (S-MWAT) (Fig. 27.1) which permits recording of patient demographic information, oncology diagnosis and treatment, symptoms, physical examination, and management.

> Mrs J.L.'s S-MWAT revealed that she had prior surgery and radiation and does not have other metastases. She first noted the wound 2 months earlier and it has been growing rapidly, doubling in size each month. She is taking care of the wound herself, changing gauze dressing three times daily, and is reluctant to wash it. She is conscious of the appearance of the wound dressing and no longer goes out of the house.

Continued

Mrs J.L. has been a 40 pack-year smoker and consumed alcohol regularly. She has chronic lung disease, ischaemic heart disease and hepatic cirrhosis. She has pain and bleeding in her wound only with dressing changes. Mrs J.L. has good support from her family and friends, but has had no assistance with managing the wound from health care providers. She is not depressed, but is embarrassed and afraid of the future. The return of cancer in such an obvious location bothers her the most. Since surgery, she has had difficulty opening her mouth normally, although she can eat some foods and drinks liquids quite well. On examination, she has a shallow ulcer that is 75% covered with adherent necrotic tissue with areas of bleeding from the removal of the adherent gauze, causing increased pain. The wound edges are flat, there is no odour, and the wound is moist with serous exudate that drips onto her clothing. It is located along the incision line, just above the angle of the jaw on her right. It measures 2.5 cm × 1.0 cm × 0.5 cm and the peri-wound skin appears pale, consistent with previous surgery and radiation. (Note: Dimensions are universally stated as length × width × depth.)

Question 5. How will you manage Mrs J.L. and her malignant wound?

In keeping with a palliative care approach, patients with malignant wounds are best managed by focusing on the uniqueness of each individual[8,9,15] to improve quality of life.[8,18] Oncology care is a balance between toxicity and benefit. It includes optimizing symptom management and offering appropriate chemotherapy, radiation therapy, photodynamic therapy, and surgery. There is a paucity of evidence-based treatment strategies.[10] Most of the published management strategies comprise case-based reports.[19] Impeccable symptom management should aim at reducing physical, functional, social, and emotional concerns.[1,20,21] The patient's primary concerns provide a starting point for treatment.[21] General principles of benign wound care have been cautiously adapted to patients with malignant wounds.[8,10]

Management of clinical problems for patients with malignant wounds[22]

Pain

Pain during dressing changes Pain caused by adherent dressings (dressings stuck to the wound bed) can be reduced by using non-adherent dressings[8–10] such as gels, moisture barriers, skin protectant pastes (use in dry wounds), calcium alginates (use in moist or bleeding wounds), contact layers such as silicone-based dressings (for painful dry or moist wound beds), foams and composite dressings, and hydrofibres (moist wounds). Appropriate adhesive dressings will stay in place without adhering to the wound bed.

Pain on exposure to air can be reduced by using saline or sterile water at a comfortable temperature prepared to cover the exposed wound. Also consider premedication prior to dressing changes.

Pain often occurs around the wound in the peri-wound skin. The skin can be compromised by subcutaneous infiltration of tumour, cellulitis, repeated dressing applications, previous surgery, radiation, and maceration from wound exudate. Therefore the peri-wound skin should be protected and treated. Potential options include barrier film sprays, ointments and creams, skin protectant pastes, mesh to hold dressings to avoid tape, adhesive removers to remove adhesive dressings, and placing a hydrocolloid around the wound to which the tape can be attached. Attempt to prevent peri-wound skin problems.

Date_______________________________ Chart Number_______________________

Name_______________________________________Date of Birth_______________

Cancer Diagnosis +/– recurrence____

When was wound first noted___________________ Rate of change/month_____________
Chemotherapy, Radiation, Surgery____

Past Medical History____

Meds Allergies

Symptom	Patient Report	Exam
Pain	How servere? Pain feels like?	Location: in wound____around wound___ With or between dressing changes?
Odour	Does it smell?	Describe: Odour Cause
Exudate	How much drainage? Do dressings work?	Amount Appearance
Bleeding	Contant or occasionally?	Location Quantity
Oedema	Any swelling?	(Circle) in, around, distal to wound Location
Function Change	Head and neck, extremities...	
Social	Does it affect social activities? Describe support from: Healthcare Family Friends	
Emotion	How does the wound make you feel? anxiety, depression, embarrassed, fear, frustration	
What bothers patient most?		
Wound bed % Pink % necrotic tissue, Describe		
Wound Location		
Classification (Circle) Subcutaneous Fungating Nodules Ulcers Zosteriform		
Measurement (Circle) Tracing Photograph Record measurements [cm -/× *w* × *d* (*h*)]		
Peri-wound skin Describe treatment effects from surgery, radiation, dressings...		
Management Previous_______________________________ Suggested		

Fig. 27.1 Schulz Malignant Wound Assessment Tool

Pain between dressing changes may be related to cancer pain or infection. It is important to find the cause and treat appropriately.

Odour from the wound

Always treat odour if it concerns the patient.

Odour from tumour necrosis can be reduced by regular wound cleaning and showering; normal saline, sterile water, and wound-cleansing products are useful. General measures to control odour include charcoal[8,10] within or on top of absorbent dressings, frequent dressing changes, bedding changes, and adequate ventilation. Autolytic or chemical debridement may reduce the amount of odour-producing necrotic tissue. Consider debridement of loose necrotic slough where the wound bed will not be disrupted. Avoid aggressive surgical debridement as abnormal blood vessels in malignant tissue may bleed profusely.

Wound infections are common and may occur with odour (e.g. infection in the wound bed) or without odour (e.g. cellulitis and abscess). Treatment of wound infections includes:

- cleanse the wound
- obtain a wound swab
- antimicrobials
- consult the surgeon if the patient appears to have an abscess.

Cleansing may include dilute acetate soaks (vinegar) in wounds with *Pseudomonas* spp and Iodosorb (cadexomer–iodine) as an effective topical disinfectant. Review the antibiotic of choice following recommendations in the benign wound infection literature.[23] Topical antibiotics have been used for mild wound infections without cellulitis; topical metronidazole gel, silver sulphadiazine (flamazine), bacitracin, fucidin, polysporin, and antifungals have been used where appropriate. However, a literature review of topical metronidazole in fungating wounds[24] reported that no randomized controlled trials were found to determine delivery method, dose, and length of treatment or effectiveness in odour reduction. The use of topical antibiotics is only supported with case-based literature. Systemic antibiotics should be used for significant infections.

We have obtained wound swabs and provided prophylactic topical antibiotics for patients receiving chemotherapy where neutropenia is anticipated. Wound culture results are then available if neutropenic sepsis develops.

Exudate

Potential causes of exudate include exudate-producing tumours, thick necrotic slough, infection, and fistulae. Treat the cause directly if possible.

Quantify the amount of exudate as moist, moderate, large, or copious amounts of exudate. Manage exudate with non-adherent dressings. Evaluate the dressing's ability to control the exudate,[11] as the absorbency of the dressing should correspond to the quantity of exudate. Absorbent dressings include foams, composite dressings, alginates and hydrofibres, wound fillers, and pouches. Dressings with salt have been shown to help dry a wound; however, they must be evaluated for risk of adherence.[12]

The quality of the exudate can be described as:[22]

- serous (clear or golden)
- serosanguinous (thin blood tinge)
- sanguinous (bloody)

- purulent (thick yellow or tan)
- brown exudate.

Bleeding

Management of bleeding in a malignant wound is directed at resolving the cause.[8,10,22]

Bleeding is most commonly related to abnormal tumour vasculature. This bleeding is typically controlled with non-adherent dressings so that it is not promoted, gentle pressure, and calcium alginates with coagulant properties. If necessary, bleeding may be reduced with topical haemostatic agents (e.g. thrombostatin on small vessels), radiation therapy, or surgery as tolerated. If coagulation abnormalities exist, treat accordingly. Tranexamic acid is an antifibrinolytic agent, which increases the risk of thrombosis and disturbances in colour vision. It may be considered if bleeding persists despite first-line treatment and the potential benefits outweigh the potential risks.

Iatrogenic causes of bleeding include adherent dressings (e.g gauze) and anticoagulant therapy. As a general rule, loose woven gauze should only be used in malignant wound beds while cleaning. Re-evaluate the use of anticoagulant therapy if bleeding in the wound bed persists despite appropriate local treatment.

Oedema associated with the wound

The oedema is often located distal to the wound.[22] Clinical experience has demonstrated that gentle compression with massage therapy may be helpful for oedema in extremities. Head and neck oedema from surgery, radiation, and then lymphatic spread of disease with malignant wounds on the neck is usually decreased with elevation of the head 24 h per day, although this needs to be balanced with the increased risk of developing pressure ulcers.

Functional compromise due to the location of the wound

Identify the patient's functional compromise and design patient-specific management aimed at restoring function and controlling the related symptoms; for example, feeding tubes may be placed when fistulae or anatomical changes in the oral cavity prohibit eating and drinking, and reduced mobility of limbs or altered head and neck function may be decreased by management of lymphoedema.

Complications

Fistula formation in malignant wounds is caused by tumour breakdown of the skin, permitting external communication of an internal organ. Fistulae alter normal function and occur most commonly in the head and neck region or on the abdominal wall. Based on clinical experience, some fistula openings in the head and neck region may be covered with occlusive dressings such as hydrocolloid dressings, in addition to reducing saliva with glycopyrrolate, scopolamine patches, or low-dose tricyclic antidepressants if well tolerated. Ostomy appliances can be applied to abdominal wall fistulae, but tend to inflate in the head and neck region. Consider referral to surgical colleagues to review potential closure of the fistula.

Emotional stress and social concerns

The emotional stresses of watching tumour growth, including fear, anxiety, frustration, embarrassment, and depression, are common patient concerns. It is important to acknowledge this stress.[8,10,13] Patients have altered relationships with family, friends, and health care providers, often creating social isolation and dependence on others for management.

Management includes the following.

- Referral for oncology treatment.
- Improve function.
- Effective cosmetically acceptable dressings play a fundamental role in improving emotional well-being. Wound dressings are often a patient's link to society. A cosmetically acceptable dressing, in addition to control of odour, exudate, and bleeding, is required for comfortable socialization. The value of socially acceptable dressings cannot be overemphasized.
- Consider involving the family, social worker, and psychology or psychiatry assistance.

Mrs J.L.'s malignant wound is growing rapidly and so she will need frequent assessments as complications can arise quickly.

The S-MWAT assessment reveals that Mrs J.L. requires adjustments to her wound dressing for the following reasons: she does not have assistance from health care providers; she uses adherent gauze three times a day which does not control her exudate as it leaks onto her clothing; removal of the gauze causes bleeding and pain; she is afraid to clean the wound; the wound dressing is not socially acceptable as she is embarrassed and has changed her social functioning because of its appearance. Therefore initial wound management for Mrs J.L. included involving community nursing, teaching the patient to clean the wound by showering, water, or a wound cleanser, and reducing the number of dressing changes by applying a small cosmetically acceptable self-adhesive foam dressing to control pain, bleeding, and exudate. A calcium alginate can be added under the foam as a wound contact layer if bleeding remains a problem, and a silicone contact layer can be applied against the wound if pain continues with dressing changes.

A change in dressing protocol reduced Mrs J.L.'s symptoms and she increased socializing. She learned to manage the wound herself and this permitted her to take a 4-day vacation to visit close relatives.

Unfortunately, the wound continued to grow at a rapid rate. Two months later, her dressing would become soaked when she drank liquids. Her appetite decreased and she began spending more time in bed. She stated: 'Pain and odour are present most of the time. I feel unwell and I don't want to socialize'.

Question 6. How will you assess and manage Mrs J.L. now? What are your primary concerns for her at this time?

Mrs J.L. is clearly deteriorating. Using the S-MWAT you note that she needs to change her dressings every time she drinks clear fluids. On a visual analogue scale she reports her pain as aching at 4/10 between and during dressing changes, there is a strong smell, with a lot of drainage which is not controlled in the dressing, and this bothers her the most. She is not bleeding or swelling, and she has help from health care and family. However, she can no longer socialize, and she fears that the tumour is growing quickly. On examination, the ulcerating malignant wound has a strong odour, copious purulent exudate from necrotic slough, and infection with cellulitis on the wound edges. The wound is located along the incision line on her face and measures 3.5 cm × 2.0 cm with a fistula in the centre opening into the buccal mucosa; the peri-wound skin is red. Mrs J.L. also has clinical signs of dehydration. Management discussions lead to hospital admission. Laboratory results demonstrated an elevated white blood cell count and a positive wound swab, suggesting wound infection with *Pseudomonas*.

The diagnosis of infection in a chronic wound is first and foremost a clinical skill, as there is no gold standard test for this condition at present. Microbiological data should be used to supplement the clinical diagnosis and not vice versa: '...the simplest and most commonly used method for assessing the presence of infection in a chronic wound is the nonquantitative swab'.[25]

> Appropriate opioids, systemic antibiotics, and rehydration were instituted. The fistula was cleaned, a skin sealant (e.g. No Sting, Skin Prep, Baza Cleanse, Protect, etc.) was applied to protect the peri-wound skin, and an occlusive adhesive non-adherent absorbent dressing was placed over the fistula and changed when saturated. Her diet was changed to thickened fluids. This management reduced the pain, odour, and fistula exudates and improved her effective oral intake.

Infection

Chronic wounds always harbour bacteria. Wound contamination is defined as 'the presence of non-replicating microrganisms within a wound', and wound colonization is defined as 'the presence of replicating microorganisms without host injury'.[25] *Corynebacteria* spp, which are coagulase-negative staphylococci, and viridans streptococci are colonizing flora that impede pathogenic bacteria and accelerate wound healing even under an occlusive moist wound-healing dressing.[25,26]. Wound infection is 'the presence of replicating microorganisms within a wound with subsequent host injury'.[25] Polymicrobial infections are common in chronic wounds; *Staphylococcus aureus* and β-haemolytic streptococci (groups A, B, C, G) tend to be present within the first 4 weeks, and *Enterococcus* spp, Enterobacteriaceae, *Pseudomonas* spp, and anaerobes appear later. Since palliative and chemotherapy patients have a lowered host resistance, they may be more susceptible to wound infection. Signs of infections in non-malignant granulating wounds include:

- cellulitis discharge (exudate)
- delayed healing
- discoloration
- friable granulation tissue which bleeds easily
- unexpected pain
- pocketing at the base of the wound
- superficial bridging of the wound
- abnormal odour
- wound breakdown[27]
- abscess formation.

These clinical signs may be present with or without systemic features of fever, chills, and sepsis. Clinically, these findings are present with infection in malignant as well as non-malignant wounds.

> Upon treatment and resolution of her acute event, open discussions began with Mrs J.L. and her family to determine primary treatment goals. Mrs J.L. requested comfort care, declined feeding tube interventions and further chemotherapy, and requested to be at home as long as possible. She was discharged home with community support. At home Mrs J.L. seldom complains of discomfort; she requires assistance for toileting, shifting positions, and walking. Her time is spent in bed and in her favourite chair. She never eats a complete meal and seldom consumes the dietary supplement provided. Her nurse approaches you, concerned about the risk of Mrs J.L. developing a pressure ulcer.

Question 7. What is a pressure ulcer? Why, when, and where do they develop? What is the pathophysiology of pressure ulcer development?

A pressure ulcer is any lesion caused by unrelieved pressure resulting in damage to underlying tissue.[28] Blood flow is compromised when applied pressure exceeds capillary pressure (20–40 mmHg). Muscle and subcutaneous tissue are more vulnerable to pressure damage than the epidermis. A pressure ulcer is described as 'a localized area of tissue necrosis that develops when soft tissue is compressed between a bony prominence and an external surface for a prolonged period of time'.[29] The most common areas for the development of pressure ulcers are over bony prominences including the occiput, scapulae, shoulders, spine, elbows, greater trochanters, ischial tuberosities, knees, sacrum, coccyx, malleoli, and heels.

Shearing, friction, and moisture also contribute to the development of pressure ulcers. Shearing forces occur when the skin and the skeleton are pulled in different directions. For example, when the head of the bed is elevated >30°, skin and superficial fascia remain adjacent to the bed sheets, while the deep fascia and skeleton are pulled down towards the foot of the bed.[30] Friction from sliding the patient can remove the protective stratum cornum. Moisture from perspiration, wound exudates, urine, or faeces can macerate skin or break it down.

Question 8. What is the risk of Mrs J.L. developing a pressure ulcer?

The Braden Scale for predicting risk of developing pressure ulcers has demonstrated good sensitivity and specificity with excellent inter-rater reliability.[31] It grades six patient characteristics:

1. sensory perception, from completely limited to no impairment
2. moisture, from constantly moist to rarely moist
3. activity, from bedbound to walks frequently
4. mobility, from completely immobile to no limitation to changes in position without assistance
5. nutrition, from very poor to excellent
6. friction and shear, from problem to no apparent problem.

Risk assessment for developing pressure ulcers should be considered when examining a palliative patient.

Question 9. Describe the practice of assessing the common sites of pressure ulcer formation on a regular basis designed for ulcer prevention. How will you reduce the risk of Mrs J.L. developing a pressure ulcer? What will you teach her family?

The Agency for Health Care Policy and Research (AHCRP) guidelines recommend three categories of preventative care for patients at risk of developing pressure ulcers.

1. Skin care and early treatment can be done by patient, family, and health care providers.
   - inspect skin daily, particularly over bony prominences, and avoid massaging in those locations
   - gentle bathing

- moisturize if needed
- protect skin from incontinence
- minimize friction and shearing
- consider protective covering (transparent films)
- optimize nutrition and mobility.

2. Mechanical loading and support surfaces (discussed below)
3. Education
   - The patient benefits from preventative and management education given to the patient him- or herself, family, friends, and bedside health care providers for repetitive timely interventions in the home or institutional settings. Palliative care teams can provide an education package consistent with their available resources that includes: 'etiology, risk factors, risk assessment tools and their application, skin assessment, selection and use of support surfaces, individualized skin care programs, and demonstration of positioning to decrease risk of tissue breakdown'.[32] Include methods to document, evaluate, and institute change.

Protocols for risk reduction have been developed according to the Braden Scale.[31]

- Mild risk (score 15–18): place the patient on a turning schedule; maximal ambulation; protect heels; manage moisture, nutrition, friction, and shear; pressure reduction support surface if bed- or chairbound.
- Moderate risk (score 13–14): mild risk interventions plus turning schedule; lateral turns should be approximately 30° to reduce pressure on bony prominences,[33] and the elevation of the head of the bed should be ≤30° reduce shearing (the 30° rule).
- High risk (score 10–12): mild risk interventions plus facilitate 30° rule and provide small shifts in position every 30 min (e.g. by moving support cushions).
- Very high risk (≤9): mild risk interventions plus consider optimizing pressure reduction surfaces with static air overlay or low-air-loss beds,[34] which are particularly useful for patients with severe pain exacerbated by turning.

Table 27.2 outlines the National Pressure Ulcer Advisory Panel (NPUAP)–AHCPR staging system and management recommendations for pressure ulcers.

Support surfaces are divided into preventative and therapeutic categories. Preventative surfaces are designed to lower the interface pressure. Therapeutic support surfaces distribute pressure more evenly to reduce peak pressure points and optimize capillary blood flow. Because of the force of gravity, no surfaces guarantee pressure below the capillary filling pressure.[35] Table 27.3 provides an overview of support surfaces.

In a setting where such 'high-tech' tools, dressings, and support surfaces are not available, health care providers focus on nursing care with appropriate cleansing, moisture balance in the wound, and turning schedules to reduce shearing forces, friction, and pressure over bony prominences.

> Mrs J.L.'s Braden Scale assessment was: sensory perception, 3 (slightly limited); moisture, 3 (occasionally moist); activity 2 (chairbound); mobility, 2 (very limited); nutrition, 1 (very poor); friction and shear, 2 (potential problem). Her total Braden Scale score was 13. Therefore she is at moderate risk of developing a pressure ulcer. Despite placing her on the appropriate protocol for pressure ulcer risk reduction, Mrs J.L. deteriorates. She states that she is developing low back pain, and on examination of the sacrum you discover a partial-thickness skin loss involving the dermis, resulting in a shallow crater.

Table 27.2 NPUAP–AHCPR staging system and management

Pressure ulcer stage	Description of pressure ulcer[35]	Dressing management[a 36]
Stage 1	Ulcers exhibit observable pressure-related alteration of intact skin with indicators that, compared with the adjacent or opposite area of the body, may include changes in one or more of the following: skin temperature (warmth or coolness), tissue consistency (firm or boggy feel), sensation (pain, itching)	± Film dressing
Stage 2	Ulcers present with partial-thickness skin loss involving epidermis, dermis, or both. The ulcer is superficial and presents clinically as an abrasion, blister, or shallow crater	Transparent film, hydrocolloid, adhesive foam or hydrocellular foam
Stage 3	Ulcers exhibit full-thickness skin loss involving damage to or necrosis of subcutaneous tissue that may extend down to, but not through, underlying fascia. The ulcer presents clinically as a deep crater with or without undermining of adjacent tissue	With exudate: calcium alginates or hydrocellular foam cavity or sheet dressing, or foam dressing, transparent film[b,c] Without exudate: hydrogel/ hydrogel-impregnated film dressing. Consider infection: disinfectant, cadexomer–iodine, or new gauze ribbon may be helpful
Stage 4	Ulcers present with full-thickness skin loss with extensive destruction, tissue necrosis, or damage to muscle, bone, or supporting structures Consider wound care specialist (e.g. tendon, joint capsule).Undermining and sinus tracts may also be associated with stage 4 pressure ulcers	With slough, deep cavity, moderate to heavy exudate: see stage 3 treatment[b,c] and surgical assessment and vacuum assisted closure

[a]Apply risk-reduction strategies for all stages.
[b]Involve a wound specialist for management if initial steps do not promote wound healing or wound progression occurs.
[c]Management during end-of-life care may be symptom management only when healing is not the primary goal.

Question 10. How will you assess Mrs J.L.'s pressure ulcer?

The NPUAP–AHCPR staging system for pressure ulcers (Table 27.2) is a uniform staging system to assist with communication and research. Although it does not have published validity or reliability testing, it is the most universal tool for staging pressure ulcers.[36]

> Mrs J.L. has a stage 2 pressure ulcer, measuring 5 cm × 4 cm × <0.5 cm. It is located over the prominence of the coccyx. It is oval with flat wound edges, 20% of the wound has thin mucoid necrotic tissue, the surrounding skin is normal, and there is granulation but no epithelialization in the wound bed.

Table 27.3 Support surfaces[35]

	Preventative	Therapeutic
Indications	Prevention and treatment of lesser stage wounds	Address needs of patients with advanced stage wounds, burns, and myocutaneous flaps
Mattress replacements	Complete mattress system: foam, air, gel, water, or combination; non-powered or powered	
Mattress overlays	Placed on top of existing mattress; foam, air, gel, water, or combination; non-powered or powered	
Specialty beds		Low-air-loss therapy, powered flotation, alternating pressure, air-fluidized or high-air-loss systems, hybrid support surfaces

Question 11. What are the phases of wound healing? What are the systemic and local factors that affect wound healing?

Wound healing occurs in eight phases: haemostasis, early inflammation, late inflammation, granulation tissue formation, extracellular matrix formation, re-epithelialization, remodelling, and scar formation.

Systemic factors affecting wound healing to varying degrees are age, anaemia, anti-inflammatory drugs, diabetes, systemic infection, jaundice, malignant disease, malnutrition, obesity, temperature, trauma, uraemia, vitamin deficiency, and zinc deficiency.

Local factors affecting wound healing to varying degrees are blood supply, denervation, haematoma, lack of protection, local infection, mechanical stress, radiation suture material, and surgical techniques.[27]

Palliative patients frequently have systemic and local factors that delay healing and the goal becomes preventing deterioration and providing a moist wound-healing environment in the event the ulcers can heal.

Question 12. What dressings are used to treat pressure ulcers? What types of dressing are available for malignant wounds and pressure ulcers?

The dressing selections for healing pressure ulcers are based on the principle of moist wound healing[37] and are described according to staging in Table 27.2. If available, local experts should be involved as many hospitals and regions have wound care specialists versed in dressing selections and wound management guidelines.

Dressings are classified according to categories of dressing function. Some of the most commonly used dressing categories for patients with malignant wounds and pressure ulcers are antimicrobial dressings, alginate dressings, composite dressings, contact layers, creams/oils, enzymes, foam dressings, gauze dressings, hydrocolloid dressings, hydrofibre, hydrogels, skin sealants, transparent film dressings, wound fillers, wound pouches, adhesives, adhesive removers, antibiotics, dressing covers, moisture barrier ointments, creams, skin protectant pastes, and perineal cleansing foams.[37,38]

When learning about wound care products, always ask what category the dressing is in as well as the function of that category.

Mrs J.L.'s functional status declined. She remained at home and her family followed the palliative care suggestions with excellent community support. Her appetite was reduced to tastes of favourite foods. Mrs J.L. was assisted with ambulation to the commode, and provided with thickened nutritional food supplements. Her sacral pressure ulcer was dressed with a hydrocolloid. Her malignant wound and fistula were managed with daily cleansing and skin sealant to protect the peri-wound skin, and either a composite dressing or an adhesive foam dressing was applied across the fistula. Dressings were changed as required if they became saturated.

Her activity declined and her Braden Scale score dropped to 11, placing her at high risk for worsening her pressure ulcers; she was placed on a turning schedule with the 30° rule with foam wedges and incremental position changes. Lifting rather than dragging reduced friction and shear. Her heels developed stage 1 pressure ulcers; heel pressure was eliminated by supporting her calves with a pillow. The heel relief option on a pressure relief mattress would also have been appropriate. Her stage 2 sacral pressure ulcer was cleansed with normal saline and a hydrocolloid dressing was applied. Then, Mrs J.L. developed diarrhoea.

Question 13. Mrs J.L is approaching the end of her life. Her family are becoming exhausted and want the best for her. How will you handle this situation? How will you manage the contamination of her sacral pressure ulcer with diarrhoea?

A family meeting is arranged to review current treatment options. The family requested admission to a palliative care ward because they were exhausted, the care was complicated, and 24-h nursing was not available in their community. *Clostridium difficile* infection was diagnosed as a cause of the diarrhoea. Incontinent products were required. Stool began to undermine the sacral dressing several times a day. Therefore the hydrocolloid dressing was discontinued, a perineal cleansing foam was used after each bowel movement, and a perineal skin protectant paste was reapplied to the clean perineum and pressure ulcer after each bowel movement. Antibiotics were instituted to reduce diarrhoea despite her close proximity to death. Mrs J.L.'s comfort was dependent on attentive nursing care. She died 5 days later with her family at her side. They believed that she had a comfortable death.

Conclusions

Palliative patients are very susceptible to developing pressure ulcers and, not infrequently, malignant wounds. Preventative skin care should be considered essential for all palliative patients. It is easier to prevent than treat pressure ulcers. Patients with malignant wounds require impeccable symptom management in conjunction with oncology care. Assessment is the cornerstone of management strategies and excellence in skin care can improve quality of life in palliative patients.

Future research specific to individuals with malignant and non-malignant wounds is essential to advance wound care. The Malignant Wound Assessment Tool is a specific assessment tool developed with construct and content validity, although reliability studies are still needed. It is a potentially valuable outcome measure for clinical practice and research on this patient population.

Despite wounds being a source of significant distress, there is a paucity of wound assessment and management research specifically in palliative patient populations. Research potential is vast and will guide advances in health care to reduce suffering for palliative patients.

References

1. **Schulz, V.N.** (2002) Cutaneous metastasis and malignant wounds. In: Nabholtz JM, Tonkin K, Reese D, *et al.* (eds) *Breast Cancer Management: Application of Clinical and Translational Evidence to Patient Care* (2nd edn). Philadelphia, PA: Lippincott–Williams and Wilkins, 475–88.
2. **Schulz, V.N., Triska, O.H., and Tonkin, K.** (2001) The development of a malignant wound assessment tool. Unpublished Thesis, University of Alberta, Edmonton, Alberta, Canada.
3. **Naylor, W.** (2002) Malignant wounds: aetiology and principles of management. *Nurs Stand,* **16**, 45–53.
4. **Neel, V.A., and Sober, A.J.** (2003) Other skin cancers In: Kufe D, Pollock R, Weichselbaum R *et al.* (eds) *Cancer Medicine,* Hamilton, Ontario: BC Decker, 1997–2013.
5. **Mortimer, P.S.** (2004) Skin problems in palliative medicine: medical aspects. In: **Doyle, D., Hanks, G., Cherny N, Calman K.** (eds) *Oxford Textbook of Palliative Medicine* (3rd edn) Oxford: Oxford University Press, 618–28.
6. **Swetter, S.M., Smoller, B.R., and Bauer, E.A.** (1995) Cutaneous cancer and malignant melanoma. In: **Abeloff, M., Armitage, J., Lichter, A., and Niederhuber, J.** (eds) *Clinical Oncology,* Vol 3. new York: Churchill Livingstone, 1023–45.
7. **Thiers, B.** (1986) Dermatologic manifestations of internal cancer. *CA Cancer J Clin,* **36**, 130–48.
8. **Haisfield-Wolfe, M.E.** (1997) Malignant cutaneous wounds: a management protocol. *Ostomy/Wound Manage,* **43**, 56–66.
9. **Grocott, P. and Dealey, C.** (2004) Skin problems in palliative medicine: nursing aspects. In: Doyle D, Hanks G, Cherny N, Calman K. (eds) *Oxford Textbook of Palliative Medicine* (3rd edn). Oxford : Oxford University Press, 628.
10. **Fairbairn, K.** (1998) A challenge that requires further research: management of fungating breast lesions. *Prof Nurse,* **9**, 272–7.
11. **Grocott, P.** (1998). Exudate management in fungating wounds. *J Wound Care,* **7**, 445–8.
12. **Upright, C., Salton, C., Roberts, F., and Murphey, J.** (1994) Evaluation of Mesalt dressings and continuous wet saline dressings in ulcerating metastatic skin lesions. *Cancer Nurs,* **17**, 149–55.
13. **Schulz, V.N., Triska, O., and Tonkin, K.** (2002) Malignant wounds: caregiver determined clinical problems. *J Pain Symptom Manage,* **24**, 572–7.
14. **Hallett, N.** (1995) Fungating wounds. *Nurs Times,* **91**, 81–3.
15. **Grocott, P.** (1995) The palliative management of fungating malignant wounds. *J Wound Care,* **4**, 240–2.
16. **Lookingbill, D., Spangler, N., and Helm, K.** (1993) Cutaneous metastases in patients with metastatic carcinoma: a retrospective study of 4020 patients. *J Am Acad Dermatol,* **29**, 228–36.
17. **Naylor, W.** (2001) Assessment and management of pain in fungating wounds. *Br J Nurs* **10** (Suppl), S33–56.
18. **van Leeuween, B.L., Houwerzijl, M., and Hoekstra, H.J.** (2000) Educational tips in the treatment of malignant ulcerating tumours of the skin. *Eur J Surg Oncol,* **26**, 506–8.

19. **Hastings, D.** (1993). Basing care on research. *Nurs Times,* **89**, 70–6.
20. **Collier, M.** (2000) Management of patients with fungating wounds. *Nurs Stand,* **15**, 46–52.
21. **Dowsett, C.** (2002) Malignant fungating wounds: assessment and management. *Br J Community Nurs,* **7**, 394–400.
22. **Schulz, V.N.** (2002) Retrospective review of patients referred to a malignant wound clinic. London Regional Cancer Centre, London, Ontario, Canada (unpublished data).
23. **Finlay, I.G., Bowszyc, J., Ramlou, C., and Gwiezdzinski, Z.** (1996) The effect of topical 0.75% metronidazole gel on malodorous cutaneous ulcers. *J Pain Symptom Manage,* **11**, 158–62.
24. **Clark, J.** (2002) Metronidazole gel in managing malodorous fungating wounds. *Br J Nurs,* **11** (Suppl), S54–60.
25. **Dow, G.** (2001) Infection in chronic wounds. In: Krasner, D., Rodeheaver, G., and Sibbald, R.G. (eds) *Chronic Wound Care* (3rd edn). Wayne, PA: HMP Communications, 343–56.
26. **Hutchinson, J.J., and McGuckin, M.** (1990) Occlusive dressings: a microbiologic and clinical review. *Am J Infect Control,* **18**, 257–68.
27. **Morris, H., Jones, V., and Harding, K.G.** (2001) Wound care: putting theory into practice—the Cardiff Wound Healing Research Unit in the United Kingdom. In: Krasner D, Rodeheaver G, Sibbald RG (eds) *Chronic Wound Care* (3rd edn). Wayne, PA: HMP Communications, 135–44.
28. **Bergstrom, N., Bennett, M.A., Carlson, C.E., *et al.*** (1994) *Clinical Practice Guideline Number 15: Treatment of Pressure Ulcers,* AHCPR Publication 95–0653. Rockville, MD: US Department of Health and Human Services, Agency for Health Care Policy and Research,
29. **National Pressure Ulcer Advisory Panel** (1989) Pressure ulcers: prevalence, cost and risk assessment. Consensus Development Conference Statement. *Decubitus,* **2**, 24.
30. **Krasner, D.** (1997) Pressure ulcers: assessment, classification, and management. In: Krasner D, Rodeheaver G, and Sibbald RG (eds) *Chronic Wound Care* (3rd edn). Wayne, PA: HMP Communications, 152–7.
31. **Braden, B.J.** (2001). Risk assessment in pressure ulcer prevention. In: Krasner D, Rodeheaver G, Sibbald RG (eds) *Chronic Wound Care* (3rd edn). Wayne, PA: HMP Communications, 641–51.
32. **Colburn, L..** (2001) Prevention of chronic wounds. In: Krasner D, Rodeheaver G, Sibbald RG (eds) *Chronic Wound Care* (3rd edn). Wayne, PA: HMP Communications, 67–77.
33. **Seiler, W.O., and Stahelin, H.B.** (1985) Decubitus ulcers: preventative techniques for the elderly patient. *Geriatrics,* **40**, 53–60.
34. **Whittemore, R.** (1998) Pressure-reduction support surfaces: a review of the literature. *J Wound OstomyContinence Nurs,* **25**, 6–25.
35. **Fleck, C.A.** (2001) Support surfaces: criteria and selection. In: Krasner D, Rodeheaver G, Sibbald RG (eds) *Chronic Wound Care* (3rd edn). Wayne, PA: HMP Communications, 661–71.
36. **Weir, D.** (2001) Pressure ulcers: assessment, classification, and management. In: Krasner D, Rodeheaver G, Sibbald RG (eds) *Chronic Wound Care* (3rd edn). Wayne, PA: HMP Communications, 619–27.
37. **Smith & Nephew** Inc (2001) *Physician Guide to Moist Wound Healing.* Available online at: www.smith-nephew.com
38. **Currence, S.** (2001) Product selection in the new millennium: developing strategies for your practice setting. In: Krasner D, Rodeheaver G, Sibbald RG (eds) *Chronic Wound Care* (3rd edn). Wayne, PA: HMP Communications, 321–8.

Chapter 28

Lymphoedema

Anna Towers

Attitude

To enable the student to:

- Understand the importance of a multidisciplinary approach, early referral, and long-term follow-up in the care of lymphoedema patients.

Skill

To enable the student to:

- Clinically differentiate lymphoedema from other causes of oedema.
- Perform an initial clinical assessment and referral.

Knowledge

To enable the student to:

- Identify the common causes of lymphoedema in patients with cancer.
- Describe the common symptoms experienced by the patient.
- Describe the components of combined physical decongestive therapy.
- Describe pharmacological and surgical interventions.

Case 1

Mrs A.D. is a 44-year-old woman who was diagnosed 5 years ago with carcinoma of the right breast. She underwent a lumpectomy, axillary node dissection (four nodes out of 18 positive), radiotherapy, and adjuvant chemotherapy. Two months ago she began to develop painless swelling of her right arm, of variable degree. Occasionally her right hand is also affected. She is not on any medication. On examination, she appears worried. She is afebrile and has a right lumpectomy scar with no evidence of local tumour recurrence. There is moderate pitting oedema of the right arm and dorsum of the hand with no redness, warmth, or tenderness.

Question 1. What is lymphoedema? What are the signs and symptoms? How common is this problem?

Lymphoedema is a failure of the lymphatic system. There is inadequate drainage of extracellular fluid and consequent swelling of the subcutaneous tissues. Lymphoedema most commonly occurs in the limbs; the limb swells and feels tight and heavy. If present and untreated for a long period, skin changes occur in the form of thickened skin folds, hyperkeratosis, and increased risk of bacterial cellulitis and fungal skin infections. Although uncomplicated lymphoedema is painless, there may be pain secondary to associated nerve injuries, venous obstruction, ligamentous strain from the increased limb weight, or infection. Untreated lymphoedema may become so severe that the limb becomes useless.

Lymphoedema related to cancer treatment is not the only type of lymphoedema. Primary lymphoedema is a genetically influenced condition caused by impaired lymph vessel or lymph node development. Filariasis as a cause of secondary lymphoedema is an important cause of suffering and disability in tropical countries.

Cancer treatments and their sequelae are the most common cause of lymphoedema in the industrial world. The incidence of arm lymphoedema after mastectomy differs widely in published reports depending on the definition used (how much swelling is required before one can label someone as having lymphoedema?) and differences in measurement techniques, breast cancer treatment, and length of follow-up. The more extensive the surgical procedure, the greater is the incidence of lymphoedema. Radiotherapy also increases the risk. Overall incidence has been reported as 13–62.5 per cent from series published in the last 30 years.[1,2] The greater the radiation dose, the greater is the risk of developing lymphoedema. There is some evidence that more conservative therapies in recent years may be resulting in a reduced incidence, of the order of 24–28 per cent.[2–4]

There are no equivalent data on the incidence of lower-limb oedema following treatment for genital cancers or melanoma.

Question 2. What is the purpose of the lymphatic system? What happens pathophysiologically when lymphoedema develops? What caused Mrs A.D.'s oedema?

The lymphatic system consists of an elaborate network of vessels that transport interstitial fluid and proteins from the interstitium back to the venous system. Lymphatic capillaries rely on external compression from striated muscle contraction to generate flow.[1,2] Therefore flow is helped by gentle to moderate exercise.

Lymphoedema reflects an imbalance between production and absorption of lymph. Protein-rich fluid accumulates in the interstitial space. The increased level of protein attracts more fluid into the tissues and, over time, also leads to chronic inflammation and fibrosis. Patients tend to develop episodes of cellulitis that can make the existing lymphoedema worse.

Primary lymphoedema develops in those with congenitally inadequate lymphatic systems. Secondary lymphoedema develops when there is an anatomical obstruction caused by tumour, surgery, post-radiotherapy fibrosis, or trauma. Obesity increases the risk of developing lymphoedema.

Mrs A.D.'s lymphoedema was caused by a combination of her previous axillary node dissection and the radiation therapy. As in this case, there is often a latent period that averages 18–24 months from lymphatic damage (surgery and radiation) to manifestation of oedema. Patients often wonder why this chronic complication takes time to manifest. This is though to be due to progressive fibrosis and contraction of the lymphatic vessels.

Question 3. When a patient presents with new onset of lymphoedema, what important conditions should be ruled out in the medical assessment of the patient?

Since the onset of lymphoedema may signal a recurrence of carcinoma, it is essential that the treating physician or oncologist exclude this possibility. With unilateral limb swelling it is important to consider the presence of either a deep venous thrombosis or cellulitis. Neither of these conditions is likely in Mrs A.D. as the swelling is variable and there is no associated redness or fever.

If you suspect a deep venous thrombosis an impendance plethysmograph or Doppler ultrasound scan is indicated. If cellulitis is present, a complete blood count (CBC) may reveal an elevated white blood count and an increased number of neutrophils (in patients who are well nourished). A chest radiograph or CT scan might show an apical tumour that could be obstructing lymphatic flow. A CT of the brachial plexus may also be indicated to exclude recurrent tumour.

The family physician orders a CBC and a CT scan (which are normal).

Question 4. What further assessment is indicated and what advice would you give Mrs A.D.?

The physician should assess the psychological condition of the patient, screen for depression, and evaluate the impact of lymphoedema on physical, social, and sexual functioning. In particular, some patients are unable to assume the full duties of their occupation once they develop lymphoedema, especially if the job requires holding the limb in a fixed position, certain repetitive movements, frequent contact with water or chemicals, or the lifting of heavy weights.

Lymphoedema patients are at particular risk of developing cellulitis in the affected limb. Some lymphatic physiologists believe that this is because of the increased protein content of lymphatic fluid that makes it attractive to bacteria.

Question 5. What specific advice about skin care and prevention would you give the patient?

Skin hygiene, similar to that practised by diabetic patients, is suggested and regular use of a non-allergenic moisturizing cream is indicated.

Prevention of infection and injury is important:

- no medical procedures such as injections, bloodletting, or acupuncture in the affected limb
- avoid exposure to heat (hot packs, saunas, sunburn)
- avoid insect bites
- use electric razors only.

There are specific recommendations for a lymphoedematous arm:

- wear gloves when gardening and a thimble when sewing
- do not use a sling as it further reduces mobility.

Specific recommendations for a lymphoedematous leg are:

- do not walk barefoot
- pay attention to nail and foot care and hygiene
- avoid sitting or standing for prolonged periods.

Nutritional advice is also important to help regain and maintain normal body weight, since obesity is a risk factor.

Elevation of the oedematous limb is only effective in the early pitting stage of lymphoedema. In general, it is best to encourage movement rather than elevation since muscle contraction helps lymphatic drainage. In particular, the lymphoedematous arm must not be suspended from a stand, as is the practice in some areas. This does not help the oedema and may induce a brachial plexopathy.

Atmospheric pressure also has an effect on lymphoedema. Lower barometric pressure (long aeroplane flights) would have a negative effect, whereas higher pressures (deep sea diving) would have a beneficial effect. Some therapists recommend wearing elastic garments when flying as a preventive measure.

> After clearance by the oncologist, the family physician sends Mrs A.D. to a certified lymphatic therapist for a series of physical treatments known as combined decongestive physiotherapy. Mrs A.D. receives treatments daily for 1 month. Following this intensive reduction treatment, she obtains a custom-fitted elastic sleeve and a separate open glove. She receives advice from the therapist concerning remedial exercises and general exercise measures.

Question 6. What are the elements of combined decongestive therapy (CDT) and how do they work?

The primary aims of CDT are to improve lymph drainage through existing lymphatics and to encourage collateral circulation. The physical treatments work by exaggerating normal physiological processes that stimulate lymph flow, such as the pressure from muscular activity.

There are two phases to this treatment. The first is an oedema reduction phase that usually lasts for a month (using a specific massage known as manual lymphatic drainage, followed by the application of non-elasticized bandages). If the patient does not have access to a trained therapist, the use of electric pneumatic devices is a less preferred second choice for reducing the oedema. This is followed by a maintenance phase where the patient wears a graduated pressure elastic garment or hosiery during the day and performs specific exercises. Additional manual lymph drainage and bandaging can be performed as needed in those with more severe degrees of lymphoedema.

The health professional needs to support and encourage the patient to follow a home maintenance programme. In this sense, lymphoedema is like any other chronic medical condition where daily care and regular medical follow-up are important.

Therefore the objectives of treatment are:[4]

- to educate patients and their families and to enlist their cooperation and participation in a long-term maintenance programme that may involve significant lifestyle changes;
- in moderate to severe lymphoedema, to reduce the oedema with an intensive treatment phase of a few weeks

- to prevent further oedema
- to prevent infections
- to minimize the psychosocial impact of the condition.

Manual lymphatic drainage (MLD)

The aim of this specific light massage is to increase the intrinsic contractility of the superficial lymph vessels and thus improve lymph flow. This method requires specific training. Vigorous and unskilled massage is counterproductive since it will increase blood flow, vessel permeability, and interstitial fluid. MLD begins with the neck and trunk. Clearing the trunk enhances drainage from the limb. The treatment starts in a normal area and moves distally towards the swollen area. MLD takes approximately 45 min, after which bandages are applied. Spouses or partners can often be taught to administer the treatment. Health professionals who are unskilled in this technique are best advised to rely on compression alone.

Compression bandaging

Special low-stretch bandages are applied after MLD to maintain the reduction. The effects of MLD and compression bandaging seem to be additive.[5,6] During the intensive reduction phase, these bandages are kept in place for 24 h and are removed at the time of the next daily treatment to allow skin care and MLD.

A randomized controlled trial has shown that the combination of compression bandaging for 18 days followed by elastic hosiery was more effective than the use of hosiery alone, with a 31 per cent reduction in excess volume with the combined treatment and 15.8 per cent with hosiery alone.[7] Data from case series suggest that over 60 per cent of the oedema volume can be removed within 4 weeks with the MLD and bandaging combination.[8–10] The treatment works best if the oedema is soft and pitting. Long-standing fibrotic non-pitting lymphoedema may respond less well, thus emphasizing the need for early referral and treatment.

Sequential pneumatic compression pumps

Pneumatic compression with machines is occasionally used in North America and less so in Europe and Australia. Pneumatic compression involves mechanical squeezing of the soft tissues in order to press the lymphatic fluid passively to the drainage points in the limb. The few randomized trials performed to date suggest that MLD, compression bandaging, and pneumatic compression are all effective.[11,12] Combined therapy is additive in its benefits and is more effective than using one modality alone. Treatment may need to be given for a few weeks to be effective. Machines that use sleeves with multiple compartments or cells (nine or more) may be superior to those that have only three or less compartments.

A theoretical limitation of these pumps is that they may simply push fluid proximally into the shoulder area (or groin, in the case of leg oedema).[13] Without the benefits of MLD for the trunk areas, this fluid cannot be removed. Some experts have expressed concern that repeated use of these machines may increase fibrosis proximal to the mechanical compression sleeve, and may actually worsen the lymphoedema in the long term.[8] However, in many localities, these machines are the only form of treatment available under government health insurance.

Pneumatic compression is contraindicated in patients with active deep vein thrombosis (DVT) in that limb, peripheral vascular disease, active infections, or oozing wounds. It will also make existing trunk or abdominal oedema worse. Caution is required if a patient has evidence of congestive heart failure, as any physical treatment for lymphoedema will increase venous return.

Elastic sleeves/stockings (compression hosiery)

Elastic garments are a cornerstone of lymphoedema management. Except for very mild cases, elastic sleeves and stockings should only be prescribed once the oedema has been reduced via MLD and bandaging or pneumatic compression. Elastic garments are used to maintain the size of the limb and help prevent further swelling. There is some evidence that, used alone, they will also reduce swelling.[14]

Lymphoedema sleeves and stockings provide higher pressures than garments used to treat venous disease. Ready-made supports made for venous stasis will not provide enough compression. For example, a lymphoedema sleeve is usually prescribed with a graduated compression of 30–40 mmHg, whereas garments for venous disease provide pressures of 20–30 mmHg. Do not forget to prescribe a glove as well if there is hand oedema. These are available with fingertips open to render it easier to accomplish daily tasks. The elastic garments are worn during the day, especially during exercise times, and are taken off at night. They should be replaced at least once every 6 months as they lose compressive ability with wear and washing.

Contraindications to the use of elastic garments include active skin or subcutaneous bacterial infection, deepened skin folds (the tourniquet effect; first reduce the oedema with bandages or pneumatic compression), tight fragile skin (reduce the oedema first), and skin oozing or lymphorrhoea (wrap the limb with low-stretch bandages until the oozing stops).

Exercise

Lymph flow is stimulated by contraction of adjacent striated muscle—hence the physiological basis for including exercise as part of the combined decongestive therapy regime. Specific daily remedial exercises are prescribed, and are performed while wearing a compression garment to maximize the effect of muscle contraction. Lymphoedema is often associated with muscle atrophy; any exercise that rebuilds muscles will help reduce the oedema. Lifting heavy weights should be avoided. Theoretically, vigorous exertion that increases blood flow and lymph production should also be avoided; however, there is controversy in this regard that must be resolved by further research.[15] Swimming is an excellent form of exercise for arm lymphoedema. Walking and gentle cycling are also good general exercises, especially for leg swelling. Specifically designed aquatic therapies have been the subject of case reports.[16]

> Six months later, Mrs A.D.'s arm is still swollen, although not as much as originally. She has been wearing the sleeve and glove and has been doing the remedial exercises after much encouragement. She is very concerned about the appearance of her arm and hand. The physician is aware that Mrs A.D. is recently divorced. At this visit Mrs A.D. says that she wants to start dating again. 'But who wants to be with a woman who has an arm and hand like this?' she asks tearfully. Mrs A.D. also volunteers that the lymphoedema has caused her financial hardship because she has had to pay for the treatments and the custom-made sleeve and glove herself. She has to spend more money to find clothes that fit. Although she is 'fed up' with the arm swelling and discomfort, she has no signs or symptoms of clinical depression.

Question 7. What are some of the psychosocial effects of lymphoedema? What approach would you recommend to facilitate the development of coping strategies?

A lymphoedematous limb is a constant reminder of cancer that is difficult to conceal. It is an iatrogenic disorder that is often difficult to treat effectively. Quality-of-life scores are significantly reduced in those with lymphoedema following breast cancer treatment compared with those without lymphedema.[16] Emotional distress, psychosocial maladjustment, and psychological morbidity are all significantly higher in women with lymphoedema.[18] These patients experience more anxiety, depression, sexual dysfunction, disturbance of body image, and social avoidance than cancer survivors who do not develop lymphoedema. In one qualitative study, in addition to the above issues, women with lymphoedema expressed a feeling of abandonment by the medical system. They expressed depression and anxiety in relation to physicians' limited knowledge concerning their condition. They were distressed because they received conflicting treatment information and because of the limited number of treatment centres.[19]

Patients with lymphoedema respond to basic attention to their psychosocial health. This includes acknowledgement of the condition by health professionals, a commitment to providing multidisciplinary treatment services, and follow-up. We also need to address the financial concerns expressed by these patients.

Question 8. What physical treatment options are there for Mrs A.D. at this time?

A further reduction treatment could be attempted within the next few months, now that her arm and hand have become used to their new 'remodelled' shape. As a general rule, more intensive reduction treatments can be tried on an annual basis, removing more of the fluid each time, and maintaining the reduction with a smaller size of hosiery and with remedial exercises. Close follow-up is particularly indicated when hand swelling is present, as this can cause significant handicap if not properly treated.

Question 9. What medications might be useful in this case?

Diuretics reduce the volume of the lymphoedematous tissue by haemoconcentration. More water will pass back into the blood, but stagnating plasma proteins remain in the tissues to trigger fibrosis and infection. Therefore the long-term use of diuretics is contraindicated. Diuretics may be useful in the palliative care setting where oedema may be very tense and prognosis is short. They may also be useful if there is a cardiac or venous component to the oedema.

5,6-Benzopyrone was used for a number of years; however, it causes hepatoxicity and for this reason is not recommended. We are awaiting research results on other agents that are related to the benzopyrones. At the moment, however, there are no proven effective pharmacological agents to treat lymphoedema.

Question 10. What surgical techniques are effective for lymphoedema?

Several surgical techniques are being evaluated, such as liposuction, resection operations that remove subcutaneous tissue and fat, and lymphatic vascular reconstruction. The long-term impacts of these interventions are not known. Therefore conservative therapies are the mainstay of treatment.

Case 2

Mrs A.L. is a 78-year-old woman admitted to the palliative care unit with bilateral leg swelling that was beginning to interfere with ambulation. Three months prior to the present admission a large infiltrating bladder tumour was diagnosed and she underwent a biopsy. Pathology showed transitional

Continued

cell carcinoma. She had bilateral hydronephrosis and J-tubes were placed, but she refused further surgery or chemotherapy.

Swelling of the left leg began 2 months before this admission, and has become much worse over the past 2–3 weeks. A month ago the right leg also began to swell, but remains less swollen that the left. Her abdomen occasionally feels swollen.

Mrs A.L. has decreased mobility because of the heaviness of her left leg. She has occasional pain in the left leg and the back, which are well controlled with oral hydromorphone 2 mg every 4 h. Her appetite is poor and she may have lost some weight recently. She has urinary incontinence.

Mrs A.L. lives alone in a seniors' residence. She was widowed 7 years ago. She has a courageous outlook, but wonders if life is worth living at this point. Her only son lives out of town.

On examination Mrs A.L. is a thin woman in no apparent distress. The examination of the head, neck, chest, and heart is normal; the abdomen shows no ascites or tenderness, but there is fullness in the lower abdomen. Her extremities demonstrate marked bilateral pitting oedema to the groin, left more than right, with some areas of weeping. There is no warmth or tenderness and no adenopathy. Her laboratory investigations reveal a slightly elevated creatinine at 136 μmol/l, albumin is low at 24 g/l, and haemoglobin is markedly low at 6 g/dl, for which she is transfused. Apart from the hydromorphone, Mrs A.L. takes thyroid replacement and laxatives.

The admitting physician summarizes her problems as bilateral leg oedema, of mixed aetiology, and mild renal failure secondary to hydronephrosis from a pelvic mass. He orders a Doppler ultrasound study to rule out DVT.

Question 1. What are the probable causes of Mrs A.L.'s swollen leg?

The patient has metastatic pelvic tumour and a poor prognosis. The leg oedema is likely to be primarily lymphoedema with a small contribution from hypoalbuminaemia. There is probably also a component of venous oedema; the Doppler studies are likely to show extrinsic compression of major veins even if no active DVT is present.

Question 2. What physical treatment options are there in this palliative care context?

Although life expectancy is poor, the patient could live for several months. There is much that should be done to minimize the complications of lymphoedema in the presence of metastatic tumour. Untreated lymphoedema can lead not only to massive limbs that markedly reduce mobility, but often produces skin oozing (lymphorrhoea) that can be difficult to manage. The basic techniques of combined decongestive therapy can be modified for this group of patients. Manual lymph drainage and compression bandaging can help prevent lymphorrhoea. One could try bandaging at a pressure that is lower than that used in the active reduction treatment. Over a period of days, this should improve the oozing of the legs. Pneumatic compression via mechanical pumps is poorly tolerated in the palliative population. In Mrs A.L.'s situation, it might have the effect of simply pushing oedema fluid to the groin.

Some therapists and patients express concern that complex decongestive therapy (CDT) may spread existing cancer in or near the limb. This is physiologically unlikely. CDT is a comfort measure that should be available to those with metastatic disease.

Question 3. What medications might help reduce the oedema in the situation of advanced malignancy?

This is one context where diuretics might be tried. However, large doses of furosemide and spironolactone may be required—of the order of five or six times the standard dose. In the presence of renal failure these may not be well tolerated and could lead to metabolic side effects. Although often ineffective, high-dose steroids may work by reducing tumour-associated inflammation and thereby reopening venous and lymphatic channels. If an active tumour is not present, there is no physiological rationale for using steroids. If used in large doses over many weeks, steroids may cause more fluid retention and lead to muscle wasting, especially in the proximal limb muscles.

Question 4. How would you treat cellulitis if it developed?

Streptococcal infections are the most common. Acute bacterial infections are generally treated with intravenous antibiotics for the first few days. If conservative physical treatment measures are insufficient to prevent recurrent attacks of cellulitis, long-term and perhaps lifelong prophylactic antibiotic treatment may be necessary. Tinea pedis is common with leg lymphoedema and may be treated with standard antifungals.

Future trends

Lymphoedema remains a poorly researched, undertreated, and usually incurable chronic condition.[20] The medical profession needs to be more aware of this problem and to help identify resources to deal with it. Research is required into prevention of the problem through more conservative surgery, such as sentinel node biopsy. Newer radiological diagnostic techniques may also permit a reduced extent of surgery. It is not clear why some patients develop lymphoedema after node dissection and others do not. Genetic or other risk factors that predispose to the development of lymphoedema have yet to be identified.

Further research into standardized assessment and measurement tools is also needed. The various modalities of combined decongestive therapy need to be further evaluated in controlled trials. Conservative physical treatments are the mainstay of therapy and need to be initiated early and perhaps even prophylactically. The possible contribution of safe pharmacological agents remains to be explored. Surgical techniques such as lymphaticovenous anastamosis need to be further researched.

Rehabilitation programmes are not easy to develop in these times of cost containment. Treatment modalities might receive higher funding priority if their effectiveness were better characterized through clinical research. The potential benefits of multidisciplinary lymphoedema clinics in large centres—for clinical, teaching, and research purposes—need to be evaluated.

References

1. **Weissleder, H., and Schuchhardt, C.** (eds) (2001) *Lymphedema: Diagnosis and Therapy.* Köln: Viavital Verlag, 188–9.
2. **Pain, S.J., and Purushotham, D.** (2000) Lymphoedema following surgery for breast cancer. *Br J Surg,* **87**, 1128–51.

3. **Petrek, J.A., Senie, R.T., Peters, M., and Rosen, P.P.** (2001) Lymphedema in a cohort of breast carcinoma survivors 20 years after diagnosis. *Cancer*, **92**, 1368–77.
4. **Cohen, S.R., Payne, D.K., and Tunkel, R.S.** (2001) Lymphedema: strategies for management. *Cancer Suppl*, **92**, 980–7.
5. **Beeknan, S.W., and Bland, K.I.** (2002) Long-term complications of breast-conservation surgery: can the incidence be reduced? *Ann Surg Oncol*, **9**, 524–52.
6. **Johansson, K., Albertsson, M., Ingvar, C., and Ekdahl, C.** (1999) Effects of compression bandaging with or without manual lymph drainage treatment in patients with postoperative arm lymphedema. *Lymphology*, **32**, 103–10.
7. **Badger, C.M.A., Peacock, J.L., and Mortimer, P.S.** (2000) A randomized, controlled, parallel-group clinical trial comparing multilayer bandaging followed by hosiery versus hosiery alone in the treatment of patients with lymphedema of the limb. *Cancer*, **88**, 2832–7.
8. **Casley-Smith, J.R.** (1994) Lymphedema therapy in Australia: complex physical therapy, exercises and benzopyrones on over 600 limbs. *Lymphology*, **27** (Suppl), 622–5.
9. **Boris, M., Weindorf, S., and Lasinski, B.** (1997) Persistence of lymphedema reduction after non-invasive complex lymphatic therapy. *Oncology*, **11**, 99–113.
10. **Dicken, S.C., Lerner, R., Klose, G., and Cosimi, A.B.** (1998) Effective treatment of lymphedema of the extremities. *Arch Surg*, **133**, 452–8.
11. **Johansson, K., Lie, E., Ekdahl, C., and Lindfeldt, J.** (1998) A randomized study comparing manual lymph drainage with sequential pneumatic compression for treatment of postoperative arm lymphedema. *Lymphology*, **31**, 56–64.
12. **Rockson, S.G.** (2002) Pneumatic compression in lymphedema related to breast cancer. *Cancer*, **95**, 2260–7.
13. **Boris, M., Weindorf, S., and Lasinski, B.B.** (1998) The risk of genital edema after external pump compression for lower limb lymphedema. *Lymphology*, **31**, 15–20.
14. **Megens, A., and Harris, S.R.** (1998) Physical therapist management of lymphedema following treatment for breast cancer: a critical review of effectiveness. *Phys Ther*, **78**, 1302–11.
15. **Harris, S.R., and Niesen-Vertmmen, S.L.** (2000) Challenging the myth of exercise-induced lymphedema following breast cancer: a series of case reports. *J Surg Oncol*, **74**, 95–9.
16. **Tidhar, D., Drouin, J., Shimony, A.** (2004) Aqualymphatic therapy for postsurgical breast cancer lymphedema. *Rehabil Oncol*, **22**, 6–14.
17. **Beaulac, S.M., McNair, L.A., Scott, T.E., La Morte, W.W., and Kavanagh, M.T.** (2002) Lymphedema and quality of life in survivors of early-stage breast cancer. *Arch Surg*, **137**, 1253–7.
18. **Tobin, M.B., Lacey, H.J., Mayer, L., and Mortimer, P.S.** (1993) The psychological morbidity of breast cancer-related arm swelling *Cancer*, **72**, 3248–52.
19. **Carter, B.J.** (1997) Women's experiences of lymphedema. *Oncol Nurs Forum*, **24**, 875–82.
20. **Harris, S.R., Hugi, M.R., and Olivotto, M.L.** (2001) Clinical practice guidelines for the care and treatment of breast cancer: 11. Lymphedema. *Can Med Assoc J*, **164**, 191–9.

Chapter 29

Genitourinary symptoms

Michael Downing

Attitude

To enable each student to:

- Recognize that in palliative care things never stay the same for long and therefore to adopt an attitude of vigilance and anticipation in order to look for change.
- Recognize the impacts of disease involving the urinary and genital systems on sexuality and psychosocial distress.

Skill

To enable each student to:

- Demonstrate competence in communication with patients and partners on sexual matters.
- Demonstrate competence in management of fistulae.
- Use an ethical basis for decision-making at various points in the disease trajectory.
- Be able to assess and manage various types of urinary incontinence.
- Appreciate the relationship between anatomy (innervations of pelvic structures) and therapeutic decisions.

Knowledge

To enable each student to:

- Describe the diagnostic steps to assess recto-vaginal and vesico-vaginal fistulae as well as possible treatments.
- Describe the general treatment approach for prostate cancer, particularly in the advanced stage.
- Describe the types of complications that may occur in prostate cancer.
- Recognize the indications for urinary catheterization and techniques for maintenance of indwelling catheters.

Case 1

A 63-year-old woman was diagnosed 2 years ago with squamous cell carcinoma of the upper vagina after reporting heavy vaginal bleeding. Treatment included both intracavitary caesium and external beam radiation. She maintained an active life but recently noted some bloody vaginal discharge and mild aching pelvic pain. Several weeks later, she suddenly discovered moderately heavy bleeding. She now comes to see you in the office.

Question 1. What steps in assessment and management are appropriate for this patient?

The patient is still ambulatory and doing well overall; your goal is to maintain this state. A CT scan shows local disease progression with no metastases. Her haemoglobin is 81 g/L and you transfuse her. The radiation oncologist is very hesitant to provide further radiation as her prior dose reached tolerance limits. You start her on oral oxycodone 10 mg every 4 h for pain and she begins chemotherapy. She experiences nausea and vomiting and chooses to stop treatment before a full course is completed but does benefit with cessation of bleeding.

Six months later, the patient has lost weight but is remaining ambulatory and busy. She is now registered with a palliative care programme on your advice and is supported by a home care nurse. However, pain is gradually increasing and she is now rotated from sustained release oxycodone to sustained release hydromorphone 18 mg every 8 h with good effect. A constant foul vaginal discharge, initially responding well to metronidazole, is worsening, and the patient sees you again and reports expelling stool through the vagina.

Question 2. What treatment options are available and how would you proceed?

Diagnosis is often easily made with vaginal passage of stool and flatus on defecation. However, if it is unclear whether a recto-vaginal fistula is present, possible investigations include a vaginogram, hypaque enema with contrast, or small bowel series and follow-through. Treatment options include defunctioning colostomy, ileostomy, total parenteral nutrition with bowel rest, and comfort-only care. The choice depends on extent of disease, functional status, other complications, and patient desire.

This ambulatory patient undergoes a diverting colostomy with good effect. Two months later the vaginal discharge increases significantly. It is serosanguinous and she is constantly wet. The sustained release hydromorphone is now increased to 24 mg every 8 h with attendant good pain relief. You see her and examination reveals palpable tumour extending to the vulva and a hard right inguinal node.

Question 3. What is your differential diagnosis and what investigations and treatment options would be appropriate to improve her comfort?

This vaginal discharge sounds different from that occurring earlier. There is no stool or flatus and the colostomy is functioning well, so recurrent recto-vaginal fistula is unlikely. The vaginal tumour may be progressing, although this usually produces a bloody foul discharge. The clue is constant wetness, suggesting urine. This could be stress incontinence, but there is no urgency (nor such problems earlier), or possibly bladder retention with overflow incontinence. Indeed, the patient also notices decreased volume of urination but, with no urgency or palpable suprapubic distension, a vesico-vaginal fistula becomes the provisional diagnosis.

Investigations for vesico-vasginal fistula include one or more of the following: oral pyridium, methylene blue test, intravenous pyelogram, cystogram, urinalysis and culture, urea, and creatinine.

A vaginal tampon was inserted and then the patient swallowed two tablets of pyridium. The tampon was removed about 2 h later and the presence of orange staining quickly identified the existence of a uro-vaginal fistula. An abdominal ultrasound scan showed a dilated right ureter with hydronephrosis. Thus the vaginal tumour has extended to the lower bladder, blocking one ureter and eroding surrounding tissue with a resulting fistula.

If the patient were very debilitated or dying, conservative treatment measures combining incontinence pads with a Foley catheter might reduce incontinence and provide short-term comfort. At the same time, the risk of vulvar skin excoriation often occurs, with additional pain and odour and an increased need for nursing care. The desire of this patient to remain as active as possible directs us to consider other interventions. Chemotherapy might relieve tumour pressure on the ureter but would not reverse the damage leading to the fistula. With one functioning kidney and the vesico-vaginal fistula, the insertion of a left percutaneous nephrostomy tube is the appropriate intervention and resolves the incontinence. Although a second tube could be placed in the non-functioning kidney in the hope of regaining function, this adds practical management risks with little true benefit.

The patient is grateful for the dramatic reduction in vaginal discharge and wetness. Her quality of life improves and she feels able once again to go shopping, to go to the hairdresser, and to engage in some social functions. Six months later, according to home nursing and her family, she is using a wheelchair. The nephrostomy tube had become dislodged once during this time but was easily replaced in the outpatient clinic by the radiologist.

Over the next three months, the patient has gradually become bedbound and is now very weak, with little intake, and has difficulty in swallowing medications. The vaginal discharge has worsened again with intermittent bleeding and a foul serosanginous discharge. There is marked perineal and bilateral leg oedema with some skin breakdown. She is now febrile. Low abdominal and pelvic pain remains under good control. She does not want more treatment and wishes to die at home. Current drugs include long-acting hydromorphone 36 mg every 8 h (no evidence of opioid neurotoxicity), immediate release hydromorphone 9 mg hourly as needed for breakthrough pain, dexamethasone 12 mg twice daily, lactulose, sennosides, metronidazole, and clotrimazole.

Question 4. How would you proceed in deciding a course of action?

There are several urgent issues to sort out including questions of whether to proceed with further investigations and treatments; pain control; routes for medication; whether to proceed with further investigation; and whether she can die at home. When faced with such issues, the physician needs to reflect on how these decisions will be made. Ethical models such as the Latimer model[1] focus the decision-making on considering the following: the patient's symptom distress; the illness and its anticipated progression; the patient as a person with unique hopes, goals, and plans; the overall goals of the patient, family, and health care team; and, based on these, the possible treatment options. These factors are helpful in weighing burden versus benefit decisions and in recognizing that 'what could be done' is not necessarily 'what should be done'.

At this point, the fundamental question is whether to aim for prolongation of life or acceptance of imminent death, since the management strategies will have major differences. A comfort-only approach, recognizing imminent death, would focus on stopping unnecessary drugs, changing the routes of drugs being continued, anticipation of complications, and discussion and planning for death.

After a lengthy discussion with the patient, her husband, and her adult daughter, they all feel her wish to let go and die at home is important and, although they are somewhat worried as to whether this will be possible, they want to try. You want to simplify care as much as possible and speak with the home care nurse.

Question 5. What specific changes in medications and care do you implement?

The analgesic hydromorphone is converted from the oral to the subcutaneous route using a taped butterfly needle, and the is dose established at 6 mg s.c. every 4 h with 3 mg s.c. every hour as needed for breakthrough pain. You discontinue the laxatives and metronidazole. Some physicians will stop the steroid, while others feel it important for both pain control and not precipitating sudden steroid withdrawal. You decide to continue the dexamethasone once daily at a lower dose of 4 mg s.c. If anxiety ensues or worsens, lorazepam 0.5–1.0 mg is often helpful. The vaginal discharge can be troublesome for care at home with the need for frequent changes of pads, necessity for moving and turning the patient, and odour problems. It can be helpful for this short period of several days to have home nursing insert sufficient Vaseline-soaked gauze padding into the vagina to form a seal to reduce leakage and minimize care requirements.

Case 2

John, a 68-year-old man, comes to see you in your office in August complaining of pain over the past 4 months. He describes this as mainly in the lower back with radiation down his left leg and accentuation with movement. It is presently at a severity level of 3/10 and varies from zero to 5/10. You notice that he is using two canes and, upon enquiry, he says that this is necessary mainly due to pain but also because he feels a little leg weakness. He notes having to get up twice nightly to pass urine, but otherwise voiding is normal. Examination is unremarkable apart from two things. There is mild weakness in the left leg but no sensory loss and reflexes are normal. However, rectal examination reveals an enlarged hard prostate. Pelvic and leg radiographs are normal, but a bone scan shows multiple bone metastases involving the pelvis, sacrum, lumbar vertebrae, and several ribs. A prostate-specific antigen (PSA) test is very high at 371 ng/ml (<4 ng/ml). You meet with John and his wife, Margaret, to discuss these results and treatment steps.

Question 1. What are the issues that must be identified and discussed?

In Canada, there were over 69 000 new cases of cancer in males in 2002; prostate cancer has the highest incidence at 26.1 per cent, followed by lung cancer at 17.2 per cent.[2] In approximately 20 per cent of patients, prostate cancer has already metastasized at the time of diagnosis, as was the case in our patient. There are several important and difficult issues to discuss. First, breaking such bad news as a cancer diagnosis takes time and skill. This is covered in more detail in Chapter 1. One cannot underestimate the shock and implications for any patient at any age. Secondly, the cancer is advanced and incurable. Hopes, fears, losses, and dreams are affected for John, Margaret, their two children, and their three grandchildren. Of course, the third consideration relates to his pain and weakness.

Question 2. What disease-specific treatment would you recommend for this patient?

There are many factors which influence treatment decisions, the details of which are beyond the scope and purpose of this chapter. They can be roughly categorized into three areas:

- tumour factors (stage, Gleason score, PSA level, prostate volume)
- patient factors (patient preference, life expectancy, age, bladder/bowel function, sexual function, other comorbid diseases)
- treatment factors (adverse effects, potential complications, quality of life impacts).

Metastatic prostate cancer is generally treated with one or more of hormone therapy, palliative radiotherapy, and chemotherapy. For either metastatic or non-metastatic disease, a third approach called 'watchful waiting', where no definitive treatment is started other than observation and monitoring, may be the best decision. This may be indicated where there is clinically insignificant cancer (e.g. small tumour, low PSA, low Gleason), short life expectancy due to advanced age or other comorbid illness, or the patient is unsuitable for radical therapy or has refused treatment.

John has multiple bone metastases, persistent pain, and early evidence of lumbosacral nerve involvement. The gold standard treatment with newly diagnosed widespread metastatic disease is usually orchidectomy.[3,4] The dramatic drop in testosterone levels or androgen deprivation via surgical castration or combined with additional hormone therapy will often cause marked decrease in tumour size and significant improvement in pain relief for over 80 per cent of patients.

> John is agreeable to this approach and you arrange surgical and oncology consultations. His functional performance status is good apart from the leg weakness.

There are several ways of following functional performance over time including the traditional oncology ECOG[5] performance status from 0 (full health) to 5 (death). Another rating measure is the Palliative Performance Scale (PPS)[6] which is measured in decreasing increments of 10 per cent from PPS 100 per cent (healthy) to PPS 0 per cent (death).

> John is currently at PPS 70 per cent, indicating presence of significant disease and some limitation to activities. However, the pain is clearly disabling and you decide to initiate analgesics.

Question 3. How would you manage the patient's pain at this point?

There are several good choices for opioids. You might start with an acetominaphen–codeine combination or a non-steroidal anti-inflammatory drug (NSAID), but with the pain reaching up to 5/10 and with the known bone and nerve involvement, a stronger opioid should be used. You may prescribe immediate release morphine, hydromorphone, or oxycodone at low initial doses and titrate upwards. A fentanyl patch is not appropriate with unstable pain .Since there is also evidence of nerve involvement, you should consider the possible short-term use of a steroid such as dexamethasone for its anti-inflammatory effect on the bone metastases and possible reduction in nerve compression.

> You prescribe oral oxycodone 10 mg every 4 h for pain control while referrals are being arranged. With some concern for possible nerve damage from root compression, you also begin dexamethasone 8 mg every morning. Of course, 'the hand that writes the analgesic order also writes the laxative order' and so docusate and sennosides are also started. He comes now to your office for follow-up on his pain control and discussions prior to his surgery in a few days. The pain relief is good and he appreciates sleeping better and walking more easily.

Question 4. What is another area for discussion which either the patient or perhaps even yourself have not raised yet and may have some difficulty talking about?

A fourth area for early discussion relates to the sexual implications of prostate cancer. This is a highly sensitive area for most patients, but even more so in various cultures and religions. Discussion of such matters in some cultures is totally unacceptable, and even illegal. Thus you would enter this area only if it is culturally permissible for the physician to discuss sexual matters with male patients and relatives. In view of the emotional impact of breaking the original news of advanced cancer this subject can be deferred until the next patient contact, unless raised by the patient. However, this topic is often difficult for patients, particularly men, to bring forward and so the physician needs to be proactive in ensuring that there are opportunities to do so.

Given the above cautions, to discuss sexuality is to recognize and be open to many aspects: individuality, sensuality, intimacy, sexual function, ego or gender identification, romance, tenderness, affection, mutual pleasuring, cuddling, attraction, closeness, desire, satisfaction, friendship, fear, inadequacy, fatigue, guilt, hope, physical comfort, timing, privacy, and sexual or erotic aids. These issues are not necessarily age related, and the physician must neither underestimate nor overestimate them in each patient. Listen, observe, relax, and maintain a sensitive non-judgemental attitude throughout all your discussions.

As might be expected, a study of patients with early-stage, late-stage and no cancer showed significant decline of sexual function in those with advanced cancer compared with those at an earlier stage or cancer free.[7] Patients in both cancer groups were more open and interested in talking about their hopes, fears, and realities than the general population. However, disease does take its toll on the body, the mind, and the spirit. By acknowledging that cancer does impact on sexuality, you are providing a basis for further exploration, validation, and reassurance.

One place to start may be to understand how John and Margaret have related in the past. Begin with the least sensitive questions, and move from general to specific and from past to present. It is often helpful to use third-person statements to introduce concepts or questions. For example, one might ask generally 'With such a busy world, many people find few times to be alone together. Do you find times to be close with each other?' This may be followed by 'Intimacy is sometimes, but not always, connected with sexual desire. How are you finding this after your initial surgery?' Also, providing a wide range of normality, such as 'many people experience these feelings or concerns', often helps the patient and partner not to feel that you are suggesting that 'they have a problem'.

Dispel such myths as cancer is contagious, having sex will aggravate the cancer and cause it to spread or produce 'damage' to the patient, one is 'radioactive' after receiving irradiation, and the prostate itself is necessary for an erection or ejaculation.

However, for John, the massive drop in testosterone levels after the orchidectomy will probably cause at least initial loss of libido and difficulty in obtaining an erection. However, about 20 per cent of men are able to maintain good libido and activity following medical or surgical castration.[8] Surgical nerve-sparing techniques are improved for radical prostatectomy depending on the extent of disease.

The PLISSIT model of sexual counselling has been used for many years and provides a reasonable clinical guide.[9] The first aspect is Permission (P) and includes the areas of permission to talk about and permission to resume sexual activity as noted above. Part of this discussion is related to dispelling myths and thus giving them the confidence to try again. The second aspect is providing Limited Information (LI) where you would discuss the physical impact of therapy and alterations that can be expected in sexual function. Try to allay fears of both partners. Sexual gratification is still very possible despite of absence of penile erection or ejaculation. The next aspect is Specific Suggestions (SS) which must be based on obtaining an adequate sexual history and appreciation of the couple's sexual attitudes. Suggestions are made regarding foreplay, mutual pleasuring, use of sexual aids, alternatives to vaginal intercourse, and variations in position to alleviate fatigue or weakness.

These steps may provide sufficient information for many but not all. The last aspect is Intensive Therapy (IT) and includes the use of medications such as oral sildenafil or alprostadil via urethral pellet insertion or penile injection. Devices such as the Vacuum Erection Device may be used externally, or surgical penile implants may be possible for those who are disease free. Testicular saline prostheses can be placed in the scrotum to preserve body image if desired. Professional sex therapy counselling may be appropriate. While not universally needed, most people will welcome information and appreciate being able to discuss sexual health issues with you.

Inquiry regarding sexual activity reveals that John is unable to produce erections and has no personal interest in sex, especially as his overall strength and energy are decreased. John is worried about Margaret and she about him. He inquires about sildenafil, but you have some concern with his known mild angina. You consider a urethral insertion pellet, alprostadil, which works well for some patients. Margaret reassures him that sexual intercourse is no longer important for her and that what she most enjoys are their quiet times on the chesterfield and lying close together in bed (except for his snoring, of course!). She is more worried about his overall energy for other things. This opens a door for you to explore: 'What is important now, what different goals do you have, etc.' They share the information that their grandchild has just turned 2 years old and they are hoping that the family can be together for Christmas. As you review current disease progression, it seems that this goal will probably be possible, and this discussion opens another door wherein you gently advise on the need to reflect on such things as wills, advanced directives, hopes, and realistic planning for the future.

Continued

Orchidectomy is completed without complication in September, and John subsequently receives palliative radiation to the pelvis and lumber vertebrae. You see him in October and he is pain free and voiding normally, and has had no side effects from the radiation. The dexamethasone has been tapered and discontinued. The PSA shows a dramatic reduction to near normal levels and you are able to discontinue his analgesics. His functional status has improved from PPS 70 per cent to 80 per cent or ECOG 1. However, John returns to see you in January as he is experiencing back pain rated at a level of 10. His PSA is increasing.

Question 5. How would you proceed in managing John's pain?

You restart him on oral oxycodone 10 mg every 4 h with 5 mg orally every hour as needed for breakthrough pain, subsequently switching to long-acting oxycodone once his pain is controlled. As he had responded well to the hormone ablation via surgery, additional hormone treatment may be beneficial and you refer him to the cancer centre. He is started on flutamide for additional androgen suppression, but in March the PSA has increased further and he is switched to bicalutamide. Both of these drugs are non-steroidal antiandrogens which act by inhibiting androgen uptake or binding to androgen receptors in target tissues.

By June, he has more pain and you adjust his opioid medication; you also begin an NSAID, diclofenac, with some improvement. Unfortunately, the PSA test in August, now 1 year post-diagnosis, has risen further. Thus the pain problems are consistent with disease progression, although some drug tolerance may play a small factor. Although John's quality of life has declined somewhat in the past 6 months, he is quite hopeful that more treatment will improve this since changes in therapy have helped in the past. His functional status is now decreased to PPS 60 per cent or ECOG 2.

Question 6. With disease progression evident, what strategies need to be reviewed with John and what would you do?

Anti-androgen therapy is no longer controlling the disease and you need to come back to the Latimer ethical model and meet with him and Margaret to review what is important for them and how to proceed.

After this, it is clear that he still wishes active treatment. He is seen by the oncologist and a chemotherapy course is added to the androgen suppression. He is to receive six treatment cycles of docetaxol in August. The long-acting morphine dose is increased to 90 mg every 8 h and, in discussion with the oncologist, you decide to begin monthly bisphosphonate infusions of pamidronate 90 mg intravenously every 4 weeks.

Although biphosphonates are more often used for pain control or hypercalcaemia in osteolytic metastases, there is some evidence for a role in prostate cancer pain,[10] and a number of patients have been able to stay on lower opioid doses as a result.

In the course of an office visit, you enquire about voiding function. John states that 'My underwear is sometimes wet; I just can't hold it'.

Question 7. What are the four types of urinary incontinence, and how do they relate to the anatomy and physiology of urinary function? How are these conditions managed?

Three sphincters influence urine flow (Fig. 29.1).

- The internal (vesical) sphincter is located at the base of the bladder and consists of muscles from the bladder which come together to surround the urethral orifice.
- The urethral sphincter depends upon the actions of smooth muscle in the upper urethra. This smooth muscle represents a continuation of the outer longitudinal layer of the bladder, now oriented in a circular fashion as it surrounds the upper urethra.
- The external sphincter consists of striated muscle, including muscle tissue arising from the urogenital diaphragm, and interdigitates with urethral smooth muscle.

The internal sphincter serves to control urine flow into the urethra, except during the purposeful act of voiding. For example, sudden increases in intravesical pressure, such as may be induced by coughing, will not result in inadvertent loss of urine if the internal sphincter is functionally intact.

The function of the urethral sphincter relates to the outer circular layer of smooth muscle in the upper part of the urethra which is in direct continuity with longitudinal muscle in the bladder wall. It acts in a coordinated manner with both the vesical sphincter and the external sphincter, which is subject to voluntary control. Muscles of the pelvic floor, such as the levator ani, may have an indirect controlling action.[11]

- Motor nerve fibres to the external sphincter and perineal muscles are part of the somatic (voluntary) nervous system via nerve roots emanating from S2–S4. The sympathetic nerve

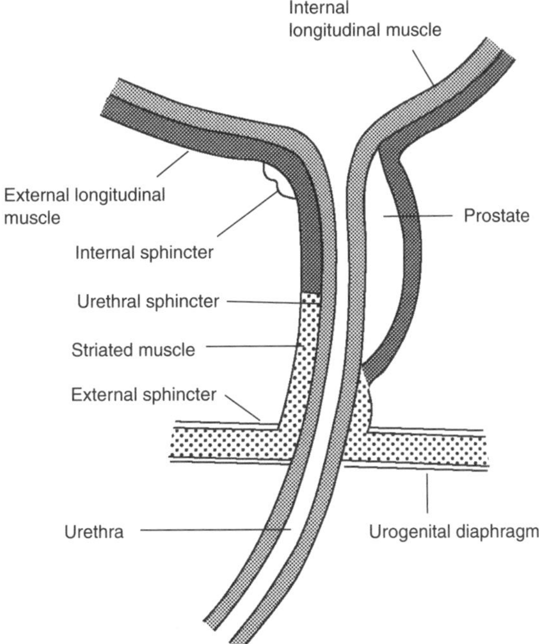

Fig. 29.1 Adapted with permission from Hutch and Rambo (1967)

supply to the bladder arises from T11–L2. The detrusor muscles of the bladder wall are innervated by parasympathetic nerves arising from S2–S4.

- Micturition occurs when the detrusor muscles contract, the bladder neck sphincter is drawn downward creating a funnel-like effect, and the sphincters relax. This is a parasympathetic function. Stimulation of the sympathetic system has a reverse effect.

Lesions causing spinal cord damage which occur at or below S1 lead to a flaccid bladder because of damage to the voiding reflex centre and/or the pelvic nerves. Injuries above S1 usually cause a spastic type of neurogenic bladder. Remember that spinal cord reflexes mediating the action of S1–S2 nerves are located at the spinal level of L1–L2.

Sensory innervation detecting stretch reaches the central nervous system via the parasympathetic system. Pain sensations travel mainly with the sympathetic fibres.

An unobstructed passage and intact bladder muscles and sphincters, controlled by balanced parasympathetic (primarily stimulating voiding) and sympathetic (primarily preventing voiding) nervous systems are required for satisfactory bladder function. In addition to anatomical and inflammatory changes, reduced awareness of bladder stimuli and drugs affecting autonomic function may interfere with normal function.

We now discuss the types of urinary incontinence that may occur:

Stress incontinence

Stress incontinence is the involuntary loss of urine with increased bladder pressure from coughing, laughing, and straining caused by functional loss of sphincter tone. The cause is usually hypermobility or displacement of the urethra and bladder neck during exertion. Also, abdominal and pelvic tumour masses may exert increased pressure on the bladder. Another cause of stress incontinence is internal urethral sphincter deficiency which may develop after prostatectomy, radiation, or a spinal cord lesion.

If the condition is not severe, management may be simply watchful waiting. Tricyclic antidepressants such as imipramine have sympathomimetic actions and, depending on the patient's medical status and current drug profile, may be a safe choice (conversely, α-adrenergic receptor antagonists such as terazosin may decrease resistance to urinary outflow and be helpful in treating the symptoms of benign prostatic hyperplasia). If drug management fails, condom drainage or incontinence pads may be necessary.

Urge incontinence

Proper control of voiding requires coordination of the detrusor muscle and the bladder neck sphincter. Local inflammatory disease or partial sphincter incompetence caused by intrinsic or extrinsic tumours may lead to a sudden loss of urine. Causes of inflammation include radiation, drugs, and infection. Involuntary detrusor contractions may also be associated with neurological disorders.

Management of this condition includes the use of anticholinergic drugs, for example oxybutinin 2.5–5.0 mg three four times daily. Alternative classes of drugs, including antidepressants or papaverine-like antispasmodics such as flavoxate, may help. Some patients with unstable bladder conditions may benefit form advice on timing of diuretic use and fluid intake, particularly those troubled primarily at night.

Overflow incontinence

Overflow incontinence is involuntary loss of urine associated with an overdistended bladder. It may present with frequent or constant dribbling or with symptoms of urge or stress incontinence. Voiding occurs in small amounts with no control. Overflow urinary incontinence may be caused by decreased detrusor contractility or by bladder outlet or urethral obstruction. The bladder may be underactive secondary to drugs, faecal impaction, or neurological problems such as low spinal cord injury or nerve injury as a result of pelvic surgery.

If medical or surgical intervention cannot correct the problem, long-term catheterization may be necessary.

Total incontinence

Total incontinence occurs when there is complete loss of sphincter function by direct tumour invasion, surgical intervention, or loss of innervation from spinal cord or nerve root damage.

If nerve root damage or spinal cord compression is considered likely, treatment such as radiation or decompressive surgery may be possible. If a reversible problem is not identified, long-term catheterization is often required.

John's urge incontinence is relieved by oxybutinin.

You receive a call from the emergency department in October stating that your patient has presented complaining of a sudden increase in back and leg pain with numbness and weakness. He says his legs 'just keep giving out' and he fell this morning at home.

Question 8. How would you proceed?

An emergency MRI scan indicates cauda equina compression from tumour in the lumbar and sacral areas. John also has new bone metastases in the ileum and inferior pubic ramus. Suprapubic ultrasound shows no urinary retention and his incontinence is worse, probably neurogenic in nature, but he refuses a catheter. He is given palliative radiation to the lumbar and sacral areas as well as being placed on dexamethasone 16 mg daily in the morning. The morphine dosage is increased to 120 mg every 8 h. Several weeks later you decrease the dexamethasone to 8 mg daily in the morning, but decide to maintain this dose as an adjuvant analgesic rather than taper it as previously.

John's pain is now under good control but the leg weakness and urinary incontinence have not improved. He now requires significant assistance to get up and must use a walker for short distances. Constipation remains an ongoing issue. Since this last acute pain episode, he has intermittent nausea, little appetite, and is tired much of the time. Although you had advised the use of incontinence pads, John finds these frustrating. His scrotum and inner thighs are becoming excoriated, especially as he is mainly chair- or bedbound. Further, it just feels 'like a diaper'. It appears the incontinence is permanent.

Question 9. Are indwelling urinary catheters appropriate and safe in palliative care?

Although there are some concerns that long-term (>4 weeks) use of Foley catheters often contributes to bacteriuria and even sepsis,[12] one must weigh other quality-of-life and comfort factors in deciding whether and when to pursue catheterization. Fainsinger and Bruera,[13] in a study in a palliative care unit where catheter use was approximately 75 per cent, concluded that there was no increased mortality and that morbidity, while not insignificant, was outweighed by patient comfort. The most common indications for inserting a Foley catheter were patient comfort (asthenia, pain, dyspnoea, nausea, delirium), frequent changes in bedlinen; psychological distress associated with incontinence, management or prevention of decubiti and other skin wounds, overflow incontinence, and urinary retention.

In addition to bacteriuria, indwelling catheters can also cause other problems such as encrustation, bladder spasms, stones, urethritis, chronic renal inflammatory changes, haematuria, and urinary leakage. To avoid these complications, catheters should be examined regularly and changed if encrustations are detected when the catheter is rolled between the thumb and index finger. Catheters can become blocked by mucus and other debris, necessitating occasional irrigation. If haematuria is present and leads to blood clotting, irrigation may be required at least daily. If the patient develops an infection, the system should be changed and a culture obtained when the new system is inserted. Fainsinger and Bruera[13] found that bacteriuria was present in 44 per cent of patients at 7 days, 75 per cent of patients at 14 days, and 92 per cent at 28 days. Interestingly, there was a 'dynamic' change in the bacteria at 10 days when the actual type of bacteria cultured changed; as a result, Fainsinger and Bruera[13] recommend a urine culture at insertion which is repeated after 2 weeks to assess the need for antibiotics. When, or even whether, to initiate antibiotics is controversial in these situations; treatment of asymptomatic bacteria is not usually recommended. A short course of a fluoroquinoline (24–48 h) in association with a difficult catheter change is appropriate. The general indications often include ascending infection causing pyelonephritis, fever, or major continuing problems with catheter blockage due to infective debris.

Condom catheters can work well for some patients who are quite immobile. Practical problems, especially if the patient is moved frequently or with smaller penises, are the condoms falling off and local skin irritation or infection.

> In John's case, several of the above indicators are present and perhaps the one which stands out most is his feeling of lack of dignity. The decision must be individualized, since the opposite is true for other patients where the presence of a catheter itself is viewed as an indignity. You make a referral to home care nursing, requesting that a condom catheter be tried. This does not work out well and so a Foley catheter is inserted. The next day you are called with the report that John is having sharp suprapubic pains and feeling that he has to void all the time. This appears to be bladder spasm.

Question 10. How would you manage these bladder spasms?

McGregor[14] recommends several practical things which can be done. Of course, removal of the catheter will solve the acute spasms but returns one to the original reasons for insertion. Patients who require ongoing use of a catheter should have it changed periodically and the bladder irrigated with normal saline to clear mucus and prevent blockage and resulting spasms. Reducing the volume of the balloon is sometimes sufficient; a common cause of bladder spasm is excess balloon size. Opium and belladonna (O & B) suppositories can be used every 4–6 h as necessary for bladder spasms, often with good relief. If this is the first time a catheter has been inserted, it may be possible to reduce the frequency of the suppositories or even discontinue them, after a few days in some patients. An anticholinergic drug, such as tolterodine 1–2 mg twice daily, oxybutynin 2.5–5.0 mg three times daily, or propantheline bromide 15 mg three times, daily could be tried. A urine culture should be obtained as acute cystitis will increase bladder sensitivity and spasm.

Bladder spasms could be caused by more ominous problems. Tumour invading the bladder can cause pain and urgency. Other causes include radiation fibrosis, extra-vesical nerve damage, and blood clots.

The use of a urinary catheter has considerably helped John's comfort and sense of dignity. He requires use of O & B suppositories for several days until the bladder adjusts to the presence of a foreign object, and they are then discontinued. He recognizes that this has also reduced some burden on his wife as it is hard for her to assist him to the commode frequently enough to avoid wetting the bedlinen. You check on his physical comfort, but also inquire how this affects his self-image and any impact on their intimacy. John says the catheter is fine and has resolved the wetness, odour, and skin irritation. He shares that of course there is no sex now, but that it has not been important for them for some time. Both feel tired much of the time, and what is of most value are the times that they can lie together and feel close. They now sleep separately since he has to change position frequently in the night and so they have rented an electric bed.

Christmas arrives and John is delighted that his family is able to spend time with them over the holiday season. It is hard for the children to see the overall decline in their father's condition. He is now bedbound, he has lost a lot of weight, and his appetite is poor. He even needs help with eating some of the time. They also see that Margaret looks very tired. John's functional performance level has declined further to PPS 30 per cent or ECOG 3–4. He dies at home in February, approximately 18 months after his diagnosis.

Question 11. What other complications might you see in advanced prostate cancer?

Other complications which commonly arise in advanced prostate cancer are:

- leg oedema due to pelvic lymphadenopathy or pelvic vascular blockage
- haematuria
- renal failure due to obstructive uropathy
- disseminated intravascular coagulapthy
- hepatic metastases, hypoalbuminaemia, ascites
- pathological fractures
- bone marrow failure with infection and bleeding issues
- sepsis
- pulmonary metastases are uncommon in earlier stages but may occur in up to 25 per cent of patients in advanced stage
- bowel obstructions are uncommon and brain metastases are rare.

Although our patient did not have obstructive uropathy, this is a reasonably common complication in metastatic pelvic tumours in both men and women. Decreased urine output may arise from blockage in one or both ureters, at the bladder outlet, or in the urethra. Urinary retention may also be caused by drugs or nerve damage such as cauda equina syndrome. Unilateral obstructive uropathy may have few or no symptoms. Bilateral blockage will result in oliguria and eventually anuria, elevated and rising creatinine with normal or increased potassium levels, and progressive renal encephalopathy. Pain may or may not be present in the abdomen or flank. The bladder, which is empty, can be checked by an 'in and out' catheterization or, if available, by simple bladder ultrasound. If available, a diagnostic pyelogram (caution if bilateral) or ultrasound, CT, or MRI scans will confirm uni- or bilateral obstruction.

Management options include no intervention, delayed intervention, retrograde endoscopic ureteric stents, or percutaneous nephrostomy/urostomy stents in addition to any possible further anticancer treatment. If the patient has advanced disease and is very ill, an appropriate and ethically sound decision between you and the patient may be to make no active intervention to reverse bilateral obstruction. In this case, close attention to symptom relief through to death over the next few days to weeks is paramount, including relief for confusion, drowsiness, nausea, and pain. Delayed intervention is often recommended by urologists for unilateral obstruction if creatinine and potassium levels are normal, especially if other treatments to modify tumour invasion are being undertaken. Other urologists press for early stent insertion. Transvesical ureteric stents are generally preferable since they are internal and require no regular management. Depending on the extent of tumour invasion, another option is external urostomy or nephrostomy tube placement. These are reasonably tolerated but there are increased risks of dislodgement, infection, and local discomfort.

Future directions

There is obvious anticipation that continued research in genomics and proteomics will result in better drug treatments, thereby improving both survival and quality of life. Prostate brachytherapy is demonstrating significant value but is not yet widely available. There is reasonable evidence for use of bisphosphonates[15] for treatment of hypercalcaemia and also for metastatic bone pain. Another advance may be vertebroplasty using bone cement or polymethylmethacrylate for vertebral fractures.[16,17] This has been done by percutaneous injection under ultrasound guidance mainly for osteoporotic fractures, but a few studies are focusing on tumour infiltration.

Acknowledgements

The author gratefully acknowledges and appreciates information and support from several staff from the British Columbia Cancer Agency, including Dr Judith Pike, oncology nurse Theresa Downing, and Counsellor Michael Boyle, as well as from Dr James McGregor, Queens's University, the author of this chapter in the first edition of this book.

Bibliography

Berger, R.E., and Berger, D.B. (1990) *Biopotency: A Medical Guide to Sexual Success.* New York: Avon Books.

Boston Women's Health Book Collective (1998) *Our Bodies, Ourselves for the New Century: A Book by and for Women.* New York: Touchstone Books, New York.

Bostwick, D.G., MacLenna, G.T., and Larson, T.R. (1999) *Prostate Cancer: What Every Man—And His Family—Need to Know* (revised). New York: Vilard Books.

Goldstein, I., and Rothstein, L. (1990) *The Potent Male: Facts, Fiction, Future.* New York: Berkley Publishing.

Heiman, J., and LoPiccolo, J. (1998) *Becoming Orgasmic: A Sexual and Personal Growth Program for Women.* New York: Simon and Schuster.

Holland, J.C. (ed) (1998) *Handbook of Psycho-Oncology.* Oxford: Oxford University Press.

Hollis, J. (1994) *Under Saturn's Shadow: The Wounding and Healing of Men.* Toronto: Inner City Books.

Kabat-Zinn, J. (1990) *Full Catastrophe Living: Using the Wisdom of Your Body and Mind to Face Stress, Pain and Illness.* New York: Delacorte.

Korda, M. (1997) *Man to Man: Surviving Prostate Cancer.* New York: Vintage Books.

Lerner, M. (1994) *Choices in Healing: Integrating the Best of Conventional and Complementary Approaches to Cancer.* Cambridge, MA: MIT Press.

Levine, P.A., and Frederick, A. (1997) *Waking the Tiger: Healing Trauma.* Berkeley, CA: North Atlantic Books.

Norman, R.W., and Bailly, G (2004) Genitourinary problems in palliative medicine. In: Doyle D, Hanks G, Cherny N, Calman K (eds) *Oxford Textbook of Palliative Medicine* (3rd edn) Oxford: Oxford University Press, 647–58.

References

1. **Latimer, E.J.** (1991) Ethical decision-making in the care of the dying and its application to clinical practice. *J Pain Sympt Manage,* **6**, 329–36.
2. **Canadian Cancer Society Annual Cancer Statistics.** Available online at www.cancer.ca
3. **Hussain, H., and Crawford, E.D.** (1997) Androgen deprivation strategies of metastatic prostate cancer. In: Raghavan D, Scher HI, Leibel SA, Lange P (eds) *Principles and Practice of Genitourinary Oncology.* Philadelphia, PA: Lippincott–Raven.
4. **Gleave, M.E., Bruchovsky, N., Moore, M.J., and Venner, P.** (1999) Prostate cancer: 9. Treatment of advanced disease. *Can Med Assoc J,* **160**, 225–32.
5. **Oken, M.M., Creech, R.H., Tormey, D.C., *et al.*** (1982) Toxicity and response criteria of the Eastern Cooperative Oncology Group. *Am J Clin Oncol,* **5**, 649–55.
6. **Anderson, F., Downing, G.M., Hill, J., Casarso, L., and Lerch, N.** (1996) Palliative Performance Scale (PPS): a new tool. *J Palliat Care,* **12**, 5–11. Available online at: www.victoriahospice.org.
7. **Ananth, H., Jones, L., King, M., and Tookman, A.** (2003) The impact of cancer on sexual function: a controlled study. *Palliat Med,* **17**, 202–5.
8. **Singer, P.A., Tasch, E.S., Stocking, C., Rubin, S., Siegler, M., and Weichselbaum, R.** (1991) Sex or survival? Trade off between quality and quantity of life. *J Clin Oncol,* **9**, 328–34.
9. **Annon, J.S., and Robinson, C.H.** (1978) The use of various learning models in the treatment of sexual concerns. In: Piccolo JL (eds) *Handbook of Sexual Therapy.* Plenum Press, New York.
10. **Bloomfield, D.J.** (1998) Should bisphosphonates be part of standard therapy of patients with multiple myeloma and bone metastases from other cancers? An evidence-based review. *J Clin Oncol,* **16**, 1218–26.
11. **Hutch, J.A., and Rambo, O.N.** (1967) A new theory of the anatomy of the internal urinary sphincter and the physiology of micturition. III. Anatomy of the urethra. *J Urol,* **97**, 696–712.
12. **Kunin, C.M., Chin, Q.F., and Chamber, S.** (1987), Morbidity and mortality associated with indwelling urinary catheters in elderly patients in a nursing home: confounding due to presence of associated diseases. *J Am Geriatr Soc,* **35**, 1001–6.
13. **Fainsinger, R., and Bruera, E.** (1991) Urinary catheters in palliative care. *J Pain Symptom Manage,* **6**, 449–51.
14. **McGregor, J.** (1998) Genitourinary symptoms. In: MacDonald N (ed) *Palliative Medicine: a case-based manual.* Oxford: Oxford University Press.
15. **Garfield, D.** (2001) New bisphosphonate shows promise in bone metastases. *Lancet Oncol,* **2**, 525.
16. **Peters, K.R., Guiot, B.H., Martin, P.A., Fessler, R.G.** (2002) Vertebroplasty for osteoporotic compression fractures: current practice and evolving techniques. *Neurosurgery* **51**(Suppl), 96–103.
17. **Jensen, M.E., Kallmes, D.E.** (2002) Percutaneous vertebroplasty in the treatment of malignant spine disease. *Cancer J,* **8**, 194–206.

Chapter 30

Home care of dying patients

Anna Wreath Taube

Attitude

To enable each student to:

- Consider the satisfaction and sense of accomplishment that all caregivers justifiably experience after successful care of a dying patient in the home.
- Recognize the burden of care which falls on lay caregivers.
- Recognize the ongoing needs for educational, physical, and emotional support of significant others in their caregiver role.
- Recognize that these needs may differ between caregivers.
- Recognize the need to keep management simple.
- Recognize potential financial costs to home patients.
- Recognize potential loss of privacy and control for patients and families.
- Recognize the need for professional proactive care and regular visits.
- Recognize the need for prompt physician response to home care personnel.
- Recognize the need for physician access in times of crisis.
- Recognize the reality of lessened professional control in the home setting.
- Recognize that institutional admission is not 'failure'.

Skill

To enable the student to:

- Perform a systematic holistic assessment of a home patient.
- Assess and support patient and caregiver emotional needs.
- Ensure timely communication between all caregivers.

Knowledge

To enable the student to:

- Describe the community resources needed to sustain medical care of the dying home patient.
- Describe physician legal responsibility after home death.

This chapter is offered in loving memory of Maggie, who graciously and gladly permitted use of her case, hoping to help others wishing to receive care at home. At the time of writing, Maggie was still alive but her anticipated survival was weeks only.

Maggie is a 56-year-old woman diagnosed with a localized duodenal adenocarcinoma, treated by surgical excision. Three years after diagnosis, CT scanning showed extensive intra-abdominal adenopathy. Chemotherapy was initiated but discontinued after 8 months due to lack of efficacy and side effects, particularly severe nausea.

Some months after discontinuation of chemotherapy Maggie presented with neuropathic left lower back pain radiating into the anterior left thigh. MRI scanning of the pelvis and lumbar spine demonstrated new left-sided metastatic lymphadenopathy invading the L2 vertebral body. The area was irradiated, with good effect for 2 months.

As the pain eventually returned, various opioid therapies were initiated and doses raised with modest effect and accentuation of chronic nausea. Trials of both gabapentin and dexamethasone provided ineffective adjuvant analgesia.

Six months after radiation she was referred to the community-based palliative consult team for assessment and management advice. Again, her primary complaints were low back/left leg pain and severe chronic nausea, now present for >2 years and accompanied by gradual weight loss.

Maggie was admitted to the acute palliative care unit (APCU) for further investigation and symptom management. Abdominal CT scanning showed enlargement of the left paraspinal mass and increased erosion of the L2 vertebral body. A second course of radiation to the area was advised but declined. For Maggie, the fear of severe exacerbation of nausea, such as she had experienced with the first course, outweighed the potential analgesic benefit. Her medical oncologist advised no further chemotherapy.

Augmented CT imaging of the brain showed no metastatic disease to explain her nausea. Serum calcium levels and renal function were normal. A supine abdominal radiograph showed severe stool accumulation in the large bowel. Previous radiographs taken every few months had demonstrated similar faecal overload, and each time she received one-time bowel cleansing care.

The APCU physician wished to switch Maggie's opioid from oxycodone to methadone, but she requested discharge home, because of difficult family circumstances, before this was initiated. Her oxycodone dose was increased. Three months after discharge the community palliative consult team was reconsulted regarding her poor pain control and intractable nausea.

At this point, imagine yourself as a family physician who has just assumed her care and is seeing her for the first time. Her previous physician has indicated that she cannot provide home visits. Maggie's performance status still allows her to leave home, but this activity now exhausts her.

Question 1. Can you outline a systematic scheme for assessment of a home palliative patient?

Holistic assessment is considered a cornerstone of palliative care in all settings, and some aspects are particularly important in the home setting (Table 30.1). Although all areas outlined below should be included, we have found that the order of assessment is best customized to each individual situation, adapting to the responses of the patient and significant others and their informational and emotional needs. Assessment may be accomplished in a single visit, but you may require repeat visits.

Table 30.1 Systematic assessment of home palliative patients: areas to be assessed

- Current symptoms
- Patient emotional status
- Patient spiritual status
- Medication profile
- Physical examination
- Patient understanding of the extent of disease, options for treatment, and prognosis
- Patient wishes with respect to medical information and participation in decision-making
- Patient wishes with respect to information release to significant others and their wishes with respect to medical information and participation in decisions
- Patient wishes with respect to care setting; lay caregiver wishes with respect to care setting
- Patient goals
- Current formal home care support services
- Lay caregiver educational, physical, and emotional supportive needs
- Home physical arrangements
- Clarify existence/absence of a personal directive
- Resuscitation status
- Patient financial picture
- Patient medication insurance plan(s)

Current symptoms

In Maggie's community the following symptoms are routinely assessed (0 = best, 10 = worst). Her results were: pain, 2–8; fatigue, 7; nausea, 9; depression, 0; anxiety, 0; drowsiness, 0; appetite, 8; best feeling of well-being, 5; shortness of breath, 0.

Maggie's pain depiction was consistent with previous descriptions. It originated in the upper lumbar spine and radiated into the left flank and anterior thigh, with severe burning and lancinating characteristics and associated thigh numbness and allodynia. At best, the pain rated 2–3/10, but was generally 8/10. She had been on oxycodone analgesia for some time but had no symptoms of oxycodone neuropsychiatric toxicity (see Chapter 6).

Nausea was continuous, at best 5/10 and at worst 9/10. Over the preceding 2 years trials of adequate dose metoclopramide, domperidone, dimenhydrinate, haloperidol, prochlorperazine, omeprazole, dexamethasone, ondansetron, megestrol acetate, transdermal scopolamine, methotrimeprazine, and olanzapine had all proved ineffective.

She gave a lifelong history of constipation. Currently her bowels were moving infrequently, most often only after enema administration, despite generous stool softener and stimulant laxative use. She noticed reduction of nausea after bowel evacuation.

Functional inquiry revealed no further concerns. Past medical and family history was unremarkable.

Patient emotional status

Maggie rated her level of depression and anxiety as 0/10. During the short APCU admission the possibility that psychosocial distress influenced Maggie's pain and intractable nausea was considered. The distress stemmed from concerns with respect to her severely mentally handicapped adult son, David.

Continued

On reconsultation, the palliative physician fully explored possible clinical depression or anxiety disorder but found no evidence for either. The social worker and chaplain on the unit had spent fruitful supportive time with Maggie, providing ideas as to how to discuss her situation with David and how to arrange for David's guardianship and trusteeship. Maggie later indicated that this planning afforded great psychological relief, but did not lessen her pain or nausea.

Patient spiritual status

Maggie's Druse faith gave her enormous spiritual sustenance. She accepted her disease as the will of God and consistently expressed confidence in His ability to minimize her suffering and facilitate her wish to remain at home.

Medication profile

Maggie's medications were oral oxycodone every 4 h around the clock (ATC), oxycodone every hour as needed for breakthrough pain (generally four breakthrough doses in 24 h), dexamethasone, omeprazole, dimenhydrinate ATC, methotrimeprazine ATC (for nausea), docusate sodium, sennosides, suppositories/enemas as needed, and clonidine.

Physical examination

Maggie was cachectic but independently mobile and able to move freely around the house. She was not able to perform any household tasks. She appeared in moderate physical distress. Blood pressure, 90/60 mmHg; heart rate, 100 beats/min, regular; respiratory rate, 12 bpm, unlaboured. She was alert. There was no myoclonus or jaundice. Tissue turgor was adequate. Head and neck and cardiopulmonary examinations were unremarkable. Her abdomen had no distention, organomegaly, or ascites. Epigastric tender firmness was present. Bowel sounds were infrequent. There was no musculoskeletal tenderness except over the upper lumbar spine. Neurological examination was intact except for left anterior thigh allodynia. There was no peripheral oedema.

Patient understanding of the extent of disease, options for treatment, and prognosis

Since a patient's grasp of these issues may not mirror previous explanations outlined in specialist or attending physician notes, it is important for the professionals involved to clarify patient understanding. All discussions are predicated on this understanding.

Maggie clearly understood and accepted the extent of her metastatic disease and the lack of further chemotherapy options. She had questions relating to her life expectancy, and the palliative physician answered these as honestly as possible.

Patient wishes with respect to medical information and participation in decision-making

Maggie expressed the need to remain fully informed at all times and to be a full partner in treatment decisions.

Depending on individual coping strategies, patients vary considerably in their desire for depth of detail of information and extent of participation in decision-making. Honouring these wishes may go a long way towards enhancing patient sense of personhood and dignity, compliance, and sustainable relationships between professionals, patients, and significant others. Such enhancements are important in all care settings, but perhaps particularly so in the home setting.

Patient wishes with respect to information release to significant others and their wishes with respect to medical information and participation in decisions

> On the palliative physician's first visit only Maggie herself participated in the assessment and discussion, although, once her decisions regarding change in management were complete, she requested reiteration of the discussion for her adult daughter who was present in the house. At no time did she appear to wish her husband John to be included in the discussion. It became clear during early visits that John, although loving and concerned, was 'taking one day at a time' and did not wish to know details of her condition or management. He particularly absented himself from all discussions regarding her emotional needs. Maggie honoured this coping mechanism. Her involved professionals did likewise, although always affording him the opportunity to ask questions. Her daughters, on the other hand, wished the same degree of full information as their mother, for which Maggie gave full consent, but deferred to her decision-making. Maggie was clearly the decision-maker in this household.

At best there may occasionally be a need to facilitate changes in these informational and decisional wishes, at worst a need to override them gently and sensitively if they threaten sustainability of care in the home. The variability between significant others in information needs and coping styles must be appreciated and adjusted to.

Patient wishes with respect to care setting; lay caregiver wishes with respect to care setting

> Maggie's wishes for her care setting were clearly reasoned. John was disabled by cardiac disease and unable to contribute to any heavy physical care. They felt well supported by their adult daughters, but both were married and had young families. David lived with his parents.
>
> Given her husband's chronic medical condition and her daughters' family responsibilities, she requested admission to a residential hospice setting once she required total care. She did not wish a home death; she was concerned about David's reaction if this were to occur. However, until the time of development of total dependence, she requested management in the home and avoidance of acute care hospital admission; her family fully supported her wishes.
>
> Her professional caregivers indicated that they would honour these wishes, with the understanding that some crises cannot be managed in the home.

In the vast majority of Western world communities, the minute-to-minute burden of nursing dependent home patients falls on the shoulders of lay caregivers—whether family, friends, or other partners. In Maggie's community there is a specialized palliative home care programme. Nevertheless, except in extenuating circumstances such as impending death or short-term reversible crisis, this relatively well-resourced home care service offers a maximum of only 20 h of in-home professional care per week through a variety of services, as outlined below.

Patients and lay caregivers often have no understanding of what provision of care in the home truly entails. They must understand what their community home care services can and cannot offer and what their lay caregiving responsibilities would be. Much patience and effort in educational discussions may be needed by involved professionals to facilitate this understanding and establish that the lay caregivers can realistically commit to and fulfil this role. In our experience, both patient and caregivers must be committed to the goal of care in the home setting.

A further issue is the inability of most home care programmes to maintain a dependent patient at home in the absence of lay caregivers. This can be difficult for such patients to understand or accept. Unless they can fund private nursing care, these patients require emotional support and discussion to facilitate their acceptance of institutional admission.

Patient goals

> Maggie's goals were good symptom control and a desire to remain at home as long as possible.

Patient goals can be as varied and many as there are patients. Professional appreciation and help towards gaining them may be greatly valued.

Current formal home care support services.

> Maggie's home care services included monitoring of her condition and needs and coordination of her care by her assigned coordinator, a registered nurse (RN). On-call assistance 24 h per day, 7 days per week ('24/7 coverage') was provided for concerns such as the need for changing of subcutaneous needle sites or symptom issues. Occupational therapist assessment and provision of medical equipment, respiratory therapist assessment and provision of supplemental oxygen, and physiotherapist and social worker services were available. Some home cleaning services were provided. At this point Maggie did not need respite services for her family or personal care services. She did need frequent enema administration by her RN.

The existence of a specialized palliative home programme and 24/7 availability, as illustrated by Maggie's care in a Canadian city, is the ideal but is rarely present throughout the world.[1] Even with Maggie's level of home care support, it is physically and emotionally exhausting for lay caregivers, however committed, to provide ATC nursing care for a dependent patient.

Educational, physical, and emotional supportive needs of lay caregivers

The educational needs of lay caregivers are extensive. Critical issues to be reviewed with them include:

- patient physical care
- emotional care
- symptom assessment
- use of as-needed medication
- medication and hydration administration
- signs of possible complications
- changes in condition before death
- who to contact in a crisis or after death.

Research has shown that lay caregiver sense of incompetence is devastating and significantly contributes to the caregiver's sense of burden.[2]

The simplest symptom management should be sought—minimizing polypharmacy, using long-acting opioid formulations or continuous administration analgesic pumps when appropriate, and using subcutaneous rather than intravenous or intramuscular routes of administration

Physical support may relate to the need for patient personal care attendant services, day or night respite service, or increased medical equipment to facilitate caregiving.

Most importantly, patient and lay caregiver emotional distress, sometimes exhausting in the extreme, must be assessed and dealt with. Caregivers' ability to find meaning in this experience and enhancement of their relationships with the patient and each other is central to reducing their sense of burden and psychological distress.[2]

In Maggie's case it was possible to discontinue a number of medications, and the switch to methadone, requiring administration only every 8 h, simplified her pharmacological management. As her condition declined, both daughters and eventually even John sought and received ongoing updates as to how they could best meet her increasing care needs. More medical equipment (walker, commode, hospital bed) was added for both Maggie's comfort and facilitation of caregiving. The family consistently refused respite services.

All professional caregivers provided medical information as needed or requested, sometimes repeatedly. They provided strong listening support. They attended to the emotional states of Maggie and her family members, reflecting understanding of these back to each individual to ensure that they felt understood, respected, and supported. They explored the need for difficult conversations between Maggie and family members, and facilitated them as the need arose. They sought to validate and support Maggie's and her family's search for meaning, hope and spirituality in her illness and pay tribute to the family's commitment to her.

Caregiver exhaustion and possibilities to lessen sources of exhaustion must be monitored and addressed continuously.

Home physical arrangements

Maggie did not have to manoeuvre stairs in her bungalow. Her corridors were wheelchair compatible. Her living room, the location in the house where she wished to spend her daytime hours surrounded by her family, was large enough to accommodate a hospital bed if needed.

Clarify the existence/absence of a personal directive

In Maggie's jurisdiction, the province of Alberta, the Personal Directives Act[3] allows patients to designate an 'Agent' of their choice, who becomes the legal proxy decision-maker in areas of medical and social decision-making in the event of patient mental incapacitation. The Act also permits patients to specify their wishes with respect to desired care measures. Agent designation is extremely useful in situations of conflict between significant others regarding their goals for patient medical or social care. Such conflict can become a crisis of huge proportions if a patient's ongoing care is in such hands. Whether or not a jurisdiction legally recognizes personal directives, they should be obtained as they will help to resolve family conflicts.

As Maggie's disease progressed, her physicians discussed the advisability for her to discuss with her family the possibility of future mental incapacitation and her wishes for comfort measures only in this event. Ultimately she completed a personal directive, not because of potential conflict in her family but rather to empower them in assuming decision-making. She appreciated their difficulty in assuming this function, if needed, given their pattern of deferral to her decision-making.

Resuscitation status

Maggie had determined by this stage that she did not wish resuscitative measures and had communicated this to her family. However, the Emergency Response Department in her community had not been formally notified of this decision. The palliative physician remedied this immediately.

If the patient's condition warrants initiation of this discussion, it is crucial to do so and, given the notorious difficulty of predicting time of death, crucial to formally record a Do Not Resuscitate (DNR) decision. At times, of course, much discussion may be needed to facilitate patient and family acceptance of DNR status when this is clinically appropriate.

In Maggie's community a DNR form is available for notification to the Emergency Response Department; alternatively, written documentation of this decision must be in the home. In the absence of either of these, if her family were to call emergency services in the event of cardiorespiratory arrest, resuscitation is legally mandated. This measure can be enormously distressing to the family. Physicians caring for home palliative patients must be aware of the pertinent circumstances in their community.

Patient financial picture

Maggie and John lived in a comfortable bungalow, for which, fortunately, they had no outstanding mortgage. They and David were on disability pensions through their province's Assured Income for the Severely Handicapped (AISH), with a tight combined monthly income. When the time came for need of a hospital bed in the home Maggie would have dearly loved to have an electrically controlled bed, to enhance her independence. They could not afford the monthly co-payment of $150 CDN.

This assessment is important since individual tailoring of medical and supportive care may be constrained by financial resources. Appreciation of such constraints is necessary for professionals managing care in the home.

Patient medication insurance plan(s).

In Maggie's situation the AISH disability plan covered the full cost of medications deemed necessary.

Physicians must know their patients' coverage for drugs and hydration supplies since limited coverage may constrain pharmacological options.

Question 2. Can a patient be safely switched to methadone in the home?

Given its unique pharmacology, methadone is useful in the control of pain syndromes that generally require higher dose opioid therapy, such as neuropathic pain (see Chapter 3). It has the advantage of a longer half-life than non-methadone opioids, but the disadvantage of unpredictable and clinically non-measurable inter-individual variability in half-life. This leads to non-predictability of timing of risk of respiratory depression on initiation of methadone therapy. There are a number of protocols for initiation of methadone analgesia. In our setting it is standard to make the switch to methadone over a minimum of 3 days.

Because of the risk of respiratory depression, many physicians are reluctant to initiate opioid rotation to methadone in the home setting. Maggie's palliative physician, who had years of experience with methadone, was comfortable to do so at home as there were no concerns regarding patient and/or family competence/reliability. However, the rotation is usually done over a minimum of 5 days in the home setting.

Maggie was greatly relieved at the prospect of improved pain control with methadone and appreciated the willingness of her caregivers to carry out the rotation in her home.

Over the course of 5 days her oxycodone doses were gradually decreased and doses of methadone increased. Her condition was monitored daily by a combination of visits from the palliative physician and home care nurses and telephone assessment by the palliative physician. There were no associated problems.

She experienced dramatically improved control of her neuropathic pain for some 2 months, with her pain rating generally 0–2/10, and never exceeding 4/10.

Although only physicians trained in its use should prescribe methadone, it is important to illustrate the viability of home rotation from a non-methadone opioid to methadone if conditions permit. In Maggie's community the consult palliative physicians work closely with primary care physicians to afford them development of expertise in methadone use.

Question 3. How would you address her nausea?

Given Maggie's long history of constipation, her description of nausea relief after bowel evacuation, and the high frequency of this aetiology contributing to nausea in this patient population, constipation was thought to be a major factor causing nausea. The most definitive method of establishing this aetiology is a supine radiograph of the abdomen.

At this stage Maggie was still able to leave her home to visit a radiology facility. The radiograph again demonstrated a colon packed with stool. Maggie's home care RN administered an oil-retention enema that evening, followed by saline enemas daily for 3 days. The results were gratifying. A repeat radiograph confirmed total bowel clean-out. Her bowel regime was augmented with the addition of an osmotic stimulant. Her bowel pattern was maintained at evacuation of soft stool every 2–3 days either spontaneously or occasionally with enema administration. With one exception, Maggie's nausea never again rated higher than 2/10, and usually remained around 0–1/10.

Over time Maggie's neuropathic pain escalated and left leg paresis ensued. A second course of radiation to the paraspinal tumour mass was indicated. Again Maggie was extremely reluctant to consider this for fear of increased nausea. After much discussion of the fact that possibly the previous radiation-induced nausea had been significantly exacerbated by concurrent faecal overload, she agreed to further treatment. She underwent 10 fractions of outpatient radiation with nausea levels reaching only 5/10.

This discussion highlights the extreme importance of close monitoring of bowel behaviour and aggressive appropriate action by the home care team.

Question 4. What crises could Maggie be at risk for?

Crises in the home can be challenging in the extreme for lay caregivers; one crisis too many may lead to a visit to the emergency department. Proactive monitoring enabling early problem detection and abortion of crises is crucial. Common home crises include:

- development of acute severe pain
- onset of agitated delirium
- onset of severe dyspnoea
- onset of seizure activity
- development of acute urinary retention
- development of spinal cord compression
- development of deep venous thrombosis with or without symptomatic pulmonary embolism
- onset of malignant bowel obstruction
- development of malignant ureteric obstruction with renal failure
- sudden severe haemorrhage.

Maggie was potentially at risk for all of these. Two months after referral to the palliative consult team the home care RN noted unilateral lower extremity painful swelling and alerted Maggie's family physician. Immediate outpatient Doppler examination of her leg was obtainable and confirmed the presence of deep venous thrombosis. Pharmacological management with low molecular weight heparin (LWMH) was initiated in the emergency department and continued indefinitely in the home. Maggie's RN instructed her in the subcutaneous administration of LMWH and she was able to take on this administration herself. This home care nurse's proactive care and the family physician's immediate response maintained patient mobility and avoided the possible crisis of pulmonary embolism.

Over time Maggie's methadone dose required increasing; 4 months after its initiation the dose was 250 mg orally every 8 h. Within days of this dose initiation the palliative physician specifically reviewed the possibility of opioid toxicity. Maggie was now experiencing nightmares, myoclonus, and decreased clarity of thought. The physician would have preferred a palliative care unit readmission for management of this complication of opioid toxicity, but Maggie was adamantly opposed. Her methadone dose was reduced and the physician monitored her daily by telephone for several days; fortunately the symptoms of toxicity resolved. Again, proactive monitoring aborted a crisis of opioid-toxicity-induced agitated delirium and hyperalgesia.

The importance of proactive care and prevention of crises cannot be overemphasized.

Question 5. In addition to the challenges above, what other stresses might Maggie and her family experience?

Even when patients and families appreciate the support of visiting physicians, home care personnel and other community service providers, the number of individuals and the time-consuming nature of their visits may take its toll. Loss of control and privacy may be real sources of (di)stress. Coordination of visits and their timing by professionals to accommodate the patient, when possible, may alleviate this to some extent.

Question 6. What other areas need to be monitored regularly?

Important areas to monitor regularly and systematically are:

- general symptomatology
- hydration status
- dysphagia (onset of which may require initiation of the subcutaneous route for medication and hydration administration),
- skin integrity
- development of ascites that might require symptom-relieving paracentesis
- need for supplemental oxygen
- need for increased home care services or equipment.

For most of her course at home Maggie required subcutaneous hydration, provided overnight to free her from constraining equipment during the day. She or one of her daughters was able to (dis)connect the hydration bag tubing to the indwelling needle placed by her RN.

She did not develop ascites, but if this had happened the consult palliative team physician would have offered home paracentesis for symptom relief.

Four months after the palliative consult her condition had deteriorated significantly and she was spending the entire day in a chair or bed. Home care carefully monitored areas at risk for decubitus ulceration and provided protection products or cushioning appliances as necessary. Skin breakdown did not ensue.

Oximetry was obtained periodically; she did not require oxygen supplementation. Periodic blood testing was obtained, as symptomatology dictated.

By this time home care was providing 5.5 h of weekly home-making services, 0.5 h of daily personal care, and three weekly RN visits. A hospital bed had been placed in the living room and a walker and commode provided.

Question 7. What community services are necessary to maintain a dying home patient?

Several other services are required in addition to physician and home care services. Community pharmacies (or hospital pharmacies that supply home patients) providing subcutaneous medications and hydration supplies are necessary. Other helpful pharmacy services are provision of preloaded medication syringes or syringe-drivers, pre-programmed pumps, and home delivery. 'Twenty-four/seven' drug availability, either through a community pharmacy or a palliative consult team 'Emergency Drug and Supply Kit' is paramount in times of symptom crisis and need for urgent change in drug management.

A laboratory home collection service is valuable, as is a portable radiology service. If available, the latter can usually only be used if the patient's home has a wheelchair ramp and the patient is accessible on the ground floor, given the weight of current portable machines. Access to specialist palliative care and oncology consultation, even if only by telephone, is useful. Clearly, physicians caring for home patients must be aware of these services and how to access them.

Question 8. What financial costs might home patients incur?

Home patients can incur significant out-of-pocket costs. Co-payments for medication, medical equipment, and oxygen, costs of a privately hired nursing service, costs of ambulance transportation to/from an acute care setting for day procedures or admission, and loss of income for lay caregivers who take unpaid leave can amount to thousands of dollars.

Professionals, patients, and families (and governments) need to be aware of these potential financial outlays for home patients. The recent Commission on the Future of Health Care in Canada recommended compensation for such costs,[1] a policy in place in too few countries.

Question 9. What physician services are necessary for care of the dying patient in the home?

Care of the dying patient in the home requires a primary care physician who is committed, knowledgeable, and willing to seek specialist care (when available) if problems beyond his or her capability arise, who provides proactive home visits, who responds in a timely fashion to home care telephone calls and requests for physician assessment, and who provides '24/7' accessibility. Physician response to crises is mandatory to avoid unnecessary emergency department visits. Since most global consult palliative services do not have the personnel to function as first responders and primary care physicians, nurses or community health workers must endeavour to provide this service.

> Maggie was extremely fortunate in having a family physician who provided all these attributes of care and who made good and appropriate use of the palliative consult team. The palliative physician remained closely involved throughout Maggie's care and provided first-responder service for methadone-related issues.

Question 10. Are there other challenges for physicians caring for dying home patients?

The home setting is not a controlled environment comparable with an institutional setting. The reality of less control for health professionals is one potential challenge. There is no daily nursing charting to depend on, and lay caregivers vary immensely in their ability to assess and report on patient symptoms or intervention outcomes.

Many homes become 'grand central station'; children's needs, telephone calls, or visitors may interrupt professional visits. Professionals must accommodate to these challenges. However, the other side of this coin can be the immense satisfaction of knowing that maintenance of patients in these environments may also be maintaining a desired quality of life.

Physician financial costs may be an issue. This care is plainly time consuming. In Maggie's location the provincial government has created time-based physician fee schedules for visits and some remuneration for physician time spent in telephone communication with home care personnel. Physician travel time is not compensated. The palliative consult team tries to ensure that primary physicians are aware of these helpful schedules.

Question 11. How can communication between all parties be maintained?

Timely communication with respect to changes in patient status or management or caregiver concerns is paramount. In Maggie's region a formalized home chart system exists and documentation is recorded by all visiting health disciplines. In additional, telephone and fax communication between consult personnel, attending physician, and home care personnel is rigorous.

Question 12. What is the physician's responsibility when the home death occurs?

This may vary between jurisdictions. In Maggie's jurisdiction registration with the Medical Examiner's Office by the home care coordinator at the time of patient referral to the home care programme permits removal of the body from the home after death without requirement of an immediately signed death certificate or Medical Examiner notification. Attending physicians are not legally required to visit the home after patient death, although many choose to do so. All physicians should be aware of the requirements surrounding home death in their own jurisdiction.

Question 13. Was Maggie's desire for death outside home a 'failure'?

As discussed above, Maggie had limited lay caregiver practical support. However, principally, she did not wish a home death because of the emotional needs of her son David. Was the impossibility of home death in any sense a failure? Clearly not from Maggie's perspective.

In some cases, however, failure and guilt overwhelm lay and even professional caregivers if complex medical care or lay caregiver burnout leads to institutional admission, especially if care in the home until death has been promised. Lay caregivers must never be pressured to continue care beyond their safe capabilities. Perhaps decisions for admission are better viewed as proof of healthy flexibility and vibrant concern for patient welfare. Following residential hospice admission the author has often encountered patient and lay caregiver expression of 'Why didn't we do this sooner?'.

Conclusion

This chapter has tried to highlight issues that characterize care of home dying patients. Although often challenging, this care can be enormously satisfying to both lay and professional caregivers.

It is hoped that future research will investigate how to empower and support lay caregivers better, how to provide home care service cost effectively and meaningfully, and how to improve financial support for home patients.

Bibliography

Cantwell, P., Turco, S., Brenneis, C., Hanson, J., Neumann, C.M., and Bruera, E. (2000) Predictors of home death in palliative care cancer patients. *J Palliat Care*, **16**, 23–8.

Doyle, D. (2003) Palliative medicine in the home. In: Doyle D, Hanks G, Cherny N, Calman K. (eds) *Oxford Textbook of Palliative Medicine,* (3rd edn). Oxford: Oxford University Press, 1097–1114.

Macmillan, K., Hycha, D., Peden, J., and Hopkinson, J. (2000) *A Caregiver's Guide. A Handbook About End of Life Care.* Edmonton, Alberta: Military and Hospitaller Order of St. Lazarus of Jerusalem.

Stajduhar, K. (2003) Examining the perspectives of family members involved in the delivery of palliative care at home. *J Palliat Care,* **19**, 27–35.

Strang, V.R., and Koop, P.M. (2003) Factors which influence coping: home-based family caregiving of persons with advanced cancer. *J Palliat Care,* **19**, 107–14.

Taube, A.W. (2003) Practical aspects of home care. In: Fischer M, Bruera E. (eds) *Cambridge Handbook of Advanced Cancer Care.* Cambridge: Cambridge University Press, 108–12.

Thielemann, P. (2000) Educational needs of home caregivers of terminally ill patients: literature review. *Am J Hosp Palliat Care,* **17**, 253–7.

References

1. **Romanow, R.** (2002) *Commission on the Future of Health Care in Canada.* Ottawa: Government of Canada.
2. **Dumont, S., Dugas, M., Gagnon, P., Lavoie, H., Dugas, L., and Vanasse, C.** (2000) Le fardeau psychologique et emotionnel chez les aidants naturels qui accompagnent un malade en fin de vie. *Cah Soins Palliat,* **2**, 17–48.
3. Personal Directives Act, S.A. 1997, c. P-4.03.

Chapter 31

'I found this on the Internet': palliative care in the information age

Jose Pereira and Alejandro R. Jadad

Attitude

To enable each student to:

- Recognize that, notwithstanding some limitations, the Internet serves as a useful source of information for patients, families, and health professionals.
- Be open to and understand patients' and families' requests to discuss information that they have found on the Internet.
- Recognize that the requests by patients and families to discuss information that they have located on the Internet serve as opportunities to explore their understanding and experience of their illnesses and to develop collaborative care plans.

Skill

To enable each student to:

- Engage patients and families in a constructive dialogue that strengthens the patient–health professional relationship when approached with Internet-derived information.
- Guide patients, their families, and other caregivers to useful information on the Internet.
- Demonstrate a respectful and professional communication manner that allows patients to discuss alternative and complementary therapies.

Knowledge

To enable each student to:

- Describe the reasons why patients, families, and health professionals use the Internet in the context of receiving or providing palliative care.
- Describe potential pitfalls for patients and families who use the Internet.
- Describe potential useful roles of Internet for patients and families.
- List resources available on the Internet for patients and their caregivers.

Mrs R.M. visits you in your office. She is a 66-year-old retired teacher and widow who was diagnosed with metastatic colon cancer 1 week previously. She had been experiencing right upper quadrant pain for several weeks prior to the diagnosis. She was admitted to hospital when she presented with an episode of massive rectal bleeding. A colonoscopy revealed a large ulcerating mass in the sigmoid colon. The histology report a few days later confirmed that the mass was indeed a poorly differentiated adenocarcinoma. Numerous lesions in the liver consistent with metastatic deposits were noted on a CT scan of the abdomen, as was extensive abdominal lymphadenopathy. The attending physician in the community hospital had informed her of these findings and discharged her with an appointment to see a medical oncologist the following week.

Mrs R.M. presents now to you, her primary attending physician, with a request for more information about her illness. Her daughter, who is a lawyer and lives in a small community outside the city limits, accompanies her. Mrs R.M. is tearful and anxious. She admits that she is fearful of the upcoming visit with the 'cancer specialist'. Apart from telling her that it was 'bad news' and there was 'no cure', she states that the doctor at the hospital had not provided her with much information about the cancer and had not discussed treatment options or prognosis with her. She admits that, because of the shock of the diagnosis, she had not asked many questions either and may have forgotten some of what she was told. Her daughter leans over to her mother, holds her hand and says: 'Mum, we will fight this. There are treatments that can cure cancer. We will search the Internet for that information'.

Question 1. What underlies the patient's request for more information?

A growing consumer orientation has fostered a general awareness of the importance of patients' involvement in issues of their own health and health care. The best medical outcomes occur when patients are fully informed and involved in decisions about their care.[1] The majority of patients value having as much information as possible from their physicians about their illness and the treatment options.[2,3] Provision of information to patients with chronic and life-threatening illnesses has been shown to benefit them by allowing them to gain control, improve compliance with treatments, reduce anxiety, create realistic expectations, and improve quality of life.[4,5]

Most prefer a collaborative decision-making model where patient and health professional cooperate with each other in making the decisions.[6–8] Lack of involvement may contribute to poor decisions in which patients are exposed to treatments that do not meet their needs or are associated with more risk of harm than potential benefit.

The lack of information (and increasingly information overload) may be the source of significant distress for many patients. A significant part of a traditional patient–physician encounter is dedicated to providing patients with information.[9] Furthermore, providing patients with additional information may alleviate future distress. Fallowfield *et al.*[10] reported that cancer patients who felt that the information given to them at the time of diagnosis was inadequate adjusted less well than those who were satisfied with the information they received.

Ultimately, adult patients have the legal and ethical right to access to information related to their illness and treatment options and to participate in making choices about their health care. When patients do not have the capacity to make their own health care decisions, a surrogate decision-maker may take on that role.

Unfortunately, health professionals frequently fail to meet all their patients' information needs. Between 20 and 48 per cent of cancer patients in one study indicated that the information they had received from their physicians was inadequate.[11,12] In another study,[13] women with breast cancer who had used the Internet were less satisfied with the amount of information they received from their physicians than those patients who had not used the Internet, suggesting that the dissatisfied patients were turning to the Internet for more information.

Question 2. How should the physician convey the information that the patient needs?

Trust plays a central role in the physician-patient relationship. This trust is nurtured when there is concern with the patient as a person, emphasis on the patient's quality of life, collaborative decision-making, supportive verbal and non-verbal communication, and attention to the patient's information needs.

The information should be conveyed in a sensitive, yet honest, way. What information is given, how it is given, and the extent to which it is given should vary from patient to patient. Health professionals need to explore the individual information needs of patients and their families and, where possible, provide this information in a way that is consistent with their needs and preferences.

Studies have shown that approximately 50 per cent of patients leave their doctors' offices not knowing what they have been told.[14] Physicians often use medical terms that patients do not understand or spend too little time transmitting information. Patients may lack sufficient skills to articulate their questions or feel too intimidated to ask the necessary questions. Observations of physician–patient interactions show that physicians, sometimes inadvertently, discourage patients from voicing their concerns, expectations, and requests for information, leading to further patient disempowerment.[15] Even when information is given, patients and their families may misinterpret it.[16] Therefore health professionals should review their patients' understanding of the information given to them.

However, no single health care professional can satisfy all the information needs of patients and their families. Professionals should be aware of information resources available to them and either avail themselves of these resources or direct their patients to them.

Patients and families may be provided with relevant reading materials such as pamphlets, booklets, or even books. Audiocassette recordings of the consultations, given to patients, have been shown to increase their overall recall of the specific advice given during the consultation.[17] Increasingly, patients, their families, and health professionals are using the Internet to address some of their information needs.[18–23]

Question 3. To what extent are cancer patients using the Internet?

Efforts to estimate the proportion of North American patients with cancer using the Internet to gather information regarding their illness and treatment report a wide range, from 4 to 58 per cent.[24,25] Estimates put the number of cancer patients worldwide using the Internet at any one time at 2.2 million. Obviously, these numbers will vary depending on where in the world or from which socioeconomic stratum the study is conducted. Internet access is much more prevalent in high-income countries and in wealthier communities.

Although the Internet is cited as an important source of information for many cancer patients, it appears to play a smaller role when it comes to making important treatment decisions.[24] The majority of patients indicate that physician recommendations influenced their treatment decision, followed by advice from their families and friends.[26] Only a small minority indicate that information from the Internet was the main factor in the decision-making.

Question 4. Why are patients and their families using the Internet?

The Internet has much to offer patients and families. In a relatively short period of time, the Internet has become a widely used source of information. The ubiquity of Internet access (especially in developed countries) and the relative ease of access to the world's largest repository of information have contributed to this phenomenon. The Internet and its vast stores of accessible information are empowering patients and families and providing them with a sometimes real, and occasionally perceived, sense of control of their own health care. Whether viewed negatively or positively, it is a phenomenon that is here to stay.

The reasons why patients with life-threatening and terminal illnesses go online are diverse.[27] Some desire more information about their illnesses and treatment options, either traditional or alternative/complementary. Others seek second opinions.[28] The search for a potentially curative treatment or treatment that can control the disease appears to be a common motivation.[13,18] Online purchase of treatments, often in the form of complementary or alternative therapies, appears to be on the increase.[29] Some Internet-based applications such as online discussion groups and listservs enable patients and families to find support online (see www.acor.org).

The Internet may enable and empower patients and their families and provide them with support.[30] In one study, the majority of breast cancer patients using the Internet reported that they used the information they had found online in discussions with their physicians and that it had proved very useful in these discussions.[13] (Interestingly, over half of them were undecided about the trustworthiness of the information they had found online.) The family of a patient with extensive bone metastases from breast cancer was able to persuade their primary health professional to initiate regular bisphosphonate treatments with information they had found online.[18] The physician was unaware of the benefits of bisphosphonate therapy in this context. In this vignette, the physician has an opportunity to direct the patient and family to information on different cancers and their treatments available online. Table 31.1 lists useful sites with such information.

Table 31.1 Samples of reputable websites with information about cancer

Canadian Health Network (Health Canada)	http://www.canadian-health-network.ca/1cancer.html
US National Institutes of Health	http://www.cancer.gov (contains sections for health professionals and sections for patients and the public) http://www.cancer.gov/cancerinfo/ http://www.nci.nih.gov/cancerinfo/pdq/
Association of Cancer Online Resources	http://www.acor.org/ (this site also contains links to online communities)
Department of Health (UK)	http://www.doh.gov.uk/cancer
British Columbia Cancer Agency (Canada) cancer management guidelines	http://www.bccancer.bc.ca/HPI/CancerManagementGuidelines/default.htm
American Cancer Society	http://www.cancer.org/docroot/home/index.asp
Healthinsite (Australian government)	http://www.healthinsite.gov.au/

Last accessed 12 June 2003.

Mrs R.M. returns to you 2 weeks later. This time her daughter and her son accompany her. He is a pharmacist and is visiting for 2 weeks. He lives in a distant city (4-h flight away). Since the last visit with you, she has met with the medical oncologist. Amongst other issues, he discussed with her the options of giving her either capecitabine or a combination of irinotecan, 5-fluorouracil, and leucovorin. He also stated that the likelihood of cure was very remote, but that these treatments could prolong her life and provide good symptom relief. She is considering them and will return to him in a few days. When he reviewed the CT scan and colonoscopy reports, he suggested that she also see a surgeon for consideration of palliative surgery to prevent further bleeds and bowel obstruction.

She states that the information that you directed her to on the Internet was very useful. She was able to understand what the oncologist was telling her and was even able to ask questions about specific treatments. She asked him about a new chemotherapy agent called oxaliplatin that she had found out about on a website published by a renowned cancer centre in another country. He indicated that his centre did not offer that specific treatment, but that she was eligible to be entered into a study being conducted at the cancer centre involving the chemotherapy treatments he had mentioned earlier. She is upset because she does not have access to oxaliplatin. When you explore this with her you find out that her perception is that while her oncologist is offering treatment that will probably not provide a cure, the other centre's treatment may be curative. Nevertheless, she is considering entering the study in her own centre but wants more information about what clinical trials are all about.

Question 5. How should health professionals respond to requests from patients and families about information they find online?

Increasingly, patients and families present to their health professionals with information they have found online.[31,32] Health care professionals need to remain open-minded; they need not be afraid to explore the information presented to them by patients and families.[33] In most cases, patients are not challenging their competence but rather are attempting to understand their illnesses, participate in decision-making, and gain some control over what appears to be a disorderly and overwhelming situation. The quality of information available to patients on the Internet is improving. A recent study reported that only about 5 per cent of sites with information about cancer provide inaccurate material.[34] Despite the presence of large volumes of inaccurate, misleading and scientifically unproven information on the Internet, there is an increase in the amount of legitimate information available online.

Health professionals should be proactive by directing patients and families to preselected websites with accurate and updated information. They should see electronic information as not necessarily replacing their role, but dramatically expanding it, particularly if the tool is used as part of a team approach involving other health care professionals. Table 31.2 describes some strategies to respond to patients who present with Internet-based information.

Question 6. How can the Internet support patients in accessing and participating in clinical trials and other research?

The number of websites that provide information about clinical trials has grown rapidly. Many of these sites are designed to enhance the understanding of clinical trials by the public and to

Table 31.2 How to respond to patients who present with information that they found on the Internet

Screen for Internet use	Specifically ask patients and families what their information needs are and whether or not they are using other sources of information, including the Internet
Provide opportunities to discuss the information and encourage such discussions	This will allow health professionals to explore the quality of the information patients and families have found and assess their understanding of the information. Patients and families may have inaccurate information or misinterpret information that they have found[16,84]
Do not be dismissive of information presented by patients and their loved ones	Encourage patients to discuss this information and explore their general information needs and expectations. A supportive and non-judgemental role is essential. Summarily dismissing information that patients and their families have found on the Internet, or even reproaching them, does not nurture a healthy physician–patient relationship. It also ignores the fact that there is some good information on the Internet and that patients can find it
Reassure patients of ongoing care	Reassure patients that their care by you will not be jeopardized because they are seeking information elsewhere
Be prepared to do some searching and research yourself	In many cases, it is possible to conduct the research together with the patients and their families at the clinic

provide information about the availability of trials to potential participants, regardless of their location.[35] A study of online clinical trial databases revealed that improved country-specific databases are needed to ensure patient access within those countries.[35] In response to the question about more information on the prospect of participating in a study, the physician could refer the patient to a website that provides excellent information about research methods and protocols in a language that is understandable to the lay person. Several such websites exist, including:

- http://clinicaltrials.gov/ (a service of the US National Library of Medicine)
- http://www.cancer.gov (a service of the US National Cancer Institute)
- http://nccam.nih.gov/clinicaltrials/
- http://www.acor.org/clinical.html (Association of Cancer online resources).

A large amount of appropriate, current, and accurate peer-reviewed information is now available online, and patients and families can be referred to this as part of the education process. It must be noted that the drug being offered by the 'renowned' cancer centre may well be a bona fide treatment or regimen that is in either phase 2 or phase 3 trials or is already approved for more general use. Many cancer centres and research institutions are now using the Internet to publicize legitimate research protocols that have been peer-reviewed and obtained approval from local ethics review boards. However, users are warned that there are many more sites that promote unproven alternative treatments under the mantle and guise of work that has been or is being submitted to scientific scrutiny.

This vignette illustrates both the importance of a health professional exploring what the information means to a patient and one of the risks of online information seeking by patients and families. Mrs R.M. is distressed by the fact that she has no access to a treatment that, rightly or wrongly, she perceives to be superior to the treatments she has been offered.

You invite Mrs R.M. and her daughter to discuss with you the information that they found online. They present the four pages of information on oxaliplatin that they have downloaded from the Internet. You have access to the Internet in your office and do a quick online search of oxaliplatin on the PubMed database (http://www.ncbi.nlm.nih.gov/PubMed/). (PubMed is a service of the National Library of Medicine in the United States and includes millions of citations of biomedical articles from life science journals.) You discover that it has indeed been subjected to trials and peer review. It is a third-generation platin agent and is an alternative treatment for this type of cancer, but whether or not it provides a significant advantage to the other treatments she is being offered is unclear. You discuss this with her and her family and explain that there are several chemotherapy options available, but that the effectiveness of the various options relative to one another is unclear. They seem more reassured.

Five weeks after she last saw you she returns for a follow-up visit. She has undergone successful palliative surgery that has relieved an impending bowel obstruction and has started chemotherapy (capecitabine) as suggested by her oncologist. Her son, who has returned for another visit to his mother, accompanies her. She is feeling somewhat fatigued but is otherwise tolerating the treatments very well. Her pain is well controlled on a regular opioid and antiemetic regimen. Apart from mild fatigue and difficulties in sleeping, she describes no other symptoms. When you ask her how she feels she is coping with her illness she becomes tearful and admits to being fearful of the future. You explore this further. She feels that she is losing control of her life. She admits that she has been exploring alternative treatments and wishes to discuss these with you. At this, her son interjects: 'Mother, those treatments are just quackery. They are taking advantage of your unfortunate situation. As much as I love you and want the best for you, I am concerned that you will be deceived and get unrealistic hopes. You will waste all of your life's savings on those treatments.'

You acknowledge his concerns and his desire that his mother receive the best care possible and ask her to discuss with you the 'alternative' treatments that she is using or considering taking.

She states that she has purchased a treatment called pau d'arco and is looking into treatment with high doses of vitamin C intravenously. She states that her daughter is convinced that this is effective and has read on the Internet about people with advanced cancer who have been cured with these treatments. She asks you if you would be able to inject the treatment intravenously if she were to procure it.

Question 7. How is the Internet changing the role of the health care professional in modern times?

The wide availability of online health information is impacting on the practitioner–patient relationship.[31,36–38] Health professionals are no longer the 'keepers' of medical knowledge, but increasingly need to take the role of knowledge arbitrators and guides. This role is consistent with the emerging paradigm of the shared decision-making model. The increased access to information (as a result of the Internet), together with other social drives in developed societies, is moving patients from passive recipients of health care to active consumers of health services with increased demand for information. Greater partnerships are needed between physicians and patients.[39] While this trend is positive in many ways, it is also creating new conflicts.

While most physicians report embracing the increased accessibility of health information on the Internet, a small number feel that is negatively impacting the physician–patient relationship.[24] The latter group cite the following as reasons for this: challenges to the physician's authority, requests for inappropriate treatments, and using more of the physician's time than is warranted or possible, given workloads.[40] In one study, almost all oncologists surveyed indicated that the time they are spending discussing information derived from the Internet has increased.[40] Another study reports that some physicians acquiesce to clinically inappropriate requests generated by information on the Internet either for fear of damaging the physician–patient relationship or because of the negative effect on time efficiency of not doing so.[38]

A challenge for the future is to encourage patient responsibility for care by facilitating their ability not only to locate but also to interpret health information made available to them.[41] Another challenge lies in the fact that physicians seem more sceptical than patients about the overall usefulness of the Internet.[42] This gap needs to be narrowed by research and education of both health professionals and the public.

Question 8. What are some of the potential pitfalls of seeking health information online?

Online activity may have detrimental consequences.[29,43] Despite perceived positive effects, some patients may be overwhelmed by the volume of information and perhaps even confused by contradictory advice.[40] A common concern relates to the quality of information available online.[44] Anyone with access to the Internet can potentially publish online; from specialists, experts, and alternative therapy promoters to charlatans and individuals expressing personal opinion.[33] Information that is current and accurate appears equal to outdated, misleading, and even fraudulent information to the untrained eye. Web pages with peer-reviewed information from reputable sources, such as national cancer institutes and scientific societies, appear side by side with sites publishing individual testimonials and unwarranted anecdotal experience. Mainstream search engines such as Google (www.google.com) do not distinguish between the two.

Inaccurate or outdated information or information taken out of context can lead to poor decisions and erode patients' confidence in their health professionals, especially if the information contradicts what their health professionals have said. Some patients may misinterpret or misunderstand even the most accurate information.[45] Online activity lacks many of the key components required for effective communication such as non-verbal cues. Unrealistic expectations may be promoted. Life savings can be lost in pursuit of elusive and ineffective cures. There is a danger of finding information for which a patient is not prepared.[18] Because of the uncontrolled nature of the Internet, unproven treatments with potentially dangerous side effects can be purchased online.[46]

Unexpected hazards can be found in online support groups and discussion fora, where individuals with ulterior motives may prey on vulnerable participants.[47,48] Online consultations, even by well-meaning health professionals, do not always capture all the medical and psychosocial information and nuances germane to the decision-making process. As described in the previous vignette, patients may discover treatments elsewhere that are not available in their own region, potentially leading to distress and the expectation that their health providers can procure the treatments.

Question 9. What underlies this patient's use of complementary and alternative therapies?

Patients are increasingly using complementary and alternative medicines and therapies (CAMs).[49–53] It is estimated that approximately one-third of the North American population are engaged in this practice. Patients cite the effectiveness of alternative practitioners' communication, their understanding of patients as people, and their focus on the quality of life as some of the most important reasons for seeking alternative health care.[54]

CAM incorporates several different approaches and methodologies, with techniques ranging from spiritual 'healing' to nutritional interventions. The expectations that patients with advanced cancer have of CAMs are varied.[49] Some use them to manage symptoms and improve their quality of life, while others expect remission of disease, prevention of spread, and, occasionally, the hope of a cure. Some use CAMs to make them stronger to fight the illness. Complementary therapies fulfil an important psychological need for some cancer patients. It has been suggested that the use of alternative medicine appears to be a marker for psychological distress in women with breast cancer.[55] The perception that CAMs offer non-toxic holistic options seems to be a common feature. CAMs are more often used as a supplement to, rather than a substitute for, conventional care.

The response by health professionals to this phenomenon has varied from acceptance to disdain and defensiveness. Open-ended questions and a non-judgemental attitude regarding CAMs encourage patients to discuss their questions and concerns, and their overall fears and expectations about their illnesses. It is important to establish good communication and foster a collaborative approach to this issue, without summarily dismissing patients' and families' requests for CAMs. Health professionals can play a valuable part in assisting patients to make informed choices about such therapies, thus minimizing their potential risks. Patients seeking out complementary therapies may be reluctant to disclose such information for fear of rejection by their 'conventional' health professionals. Therefore health professionals need to provide open-minded opportunities for patients and families to discuss their desire to use CAMs. They also need to explain the process required of conventional medical research and the rigours of the peer-review process, and juxtapose this with the current status of research into many of the CAMs.

It is very rare that patients reject conventional therapies in favour of CAMs. These cases present a challenge, particularly if conventional therapies such chemotherapy, radiotherapy, or surgery have a good chance of curing or controlling the disease. After excluding impaired competency and depression, the best that health professionals can do is to explore patients' understanding of their illnesses and prognoses and their concerns about conventional therapies, and explain the ramifications of not pursuing conventional therapies. These discussions should be clearly documented.

Question 10. Are there guidelines on the use of CAMs?

Many national medical associations have published guidelines on the use of CAMs. The National Centre for Complementary and Alternative Medicine (NCCAM) is the US Government's lead agency for scientific research on complementary and alternative medicine. NCCAM's mission is to explore complementary and alternative healing practices in the context of rigorous science, to train CAM researchers, and to inform the public and health professionals about the results of CAM research studies. NCCAM prompts patients to take charge of their health by being well informed and finding out what scientific studies have been done on the safety and effectiveness of the CAM that they are considering. Patients are also instructed to inform their primary health care providers if they are using CAMs (for their own safety and to allow their health care providers to develop a comprehensive treatment plan), and preferably to do this before making any decisions about treatments or care. For example, the Canadian Medical Association has published a patient's guide to choosing unconventional therapies. This is available online and can be distributed to patients (http://www.cmaj.ca/cgi/reprint/158/9/1161.pdf).

These guidelines prompt patients to ask the following key questions.

- What benefits can be expected from this therapy?
- What are the risks associated with this therapy?
- Do the known benefits outweigh the risks?
- What side effects can be expected?
- Will the therapy interfere with conventional treatment?
- Will the therapy be covered by health insurance?

What should the physician do when a patient or family make a request for a CAM for which there is little empirical support? For example, in this vignette, a search for information on unconventional therapies using the British Columbia Cancer Agency's website (see Table 31.3), a site which provides detailed information including risks and scientific references on various alternative and complementary treatments, finds the following statement with respect to vitamin C: 'There is no evidence that vitamin C has efficacy as a treatment of cancer'. The lack of evidence on the one hand and the hopes of the patient and family on the other present an ethical dilemma for the physician. Although the physician has a legal duty to treat a patient once the physician–patient relationship has been established, this does not imply that he or she must provide any treatment demanded by the patient.[56,57] If the proposed treatment clearly falls outside the bounds of standard medical care, the physician has no obligation to offer or provide it. However, in certain circumstances it is ethical to satisfy strong patient and family desires if one is convinced that harm will not ensue.

To assist in approaching this dilemma, some institutions have created guidelines. An example can be found at http://www.camline.org/protocolsGuidelines/sunnybrook.html (last accessed on 14 June 2003). Ultimately, whether or not a health care team acquiesces to requests for unproven treatments, the patient and family should be assured of and provided with the team's ongoing support.

Table 31.3 Samples of websites related to complementary and alternative treatments

ABC of complementary medicine: *British Medical Journal*	http://bmj.com/cgi/reprint/319/7211/693.pdf
A patient's guide to choosing unconventional therapy: *Canadian Medical Association Journal*	http://www.cmaj.ca/cgi/reprint/158/9/1161.pdf
National Centre for Complementary and Alternative Medicine (USA)	http://nccam.nih.gov/
British Columbia Cancer Agency (Canada)	http://www.bccancer.bc.ca/PPI/UnconventionalTherapies/default.htm
What Is Complementary and Alternative Medicine (CAM)?	http://nccam.nih.gov/health/whatiscam/
CAM Line (for health care professionals)	http://www.camline.org/about.htm
National Cancer Institute (USA)	http://www.cancer.gov/cancerinfo/treatment/cam
Understanding clinical trials	http://nccam.nih.gov/clinicaltrials/

Last accessed 12 June 2003.

Question 11. How can health professionals use the Internet in response to their patients' requests about CAMs?

The Internet abounds with websites espousing a wide variety of CAMs.[58] Although many of these appear to be misleading and even fraudulent, a growing number of sites present objective evidence-based information on these treatments. Health professionals may wish to direct their patients and families to these sites or may even use them themselves (see Table 31.3). The information in some of these can be printed and handed to patients, or forwarded to them electronically.

> During the visit, Mrs R.M.'s son asks whether or not there are guidelines on how to select a good website. He would like to review these with his family. He feels that this may guide them away from sites of poor quality.

Question 12. Is it possible to apply guidelines to judge the legitimacy and quality of health-related websites and the information contained in them?

The premise underlying this request relates to concerns about the quality of information available on the Internet. The prevalence of inaccurate cancer information on the Internet is difficult to estimate. The optimism that one study generates, demonstrating that only 5 per cent of websites on cancer contain erroneous information,[34] is tempered by reports of physicians stating that 26 per cent of the information that cancer patients present to them is inaccurate.[38] As Eysenbach[24] argues, it depends on the type of question or search strategy used. Typing in the term 'cure for cancer' may bring more sites with unproven information than simply typing in 'cancer'.

Given the concerns about quality, several tools, criteria, and codes of conduct have been proposed to assess the quality of information on websites and to ensure appropriate publishing of health-related information on the Internet:[59–61] http://www.hon.ch/HONcode/Conduct.html; Discern (http://discern.org.uk); Netscoring (http://www.chu-rouen.fr); eHealth Code of Ethics, Internet Health Coalition (http://www.ihealthcoalition.org). Several of these tools and guidelines have recently been reviewed.[62] These guidelines collectively cover issues of quality, privacy, informed consent, and confidentiality, as well as advertising, editorial policy, sponsorship, and authorship. Some criteria are short AND others lengthy. The Netscoring tool includes 49 criteria which fall into eight categories: credibility, content, links, design, interactivity, quantitative aspects, ethics, and accessibility.

The Commission of the European Communities HAS recently published a consensus-based set of criteria with which to judge health websites.[59] The criteria include transparency and honesty, authority, privacy and data protection, updating of information, accountability, responsible partnering, editorial policy, and accessibility. Readers are encouraged to review these.

Judging whether or not information on a website is applicable, accurate, and credible presents a challenge to patients, their families, and health care professionals, even when using the tools or guidelines. Limitations of the tools and guidelines have been noted.[63–65] Simply checking whether a website passes the criteria for explicit authorship and sponsorship, attribution of sources, and dating of material may not suffice to verify the quality of information. Some of the tools specifically ask one to check off whether or not the information is reliable. This would not be possible for a lay person.

Despite these shortcomings, users should look for specific elements that aid in distinguishing better websites from less credible ones. Patients and their families should be given a copy of this list (Table 31.4).

Table 31.4 Questions to consider when looking for health information online

Who runs this site?	The site should include the name, physical address and electronic address of the person or organization responsible for the site
	Does it sell advertising? Does a drug company sponsor the site? The source of funding can affect the content that is presented, how the content is presented, and what the site owners want to accomplish on the site
Who pays for the site?	All sources of funding for the site (grants, sponsors, advertisers, non-profit, voluntary assistance) should be listed
Where does the information come from?	In addition to identifying who wrote the material you are reading, the site should describe the evidence that the material is based on. Medical facts and figures should have references (such as to articles in medical journals). Also, opinions or advice should be clearly set apart from information that is 'evidence based' (i.e. based on research results)
Who is the target audience?	Clear statement of sources for all information provided and date of publication of source. Should include names and credentials of all
What is the purpose of the site?	Human/institutional providers of information, and dates at which credentials were received
Are there any sensational comments on the site?	For example: 'We offer a cure'; 'There is a conspiracy by traditional medicine to hide this treatment from ill patients…'. If so, beware of the credibility of the information on the website
How is the information selected?	Is there an editorial board? There should be a clear statement describing what procedure was used for selection of content. Do people with excellent professional and scientific qualifications review the material before it is posted?
How current is the information?	Websites should be reviewed and updated on a regular basis. The most recent update or review date should be clearly posted, with the date of update clearly displayed for each page and/or item
How does the site choose links to other sites?	Websites usually have a policy about how they establish links to other sites. Some link to any site that asks, or pays, for a link
	All efforts should be made to ensure that partnering or linking to other websites is undertaken only with trustworthy individuals and organizations who themselves comply with relevant codes of good practice
What information about you does the site collect and why? How does the site manage the information you provide about yourself?	Any credible health site asking for this kind of information should tell you exactly what they will and will not do with it
Is the site user-friendly?	Is it readable and easily searchable?
How does the site manage interactions with visitors?	There should always be a way for you to contact the site owner if you run across problems or have questions or feedback If the site hosts chat rooms or other online discussion areas, it should tell visitors what the terms of using this service are. Is it moderated? If so, by whom, and why? It is always a good idea to spend time reading the discussion without joining in, so that you feel comfortable with the environment before becoming a participant

A few weeks later Mrs R.M. requests a home visit. She has moved in with her daughter who has taken leave from work for a few weeks to be with her mother. She is feeling weaker and is finding trips out of home burdensome. She has stopped taking her alternative treatments as she feels that her disease has progressed significantly. She has lost a lot of weight and is experiencing severe abdominal pain despite a regular oral hydromorphone regimen. She also describes periods of severe abdominal cramping and emesis. In the interim, she has signed a Do Not Resuscitate directive and has expressed the goal of being kept comfortable until she dies. Before leaving to visit her at the end of your office day, you reflect on what you might expect when you see her. You are not certain how to further manage her cancer pain, nausea, and possible malignant bowel obstruction. Although you do not have your palliative care handbook at hand, you are aware of some useful websites on the Internet with just the information you are looking for. You find these sites and bookmark them for future reference in a folder called 'Palliative Care'.

Question 13. Are there websites that provide clinical information on palliative and end-of-life care for health professionals?

Numerous credible websites with high-quality information are now available with the type of information that this physician is seeking. Table 31.5 lists some useful sites for health professionals.

Table 31.5 Sample of sites with information for health care professionals on caring for terminally ill patients

Virtual Canadian Hospice	http://www.virtualhospice.ca
Ian Anderson Project (Canada) (for health care professionals)	http://www.cme.utoronto.ca/endoflife/default.htm
End of Life/Palliative Education Resource Centre- Fast Facts. (USA)	http://www.eperc.mcw.edu/educate/flash/fastfact/start.htm
Education for Physicians on End-of-life Care (EPEC) (USA)	http://www.epec.net/
Alberta Palliative Care Handbook (Canada)	http://www.albertapalliative.net/APN/PCHB/PCHBIdx.html
Edmonton Palliative Care Program (Canada) (palliative care tips)	http://www.palliative.org/PC/ClinicalInfo/PCareTips/PCareTipsIDX.html
Cochrane Pain, Palliative Care And Supportive Care Group: Summaries	http://www.update-software.com/abstracts/g380index.htm
Talaria: A Cancer Pain Resource	http://stat.washington.edu/Talaria/Talaria.html
Palliative Drugs (UK)	www.palliativedrugs.org/
StopPain.org (Beth Israel Medical Center, NY, USA)	http://www.stoppain.org/
Palliative Care Handbook, International Association of Hospice and Palliative Care (IAHPC)	http://www.hospicecare.com/manual/IAHPCmanual.htm
Pubmed (US National Library of Medicine)	http://www.nlm.nih.gov/medlineplus/tutorial.html

Table 31.5 (continued) Sample of sites with information for health care professionals on caring for terminally ill patients

PDQ Supportive Care in Cancer, National Cancer Institutes (USA)	http://www.nci.nih.gov/cancerinfo/pdq/supportivecare
Agency for Healthcare Research and Quality, US Department of Health and Human Services	http://hstat.nlm.nih.gov/hq/Hquest/db/3637/screen/DocTitle/odas/1/s/32802 Evidence Report/Technology Assessment No. 35, Vols 1 and 2: Management of Cancer Pain
Innovations in End of Life Care (USA)	http://www2.edc.org/lastacts/

Last accessed 12 June 2003.
Readers are also referred to the ABC in Palliative Care Series which is available on the online version of the *British Medical Journal*.

> Mrs R.M.'s son telephones you. He is concerned about his mother and wishes to be updated on her condition and her treatment. He feels guilty that he is so far away and not able to provide hands-on care at this time. At the end of the conversation he asks you if it would be possible for you to communicate with him by e-mail. He finds this a very convenient way of communicating. He also suggests that his sister, who lives outside town, also contact you by e-mail if she has questions about her mother and for repeat prescriptions.

Question 14. What are the considerations and implications of communicating with patients and their families by e-mail ?

In the context of an established health provider–patient relationship, e-mailing is increasingly being used as a legitimate way for health care professionals to communicate with patients, such as notifying them of scheduled visits. Although e-mail use in general is widespread, it is not often used for communicating between patients and physicians.[66] Sittig[67] suggests that, although many physicians worry that either the number or length of messages from their patients will overwhelm them, no evidence to support this could be found. In his study of five physicians using this modality, over 75 per cent of messages requested information on medications or treatments and actions on these.

Responses of physicians to unsolicited e-mail advice vary greatly and consensus on standards is still lacking.[68] Several authors have alluded to the potential benefits of this technology.[67]

E-consultation may be fraught with dangers. Although convenient for patients, it may be time-consuming for health professionals, especially when compiling responses to complex questions, and remuneration is largely lacking. There exists the danger of misdiagnosing without access to a complete patient history and physical examination. Although many questions still exist about what constitutes a therapeutic relationship between patient and care provider online,[69] it could be argued that it is unethical to diagnose and treat over the Internet in the absence of a pre-existing patient–physician relationship, and if the interaction is limited to a single e-mail.[70] Unsolicited patient questions should not be ignored but dealt with in some appropriate manner, albeit to inform the patient or family member that you do not generally provide consultations and prescriptions online. If the patient gives a list of symptoms and asks for possible diagnoses, a standard reply could be sent, which points out that it is impossible to make a remote diagnosis without a complete medical history and examination.

A distinction needs to be made between receiving e-mail messages from patients with whom you already have a relationship and receiving messages from those who are strangers to you. The latter may occur if you host a website with medical information and/or openly solicit consultations online. The following discussion applies to interactions with patients known to you.

The American Medical Informatics Association recently published guidelines for physician–patient e-mail in the context of an established relationship.[71] Guidelines on Internet-based prescribing have also been published.[72] These include the presence of a valid patient–physician relationship.

You visit Mrs R.M. at home. As expected, she is much more cachectic now and largely bedbound. A bed has been set up for her in the family room on the main floor where she is able to participate in family activities. An examination suggests a partial intermittent bowel obstruction and visceral pain from her liver metastases. Informed by the information you found on the Internet, you begin to formulate a care plan with the patient, home care nurse, and daughter. During this discussion, the daughter confesses to feeling out of her depth with her mother's care. Although home care has been very helpful, they are not able to provide 24-hr care in this rural area. The daughter would like more information on what to expect and how to care for her mother. She has been on the Internet and found the website of a local hospice. She wishes to discuss this with the family. She also found an online support group of patients and families with colon cancer. This seems a useful resource given her distance from the large cancer centre, but she is hesitant to register in the group. She has some trepidation about what to expect. She has never participated in such online groups before.

Question 15. What other resources are available for palliative patients and caregivers online?

Studies have shown that information is one of the most important support needs for families to enable them to care for their sick relative or friend effectively.[73] The provision of information lessens the patient's and family's fears and increases their sense of control, thus empowering them. Health professionals need to take responsibility in determining the information needs of patients, as well as their caregivers, and provide it at a pace and time consistent with the needs of individual families. Caregivers appreciate the spontaneous provision of this information.[74]

Information needs include details regarding the disease, prognosis, symptoms, community resources, crisis management, and what to expect in the terminal phases and at the time of death. This information can be delivered verbally or in printed form via handouts, booklets, or printouts. Studies indicate that caregivers value information delivered using a variety of media.[73] Increasingly, the Internet is becoming a source of information specifically related to being a caregiver (Table 31.6).

Virtual support groups on the Internet may provide some of the benefits that face-to-face support groups do, including improvements in coping responses, reduction of psychological symptoms, improvements in quality of life, and decreased sense of isolation.[75–83] One study of a cancer support group revealed that 80 per cent of postings contained information giving or seeking, personal opinions, encouragement, and support.[75] The remainder contained messages of gratitude and prayer. Participants in an Internet support group for women with breast cancer reported decreased levels of depression and perceived stress.[76] Despite the apparent benefits, it must be noted that this method is not appropriate for everyone. It also raises several ethical issues. One relates to the level of psychological care to be provided by the moderator and that person's responsibilities. Safeguards need to be in place to ensure that

Table 31.6 Sample of sites with information for patients and informal caregivers about caring at the end of life

Virtual Canadian Hospice	http://www.virtualhospice.ca
A Caregivers Guide. Alberta Palliative Care Network website (Canada)	http://www.albertapalliative.net/APN/CGG/CGGIdx.html
A Guide for Caregivers: The Living Lessons Project (Canada)	http://www.living-lessons.org/b.resources/secured/ Caregivers per cent20Guide per cent20English.pdf
National Cancer Institute (USA).	http://www.cancer.gov/cancerinfo/treatment/
StopPain.org (Beth Israel Medical Center, NY, USA)	http://www.stoppain.org/caregivers/
Caring for Someone with AIDS at Home. Centers for Disease Control and Prevention, National Centre for HIV, STD and TB Prevention (USA)	http://www.cdc.gov/hiv/pubs/brochure/careathome.htm
Medline Plus Health Information for the Public. US National Library	http://www.nlm.nih.gov/medlineplus/tutorial.html
PDQ Supportive Care in Cancer, National Cancer Institutes (USA)	http://www.nci.nih.gov/cancerinfo/pdq/supportivecare
Canadian Virtual Hospice (Canada)	http://www.canadianvirtualhospice.ca
Canadian Hospice and Palliative Care Association (Canada)	http://www.chpca.net/

Last accessed 12 June 2003.

virtual support groups are safe for patients and their families. Professional facilitation and monitoring is required. Secure access limits abuse and use by fraudulent users.[46]

Closing remarks

The burgeoning phenomenon that is represented by the Internet and its associated technologies is exerting significant influence on how we provide care, how patients are accessing care, and the patient–health professional relationship. Yet the Internet is only one of many new communication technologies that can change the way we practise, learn, and conduct research. These technologies include personal digital assistants (PDAs) or 'handheld computers', patient-held clinical records, and new instructional technologies for distance learning and 'just-in-time' learning. Many of the latter rely on Internet-based platforms.

We should not underestimate the impact of the Internet on health care, even in the care of terminally ill patients and their families.

References

1. **DiMatteo, M.R.** (1997) Health behaviors and care decisions: an overview of professional-patient communication. In Gochman D (ed) *Handbook of Health Behavior Research II: Provider Determinants.* New York: Plenum Press, 5–22.
2. **Mazur, D.J., and Hickam, D.H.** (1997) Patients' preferences for risk disclosure and role in decision making for invasive medical procedures. *J Gen Intern Med,* **12**, 114–17.

3. **Wu, W.C., and Pearlman, R.A.** (1988) Consent in medical decision making: the role of communication. *J Gen Intern Med*, **3**, 9–14.
4. **Mossman, J., Boudioni, M., and Slevin, M.L.** (1999) Cancer information: a cost-effective intervention. *Eur J Cancer*, **35**, 1587–91.
5. **Annunziata, M.A., Foladore, S., Magri, M.D., *et al.*** (1998) Does the information level of cancer patients correlate with quality of life? A prospective study. *Tumori*, **84**, 619–23.
6. **Cassileth, B.R., Zupkis, R.V., Sutton-Smith, K., and March, B.A.** (1980) Information and participation preferences among cancer patients. *Ann Intern Med*, **92**, 832–6.
7. **Strull, W.M., Bernard, L.O., and Charles, G.** (1984) Do patients want to participate in medical decision-making? *JAMA*, **252**, 2990–4.
8. **Deber, R.B., Kraetschmer, N., and Irvine, J.** (1996) What role do patients wish to play in treatment decision making? *Arch Intern Med*, **156**, 1414–20.
9. **Calkins, D.R., Davis, R.B., Reiley, P., *et al.*** (1997) Patient–physician communication at hospital discharge and patients' understanding of the postdischarge treatment plan. *Arch Intern Med*, **157**, 1026–30.
10. **Fallowfield, L., Hall, A., Maguire, G.P., *et al.*** (1996) Psychological outcomes of different treatment policies in women with early breast cancer outside a clinical trial. *BMJ*, **301**, 575–80.
11. **Turner, S., Maher, E.J., Young, T., *et al.*** (1996) What are the information priorities for cancer patients involved in treatment decisions? An experienced surrogate study in Hodgkin's disease. *Br J Cancer*, **73**, 222–7.
12. **Jones, R., Pearson, J., McGregor, S., *et al.*** (1999) Cross-sectional survey of patients' satisfaction with information about cancer. *BMJ*, **319**, 1247–8.
13. **Pereira, J., Koski, S., Hanson, J., *et al.*** (2000) Internet usage among women with breast cancer: an exploratory study. *Clin Breast Cancer*, **1**, 148–53.
14. **DiMatteo, M.R.** (1991) *The Psychology of Health, Illness, and Medical Care: An Individual Perspective.* Pacific Grove, CA: Brooks Cole, 185–223.
15. **West, C.** (1984) *Routine Complications: Troubles with Talk between Doctors and Patients.* Bloomington, IN: Indiana University Press.
16. **Buchanan, J., Borland, R., Cosolo, W., *et al.*** (1996) Patients' beliefs about cancer management. *Support Care Cancer*, **4**, 110–17.
17. **Bruera, E., Pituskin, E., Calder, K., Neumann, C.M., and Hanson, J.** (1999) The addition of an audiocassette recording of a consultation to written recommendations for patients with advanced cancer: a randomized, controlled trial. *Cancer*, **86**, 2420–5.
18. **Pereira, J., Bruera, E., Macmillan, K., and Kavanagh, S.** (2000) Patients with advanced cancer and their families on the Internet: motivation and impact. *J Palliat Care*, **16**, 13–19.
19. **Eysenbach, G., Sa, E., and Diepgen, T.L.** (1999) Shopping around the Internet today and tomorrow: towards the millennium of cybermedicine. *BMJ*, **319**, 1294.
20. **Jones, R.** (2000) Developments in consumer health informatics in the next decade. *Health Libr Rev*, **17**, 26–31.
21. **Kassirer, J.P.** (1995) The next transformation in the delivery of health care. *N Engl J Med*, **332**, 52–4.
22. **Goggins, M., Lietman, A., Miller, R.E., *et al.*** (1998) Use and benefits of web site for pancreatic cancer. *JAMA*, **280**, 1309–10.
23. **Eng, T.R., Maxfield, A., Patrick, K., Deering, M.J., Ratzan, S.C., and Gustafson, D.H.** (1998) Access to health information and support a public highway or a private road? *JAMA*, **280**, 1371–5.
24. **Eysenbach, G.** (2003) The impact of the Internet on cancer outcomes. *CA Cancer J Clin*, **53**, 356–71.
25. **Jadad, A.R., Sigouin, C., Cocking, L., *et al.*** (2001) Use of the Internet by cancer patients, physicians and nurses. *JAMA*, **286**, 1451–2.

26. **Diefenbach, M.A., Dorsey, J., Uzzo, R.G., *et al.*** (2002) Decision-making strategies for patients with localized prostate cancer. *Semin Urol Oncol,* **20**, 55–62.
27. **Jadad, A.R., Rizo, C.A., Enkin, M.W.** (2003) I am a good patient, believe it or not. *BMJ,* **326**, 1293–5. Available online at http://bmj.bmjjournals.com/cgi/content/full/326/7402/1293
28. **Widman, L.E., and Tong, D.A.** (1997) Requests for medical advice from patients and families to health care providers who publish on the world wide web. *Arch Int Med,* **157**, 209–12.
29. **Weisbord, S.D., Soule, J.B., and Kimmel, P.L.** (1997) Poison on line- acute renal failure causes by oil of wormwood purchased through the Internet. *N Engl J Med,* **337**, 825–7.
30. **Eysenbach, G., and Jadad, A.R.** (2001) Evidence-based patient choice and consumer health informatics in the Internet age. *J Med Internet Res,* **3**, e19. Available online at http://www.jmir.org/2001/2/e19/
32. **Potts, H., and Wyatt, J.C.** (2002) Online survey of doctors' experience of patients using the Internet. *J Med Internet Res,* **4**, e5.
32. **Pereira, J., Bruera, E., and Quan, H.** (2001) Palliative care on the Net: an online survey of health care professionals. *J Palliat Care,* **17**, 41–5.
33. **Biermann, J.S., Golladay, G.J., Greenfield, M.L.V.H., and Baker, L.H.** (1999) Evaluation of cancer information on the Internet. *Cancer,* **86**, 381–90.
34. **Eysenbach, G., Powell, J., Kuss, O., and Sa, E.** (2002) Empirical studies assessing the quality of health information for consumers on the World Wide Web. *JAMA,* **287**, 2691–700.
35. **Till, J.E., Phillips, R.A., and Jadad, A.R.** (2003) Finding Canadian cancer clinical trials on the Internet: an exploratory evaluation of online resources. *Can Med Assoc J,* **168**, 1127–9.
36. **Murray, E., Lo, B., Pollack, L., *et al.*** (2003) The impact of health information on the physician–patient relationship: patient perceptions. *Arch Intern Med,* **163**, 1727–34.
37. **Ball, M.J., and Lillis, J.** (2001) E-health: transforming the physician/patient relationship. *Int J Med Inform,* **62**, 1–10.
38. **Murray, E., Lo, B., and Pollack, L., *et al.*** (2003) The impact of health information on the Internet on health care and the physician–patient relationship: national U.S. survey among 1050 U.S. physicians. *J Med Internet Res,* **5**, e17.
39. **Jadad, A.R.** (1999) Promoting partnerships: challenges for the Internet age. *BMJ,* **319,** 761–4. Available online at at http://bmj.com/cgi/content/full/319/7212/761
40. **Helft, P.R., Hlubocky, F., and Daugherty, C.K.** (2003) American oncologists' views of Internet use by cancer patients: a mail survey of American Society of Clinical Oncology members. *J Clin Oncol,* **21**, 942–7.
41. **Anderson, J.G., Rainey, M.R., and Eysenbach, G.** (2003) The impact of cyberhealthcare on the physician–patient relationship. *J Med Syst,* **27**, 67–84.
42. **Metz, J.M., Devine, P., and DeNittis, A., *et al.*** (2003) A multi-institutional study of Internet utilization by radiation oncology patients. *Int J Radiat Oncol Biol Phys,* **56**, 1201–5.
43. **Sonnenberg, F.A.** (1997) Health information on the Internet: opportunities and pitfalls. *Arch Intern Med,* **157**, 151–2.
44. **Silberg, W.M., Lundberg, G.D., and Musacchio, R.A.** (1997) Assessing, controlling, and assuring the quality of medical information on the Internet. Caveant lector et viewor—let the reader and viewer beware. *JAMA,* **277**, 1244–5.
45. **Chen, X., and Siu, L.L.** (2001) Impact of the media and the Internet on oncology: survey of cacner patients and oncologists in Canada. *J Clin Oncol,* **19**, 4291–7.
46. **Hainer, M.I., Tsai, N., Komura, S.T., and Chiu, C.L.** (2000) Fatal hepatorenal failure associated with hydrazine sulfate. *Ann Intern Med,* **133**, 877–80.
47. **Stephenson, J.** (1998) Patient pretenders weave tangled 'web' of deceit. *JAMA,* **280**, 1297.

48. **Feldman, M.D., Bibby, M., and Crites, S.D.** (1998) 'Virtual' factitious disorders and Munchausen by proxy. *West J Med,* **168**, 537–9.
49. **Downer, S.M., Cody, M.M., McCluskey, P., *et al.*** (1994) Pursuit and practice of complementary therapies by cancer patients receiving conventional treatment. *BMJ,* **309**, 86–9.
50. **Begbie, S.P., Kerestes, Z.L., and Bell, D.R.** (1996) Patterns of alternative medicine use by cancer patients. *Med J Aust,* **165**, 545–8.
51. **Oneschuk, D., Fennell, L., Hanson, J., and Bruera, E.** (1998) The use of complementary medications by cancer patients attending an outpatient pain and symptom clinic. *J Palliat Care,* **14**, 21–6.
52. **Astin, J.A.** (1998) Why patients use alternative medicine: results of a national study. *JAMA,* **279**, 1548–53.
53. **Eisenberg, D.M., Davis, R.B., Ettner, S.L., *et al.*** (1998) Trends in alternative medicine use in the United States, 1990–1997. Results of a follow-up national survey. *JAMA,* **280**, 1569–75.
54. **Eisenberg, D.M., Kessler, R.C., Foster, C., Norlock, F.E., Calkins, D.R., and Delbanco, T.L.** (1993) Unconventional medicine in the United States: prevalence, costs, and patterns of use. *N Engl J Med,* **328**, 246–52.
55. **Burstein, H.J., Gelber, S., Guadgnoli, E., *et al.*** (1999) Use of alternative medicine by women with early-stage breast cancer. *N Engl J Med,* **340**, 1733–9.
56. **Weijer, C., Singer, P.A., Dickens, B.M., and Workman, S.** (1998) Bioethics for clinicians: dealing with demands for inappropriate treatment. *Can Med Assoc J,* **159**, 817–21.
57. **Picard, E.I., and Robertson, G.B.** (1996) *Legal Liability of Doctors and Hospitals in Canada* (3rd edn) Scarborough, Otario: Carswell, 235–69.
58. **Bower, H.** (1996) Internet sees growth of unverified health claims. *BMJ,* **313**, 381.
59. **Commission of the European Communities** (2002) eEurope 2002: quality criteria for health related websites. *J Med Internet Res,* **4**, e15. Available online at http://www.jmir.org/2002/3/e15/
60. **Health on the Net Foundation.** Health on the Net code of conduct (HONcode) for medical and health web sites. Available online at http://www.hon.ch/HONcode/Conduct.html
61. **Winker, M.A., Flanagin, A., Chi-Lum, B, *et al.*** (2000) Guidelines for medical and health information sites on the Internet: principles governing AMA web sites. *JAMA,* **283**, 1600–6.
62. **Risk, A., and Dzenowagis, J.** (2001) Review of Internet health information quality initiatives. *J Med Internet Res,* **3**, e28. Available online at http://www.jmir.org/2001/4/e28
63. **Jadad, A.R., and Gagliardi, A.** (1998) Rating health information of the Internet: navigating to knowledge or to Babel? *JAMA,* **279**, 611–14.
64. **Impicciatore, P., Pandolfi, C., Casella, N., and Bonati, M.** (1997) Reliability of health information for the public on the World Wide Web: a systematic survey of advice on managing fever in children at home. *BMJ,* **314**, 1875–9.
65. **Juhling McClung, H., Murray, R.D., and Heitlinger, L.A.** (1998) The Internet as a source for current patient information. *Pediatrics,* **101**, 1065.
66. **Baker, L., Wagner, T.H., Singer, S., and Bundorf, M.K.** (2003) Use of the Internet and e-mail for health care information: results from a national survey. *JAMA,* **289**, 2400–6.
67. **Sittig, D.F.** (2003) Results of content analysis of electronic messages (e-mail) sent between patients and their physicians. *BMC Med Inform Decis Mak,* **3**, 11.
68. **Eysenbach, G., and Diepgen, T.L.** (1998) Responses to unsolicited patient e-mail requests for medical advice on the World Wide Web. *JAMA,* **280**, 1333–5.
69. **Dyer, K.A.** (2001) Ethical challenges of medicine and health on the Internet: a review *J Med Internet Res,* **3**, e23. Available online at http://www.jmir.org/2001/2/e23

70. **Eysenbach, G.** (2002) Towards ethical guidelines for dealing with unsolicited patient emails and giving teleadvice in the absence of a pre-existing patient–physician relationship—systematic review and expert survey. *J Med Internet Res,* **2**, e1. Available online at http://www.jmir.org/2000/1/e1/)
71. **Borowitz, S.M., and Wyatt, J.C.** (1998) The origin, content, and workload of e-mail consultations. *JAMA,* **280**, 1321–4.
72. **Jones, M.J., and Thomasson, W.A.** (2003) Establishing guidelines for Internet-based prescribing. *South Med J,* **96**, 1–5.
73. **Wilkes, L., White, K., and O'Riordan, L.** (2000) Empowerment through information: supporting rural families of oncology patients in palliative care. *Aust J Rural Health,* **8**, 41–6.
74. **Sykes, N.P., Pearson, S.E., and Chell, S.** (1992) Quality of care of the terminally ill: the carer's perspective. *Palliat Med,* **6**, 227–36.
75. **Klemm, P., Reppert, K., and Visich, L.** (1998) A nontraditional cancer support group. The Internet. *Comput Nurs,* **16**, 31–6.
76. **Winzelberg, A.J., Classen, C., Aplers, G.W.,** ***et al.*** (2003) Evaluation of an Internet support group for women with primary breast cancer. *Cancer,* **97**, 1164–73.
77. **Christensen, H., Griffiths, K.M., and Korten, A.** (2002) Web-based cognitive behavior therapy: analysis of site usage and changes in depression and anxiety scores. *J Med Internet Res,* **4**, e3.
78. **Lieberman, M.A., Golant, M., Giese-Davis, J.,** ***et al.*** (2003) Electronic support groups for breast carcinoma: a clinical trial of effectiveness. *Cancer,* **97**, 920–5.
79. **Weinberg, N., Schmale, J., Uken, J., and Wessel, K.** (1996) Online help: cancer patients participate in a computer mediated support group. *Health Soc Work,* **21**, 24–9.
80. **Gustaffson, D.H., McTavish, F., Hawkins, R.,** ***et al.*** (1998) Computer support for elderly women with breast cancer. *JAMA,* **280**, 1305.
81. **Mayer, M., and Till, J.E.** (1996) The Internet: a modern Pandora's box? *Qual Life Res,* **5**, 568–71.
82. **Fernsler, J.I., and Manchester, L.J.** (1997) Evaluation of a computer-based cancer support network. *Cancer Pract,* **5**, 46–51.
83. **George, D.S.** (1998) Teleconferencing support: women with secondary breast cancer. *Int J Palliat Nurs,* **4**, 115–19.
84. **Mackillop, W.J., Stewart, W.E., Ginsburg, A.D., and Stewart, S.S.** (1988) Cancer patients' perceptions of their disease and its treatment. *Br J Cancer,* **58**, 355–8.

Index